D0857650

THE PATHWAY FOR OXYGEN

THE PATHWAY FOR OXYGEN

Structure and Function in the Mammalian Respiratory System

Ewald R. Weibel, M.D.

Harvard University Press
Cambridge, Massachusetts, and London, England
1984

LIBRARY OF CONGRESS CATALOGING IN PUBLICATION DATA

Weibel, Ewald R.
    The pathway for oxygen.

    Bibliography: p.
    Includes index.
    1. Respiration.   2.   Oxygen in the body.   I.   Title.
[DNLM: 1.   Respiration.   2.   Respiratory system — Anatomy
and histology.   3.   Respiratory system — Physiology.
WF 102 W415p]
QP121.W395   1984   612'.2   83-18622
ISBN0-674-65791-8 (cloth)
    0-674-65790-X (paper)

To André F. Cournand and George E. Palade,
who taught me how to look beyond morphology

FOREWORD

THIS BOOK is based on a series of lectures delivered by Professor Ewald Weibel in the fall term of 1979, when he was a visiting Alexander Agassiz Professor to the Museum of Comparative Zoology of Harvard University. In those sessions, Professor Weibel provided the basis for a new synthesis between the traditional fields of anatomy and physiology by applying stereological methods to quantify structures and their spatial relationships. He used a comparative approach to examine the quantitative match between structures and their function in the transfer of oxygen from the environmental air to the respiratory chain enzymes in the mitochondria. He tested the idea that there is rationality and symmetry underlying the design of structures. The lectures generated lively discussion, and the audience grew from week to week as the practitioners of the traditional fields challenged assumptions and questioned conclusions. The book stimulates the same intellectual excitement that characterized the lectures—the excitement involved in breaking new ground and formulating a new level of understanding of the relationships between structures and their function.

We hope that this publication will be the first in a series of Agassiz Lectures which preview the forefronts of comparative zoology and provide us with new syntheses. It is fitting that the first book in this Agassiz series is written by a current leader of Swiss science. When Louis Agassiz moved from Switzerland to the United States and founded the Museum of Comparative Zoology at Harvard, he set in motion research in all aspects of zoology and natural history in North

America. To Louis Agassiz, natural history museums were centers for multifaceted studies on the biology of organisms and for the training of the next generation of biologists. This was the stamp he placed upon the MCZ as he nursed it through its infancy. The endowment supplied by the Agassiz family, and in particular Louis Agassiz's son Alexander, made Louis Agassiz's early policies and administrative decisions a tradition of the MCZ. The establishment of the Alexander Agassiz professorships played an important role in the realization of this tradition. This book reflects the tradition of the MCZ's founder, and once again zoology is indebted to the land of Louis Agassiz's birth.

A. W. Crompton
C. Richard Taylor

PREFACE

UNQUESTIONABLY, most of the great advances in the understanding of living organisms have come about through the thorough and imaginative work of investigators who acquired special skills with which to solve a problem at hand: they were either morphologists, physiologists, biochemists, or molecular biologists. The field of respiration has been no different. In this book I have tried to pull together the results of these many approaches to the problems of respiration. My aim has been to explore the mechanisms by which an efficient pathway for oxygen — from the lung through the blood, the tissues, the cells to the molecular respiratory chain in the mitochondria — is established and maintained in man and animals, and how these different mechanisms are dependent on each other. I have had to consider questions of design as well as regulation, of structure as well as function, at the macroscopic as well as the cellular and molecular levels of organization. My bias as a morphologist will be clear throughout this book, but I have made a special effort to give physiology and biochemistry their due weight. The meaning of design in a functional system cannot be understood without a full consideration of dynamic regulatory mechanisms, including all the ancillary functions performed by a multitude of cells that maintain a healthy lung or an adequate distribution of blood flow to the organs of need, to mention only two problems.

The topic is vast and almost unlimited; it was impossible to deal with all aspects in the appropriate depth. Each chapter has therefore been supplemented with a bibliography where the reader can find guidance on how to deepen his understanding of some topic by further reading of review articles and textbook syntheses. But to understand the process of science — which often proceeds in leaps — one must also look at the sources of scientific information: original papers, often highly specialized and focused on a very particular question. Such references are usually large in number; for each chapter I have compiled only a small, rather personal list, from very recent publications to "classics" (marked by an asterisk) which have initiated a major step in our understanding of the system. At the end of the book there is a list of general references which make particularly worthwhile additional reading.

How This Book Came About

In the fall of 1979 I was invited by Harvard University to deliver a series of Agassiz Lectures, "Structure and Function in the Respiratory System." These lectures formed the core of this book, but they have been expanded to include background material and to be more explicit where, in the lecture, I had relied on the audience's intuition.

The lectures were built on a body of experience acquired in two decades of scientific activity. After solid training as a morphologist with Gian Töndury in Zürich and Averill A. Liebow at Yale University, I had the unusual privilege of working in two outstanding centers of respiratory physiology and cell biology: first with André F. Cournand, Dickinson W. Richards, and Domingo Gomez at Columbia University, and then with George E. Palade at Rockefeller University. My experience with these great teachers has deeply affected my thinking. I could not have taken the approach chosen for this book — and for my research — had I not been instilled, in this early period, with the desire to understand the role of structural organization in terms of the functions served, to look beyond my own trade of morphology to physiology and cell biology. I have become convinced not only that structure determines function, but that functional demand also determines structural design, be it through evolution or by modulation of design features.

To shed some light on this interdependence of structure and function has been my constant endeavor. This would not have been possible without the contributions of a large group of superb colleagues and collaborators, particularly Hans and Marianne Bachofen, Robert Bolender, Peter Burri, Luis Cruz-Orive, Peter Gehr, Joan Gil, Hans Hoppeler, Odile Mathieu, and Klaus Schwerzmann. For our group a decisive period began some years ago when a collaboration was established with C. Richard Taylor from the Museum of Comparative Zoology at Harvard University. Our scientific interests and special skills are mutually complementary, with sufficient overlap to stimulate close cooperation. This has been a most fruitful association. It has also allowed me to write a good part of this book in the stimulating Harvard environment while spending a sabbatical leave at the Museum of Comparative Zoology. I am grateful to C. Richard Taylor and Alfred W. Crompton for their hospitality.

The burden of writing a book like this must be shared. I am most grateful to my secretary of many years, Gertrud Reber, for her superb and devoted assistance, and also to Karl Babl, who did most of the graphic art for this book, diligently assisted by Marianne Schweizer. Some of the artwork was contributed by Alexandra Sänger and Reinhold Schneider.

Last, but not least, I should gratefully acknowledge the generous and continued support which our research has received, particularly from the University of Berne and the Swiss National Science Foundation.

E. R. W.

CONTENTS

1 OXYGEN AND THE HISTORY OF LIFE 1

The Cell's Oxygen Sink and Energetics 3
Getting Oxygen to the Sink 5
Evolution of O_2 Transport Systems 10
Evolution of External Gas Exchangers 13
Looking at the System as a Whole: Philosophy of the Approach 23

2 THE BODY'S NEED FOR OXYGEN 30

Levels of O_2 Consumption 36
Estimating the Limits of O_2 Consumption 41

3 LINKING STRUCTURE AND FUNCTION: MODEL, MEANS, AND TOOLS 49

How Does Structure Affect O_2 Flow? 52
Are Animals Built Reasonably? 58
The Tools 66

4 CELL RESPIRATION 80

Gaining Energy from Combustion 80
Metabolic Pathways of the Cell 87
The Cell's Energetic Balance Sheet 99

5 MITOCHONDRIA: THE CELL'S FURNACES 106

Putting Some Order into Cell Metabolism 109

Oxidation–Phosphorylation Coupling Depends on Structure   *111*
Mitochondria and the Cell's Aerobic Potential   *115*
Mitochondria in Muscle Cells   *118*

6   THE VEHICLE FOR OXYGEN TRANSPORT: BLOOD AND CIRCULATION   *138*

The O_2 and CO_2 Carrier: Blood   *140*
Moving Blood Around: Circulation   *156*
O_2 Transport by the Blood   *170*

7   DELIVERING OXYGEN TO THE CELLS   *175*

Distributing Blood to the Tissues: Design of the Vasculature   *176*
The Microvascular Unit   *178*
O_2 Flow from Blood to Cells   *195*

8   DESIGN AND DEVELOPMENT OF THE MAMMALIAN LUNG   *211*

Development of the Lung   *213*
Lung Histogenesis: Differentiation toward Gas Exchange   *220*
The Lung at Birth and Its Postnatal Maturation   *224*

9   LUNG CELL BIOLOGY   *231*

Organization of the Lung's Cell Population   *233*
A Closer Look at the Cells of the Gas Exchange Region   *248*

10   AIRWAYS AND BLOOD VESSELS   *272*

The Airway Tree   *272*
Ventilation   *282*
The Vascular Trees   *287*
Pulmonary Blood Flow   *292*
Ventilation–Perfusion Matching   *294*

11   THE LUNG'S MECHANICAL SUPPORT   *302*

External Support and Motive Force   *302*
The Pleural Cavity   *305*
The Lung's Fiber Skeleton   *307*
Surface Tension   *317*
Micromechanics and the Configuration of the Alveolar Septum   *325*
Keeping the Barrier Dry and Thin   *331*

12   THE LUNG AS GAS EXCHANGER   *339*

Design of the Gas Exchanger   *339*
Physiological Basis for Gas Exchange   *343*
Pulmonary Diffusing Capacity: Physiology   *347*
Pulmonary Diffusing Capacity: Morphometry   *351*
Structure and Function Compared   *359*
Matching the Conductance to O₂ Needs: The Emergence of a
   Paradox   *364*
Resolving the Paradox: Models and Nature   *369*

13   THE RESPIRATORY SYSTEM IN OVERVIEW   *378*

Adjusting Performance to Needs   *380*
Adjusting Potential to Needs   *394*
The Limits to Potential: The Smallest Mammal   *399*

UNITS OF MEASUREMENT   *411*

GENERAL REFERENCES   *414*

INDEX   *415*

THE PATHWAY FOR OXYGEN

1

OXYGEN AND THE HISTORY
OF LIFE

IF A CANDLE BURNS in a closed container, its flame will soon be extinguished because the O_2 required to burn the wax has been consumed. Living creatures kept in a closed box will die for much the same reason: a continuous flow of O_2 is required for maintaining the "fire of life," a most appropriate term coined by Max Kleiber and used as title for his fundamental treatise on the metabolism of animals, published in 1961.

Life is a complex phenomenon that depends on a high level of activity and on a high degree of order among the many functional units that make up an organism. No such order and no such activity can be maintained without the continuous input of energy, and for most "animals" — protozoa and metazoa alike — this energy is produced by combustion of organic compounds such as sugars, a process which requires O_2.

According to ancient, even medieval, views and beliefs, the heart was considered to be a furnace where the "fire of life" kept the blood boiling. Contemporary cell biology holds that each cell maintains a set of furnaces, the mitochondria — organelles specialized toward supplying the cell with energy by combustion, that is, by oxidation of organic substrates. As we shall see in detail later, the mitochondrion is equipped with a set of enzymes that can break up sugars into CO_2, extracting hydrogen ions in the process which are, in turn, burned with O_2 to make water (Fig. 1.1). For every four hydrogen ions one molecule of O_2 is consumed, and this liberates a lot of energy which can be utilized to drive the vital functions of the cell. This funda-

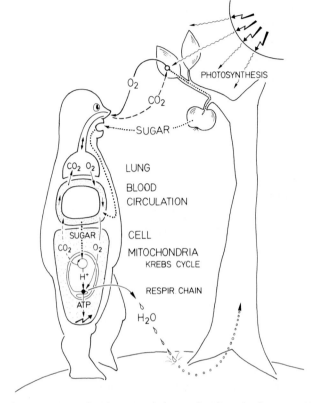

Fig. 1.1 The oxygen cycle: the energetic needs of our body are paid by solar energy.

mental process of energy production by oxidation depends totally on an adequate and continuous supply of O_2. The cells do have other means for covering their energetic needs in the absence of O_2, but they are rather inefficient and, in the long run, they all eventually need to be supported by oxidative metabolism. Thus, O_2 plays a key role in cellular energetics.

Why are O_2 and carbohydrates such convenient sources for covering the energetic needs of cells and living creatures? Why aren't these sources of energy soon exhausted? Indeed, one can easily calculate that the population of a larger city will consume most of the O_2 contained in the air column above the city's grounds in just about one life span of a human being. This does not happen, however, because the O_2 in the atmosphere is continuously replenished by the plants that surround us and, most importantly, by algae in the oceans. Drawing on part of the sun's energy radiation, plants use the CO_2 and H_2O produced by combustion in animal cells as substrates for making carbohydrates through photosynthesis (Fig. 1.1); by the same token they generate molecular O_2 which is released to the air, thus quasi reversing the process. Thus, in a broad sense, animals and plants form a large symbiotic system with O_2 and CO_2 as the two gaseous components that are exchanged in a continuous cycle through the air, a cycle that is driven by solar energy (Fig. 1.1). The energetic costs of life on earth are hence borne by the sun. Remember that all nonnuclear fuels that we burn to keep our houses warm or to run our machines and automobiles — wood, coal, and fossil oils — derive from this same process and are stored solar energy; if they are consumed at a rate greater than that by which they are regenerated, these energy sources will soon be exhausted.

The Cell's Oxygen Sink and Energetics

It is believed that the first elements of life developed when the earth's atmosphere did not yet contain any molecular O_2 to speak of. Indeed, anaerobic conditions were important for the formation of nucleotides by the "first spark" — a process that is now considered to be the origin of life since it led to the development of DNA and RNA, the carriers of genetic information. Under these conditions energy was presumably generated by anaerobic "oxidation," that is, by simple transfer of electrons to some suitable electron acceptor.

Let me explain. It turns out that the essential part of "combustion" or "oxidation" is the liberation of energy as electrons are transferred from an "electron donor" to an "electron acceptor" of higher electron affinity, a point we shall discuss in detail in chapter 4. All this can happen without O_2. But when, in the course of time, O_2 did become available in the earth's atmosphere, it became the ideal terminal electron acceptor because of its very high electron affinity, and "combustion" could now be carried to the end, that is, to true "oxidation," liberating as much energy as the substrates can give off and ending up in the formation of water (Fig. 1.1).

Now, the energy liberated in this process cannot be utilized directly, mostly because our system is not equipped to exploit the energy contained in heat; rather, it is necessary to "capture" this energy in a high-energy bond between phosphate groups that are attached to a nucleotide, mostly in the form of *adenosine triphosphate*, ATP. This energy can then be donated to most energy-requiring processes of cells, such as the contraction of muscle proteins or the metabolic activity of enzymes.

One of the fundamental steps in the evolution of cells, therefore, was the development of a complex set of enzymes or catalysts that could transfer the energy liberated by the various steps of oxidation to ATP in an efficient and well-controlled manner, a process called *oxidative phosphorylation*. In principle, it involves three steps (Fig. 1.1). Sugar which contains six carbon atoms is first split into two halves in a process called *glycolysis* (this step is different if other substances such as fats are burned). The fragments are then broken into CO_2 molecules, and this liberates hydrogen ions (H^+) which carry electrons along; this occurs in what is called the *Krebs cycle*. The third step takes place in the *respiratory chain* which ends in the reaction of H^+ with O_2 to make water. This last reaction liberates a lot of energy—remember the explosion that results if hydrogen and oxygen are reacted in the chemical laboratory—and this energy is used to make ATP. As we shall see, six ATP molecules can be generated for every O_2 molecule consumed.

These mechanisms of oxidative energy production are rather ancient in terms of evolution, as evidenced by the fact that all aerobic bacteria contain a set of enzymes by which they can generate, by oxidation of substrates, the energy-rich fuels like ATP that drive the cell's functions. These enzymes are not simply contained in the cell, but many of them are concentrated in a specialized region of the bacterial cell membrane.

In eukaryotes, the enzymes of oxidative phosphorylation, very similar to those found in bacteria, are housed in a specialized organelle, the *mitochondrion*, a small rod-shaped body bounded by two membranes and about the size of a bacterium. As in bacteria, one finds part of the enzyme system, namely the respiratory chain and part of the Krebs cycle enzymes, to be bound to the inner mitochondrial membrane, as we shall see later. Indeed the enzyme systems of bacteria and mitochondria are so similar that it has been speculated that mitochondria evolved from bacterial microorganisms which joined with protoplasmic elements in a kind of endosymbiosis where each part would contribute to and benefit from close cooperation: the protoplasmic elements would perform most synthetic functions, whereas the bacterial endosymbionts would spill off energy-rich compounds produced by oxidative metabolism. This notion is further supported by the fact that mitochondria contain their own genetic material in form of a circular strand of DNA, similar to bacterial DNA which is also circular. Furthermore, they contain their own ribosomes, again similar to those of bacteria, which can perform the synthesis of some mitochondrial proteins.

Mitochondria are fundamental constituents of all living cells beyond bacteria, from simple protozoa to all higher animals and man. When cells multiply by division, their mitochondrial complement is evenly divided between the two offspring. Cells are regarded as units of living matter not only because each contains the full set of genes, but also because each cell is self-sufficient in terms of liberating energy from substrates; when mitochondria are involved this depends on the availability of O_2.

Getting Oxygen to the Sink

During the evolution of the eukaryotic cell a first element of order or design was introduced into the respiratory system when the site of ATP generation was separated from the sites of ATP utilization: the enzyme system supporting oxidative phosphorylation became concentrated in the mitochondria, the cells' furnaces. Mitochondria act as "O_2 sinks" where molecular O_2 is removed as water, the end product of combustion, is produced (Fig. 1.1). But the "fire of life" can only be kept burning if there is a continuous inflow of O_2 from the cell's environment. In protozoa such as amoebae or paramecia, the cell's environment is the aqueous medium in which the cell lives and which either picks up its O_2 from the air or receives a continuous local supply from the photosynthetic activity of algae. In higher organisms, made of a large number of specialized cells each equipped with mitochondria, this environment is the intercellular fluid that is found in tissues. The problem is now how to ensure an adequate flow of O_2 from its store in environmental air to all the cells in the body.

The mechanisms by which a flow of O_2 into the tissues can be maintained are (1) *diffusion*, or molecular movement of O_2 through air or fluid, and (2) *convection*, or mass transport of O_2 by moving the medium in which O_2 is contained. Diffusion can be compared to people actively walking in the streets; convection to using a subway for getting a group of people from one point in town to another.

Diffusion of O_2 molecules is related to Brownian motion: in a gas, or in a fluid, molecules are in continuous motion which is random in a stationary state. If the gases are unevenly distributed, however, the molecular motion will show a preferential direction away from the higher concentration until homogeneity is achieved. Let us now see what happens in a situation such as that shown in Figure 1.2: two compartments A and B are separated by another compartment Y. Assume that the O_2 concentration in A is larger than that in B, and that O_2 can easily diffuse into and through Y; molecular motion will then drive O_2 through Y from the side with higher concentration in A to that of lower concentration. The driving force for this O_2 flow across compartment Y is the difference in O_2 partial pressures, P_{O_2} in compartments A and B, also called the P_{O_2} gradient across the barrier Y. In this case one finds that the O_2 flow rate by diffusion across Y, expressed in moles of O_2 per minute, is

$$\dot{M}_{O_2}(Y) = G(Y) \cdot [P_{O_2}(A) - P_{O_2}(B)]. \tag{1.1}$$

This flow rate achieves a constant value if the P_{O_2} in A and in B is kept constant, that is, when the inflow of O_2 into A and the outflow out of B are equal to the flow across Y. Such a situation is called a "steady state."

The coefficient $G(Y)$ is the conductance of compartment Y and depends on a number of its properties. First it depends on the

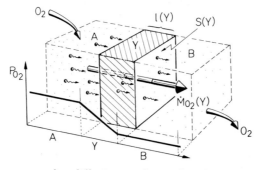

Fig. 1.2 O_2 transport by diffusion is driven by the O_2 partial pressure gradient and determined by the barrier dimensions, $S(Y)$ and $l(Y)$.

permeability properties of the material that makes up Y: O_2 diffusion through air is about 300,000 times easier or faster than that through water, for example. Then the flow rate is directly proportional to the cross-sectional area over which diffusion takes place and inversely proportional to the distance the molecules have to travel. We shall see in chapter 3 how these design properties affect O_2 flow.

A pathway for diffusive flow of O_2 in a given direction therefore needs compartments with different P_{O_2} to be established and to be separated by some structural barrier. Note that the content of the barrier is considered static; only O_2 moves by displacement of molecules in the direction of the concentration gradient, and the O_2 provides its own driving force, the partial pressure difference.

Convective O_2 flow is different. Here we assume that O_2 molecules are dissolved in a fluid or bound to some carrier which is moved by outside forces (Fig. 1.3). The amount of O_2 that can be conveyed this way depends essentially on two factors: the concentration $C_{O_2}(B)$ at which O_2 can be piled into the carrier B, expressed in mol/ml, and the volume flow rate of the carrier, $\dot{V}(B)$, expressed in ml/min, for example. It turns out that the density of O_2 loading depends again on the partial O_2 pressure and on some factor β_{O_2} called the O_2 capacitance (β_{O_2} is the quantity of O_2 required to raise the P_{O_2} by one unit), so that we have as O_2 flow rate for convective flow in a channel B

$$\dot{M}_{O_2}(B) = \dot{V}(B) \cdot C_{O_2}(B) = \dot{V}(B) \cdot \beta_{O_2} \cdot P_{O_2}(B). \tag{1.2}$$

To design a pathway for O_2 flow by convection requires on the one hand a system of tubes along which the carrier can move and on the other hand a pump that can generate and maintain the flow rate $\dot{V}(B)$. The evident example for this kind of transport is the flow of blood,

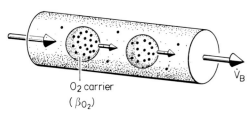

Fig. 1.3 O_2 transport by convection is determined by the mass flow rate of the carrier, $\dot{V}_B$, and its capacitance for O_2, β_{O_2}.

pumped by the heart, where O_2 can be bound at high concentration to the red blood cells, as will be discussed in chapter 6.

These two mechanisms can now be combined if two channels of convective transport, A and B, are joined over a certain area by means of a permeable barrier, Y, as shown in Figure 1.4. It is immediately evident that O_2 will flow by diffusion from A through Y to B if there is more O_2 in the fluid flowing through channel A than in that flowing through B. And it is also evident from what we have said above with respect to diffusion (equation 1.1 and Fig. 1.2) that the exchange of O_2 between A and B is essentially determined by the P_{O_2} difference between these two compartments.

There is, however, one important point to note. As the fluid A flows along the permeable barrier Y it will gradually lose some of its O_2, and its P_{O_2} will fall. Conversely, the O_2 extracted from A will be added to that in B so that the P_{O_2} in fluid B will gradually rise (Fig. 1.4). As a consequence, the P_{O_2} difference between A and B will become smaller and smaller, and may, given enough time, eventually vanish. But since the diffusive O_2 flow is proportional to the P_{O_2} difference,

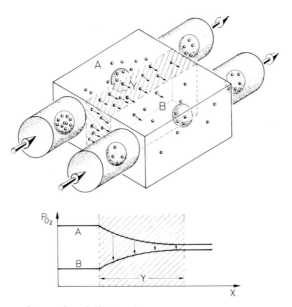

Fig. 1.4 O_2 exchange by diffusion between two compartments, A and B, which are perfused by convective flow of a carrier and separated by a barrier, Y.

the driving force, it follows that the amount of O_2 exchanged also becomes smaller as the two media pass along the barrier (Fig. 1.4). Steady-state conditions prevail if the two P_{O_2} profiles in A and B remain stable, and this is achieved if the two flows are adjusted to each other and to the diffusive O_2 flow rate through Y.

Using these elements we can now draw up a basic pathway for O_2 transport from the O_2 store in air or water—continuously replenished through photosynthesis—to the O_2 sink in the mitochondria, where it disappears in the process of oxidation (Fig. 1.5). In principle, two gas exchangers are joined by the closed circular loop of convective blood flow (B). The external gas exchanger (A-B) is related to an open loop of convective flow of either air or water by which the P_{O_2} on the A-side of the exchanger barrier is kept steady and high. The internal gas exchanger (B-C) connects the deep side of the blood flow loop with the O_2 sink. One of the important things to note is that along this pathway the P_{O_2} will fall in the form of a stepwise cascade. By that the pathway has an over-all direction, leading O_2 from the air to the mitochondria and not the other way. It is also interesting to note that this direction, this polarity, is the result of O_2 consumption in the mitochondria; if there were no O_2 consumption, the P_{O_2} would soon become even throughout the pathway. Thus the consumer itself actually sets up the driving force for O_2 flow into the system. If more

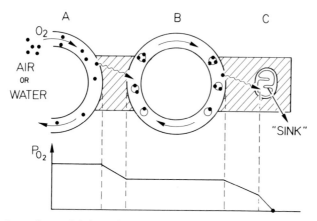

Fig. 1.5 Cascade model describes O_2 flow by diffusion and convection from air or water (A) through the blood (B) to the mitochondria in cells (C) where it disappears into the "sink." The P_{O_2} falls step by step from environmental values to eventually zero in the sink.

O_2 is consumed, the P_{O_2} cascade may become steeper and more O_2 can flow in. However, this is not enough because the pumps that drive the convective transport systems must also work harder: when we run, our heart beats more fiercely and we breathe more rapidly and more deeply. But before we look at these mechanisms in more detail, let us first see how nature has played with great virtuosity on the theme of this basic pathway, how respiratory systems have evolved that are fit to ensure adequate O_2 supply in a variety of different organisms living under different conditions.

Evolution of O_2 Transport Systems

Nature has chosen two basically different approaches to solve the problem of getting O_2 to the cells in the depths of higher organisms: (1) using air as a carrier for O_2 flow by convection and diffusion through a system of channels in insects, and (2) developing an intermediate O_2 carrier, blood, which connects the cells to an external gas exchanger.

The respiratory system of insects is rather unusual and, in many ways, surprising. Their body is pervaded by a system of air-filled tubes, called tracheae (Fig. 1.6); they are open to the outside air at lateral openings, called spiracles, and branch into the tissues, finally

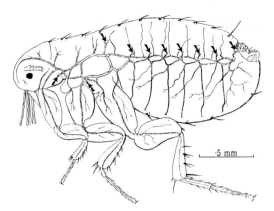

Fig. 1.6 The body of an insect is pervaded by a system of air-filled tracheae that connect to outside air through the spiracles (arrows) and penetrate into the muscles as tracheoles. (From Wigglesworth, 1972.)

penetrating into the muscle cells where the terminal tracheoles come to lie in the immediate vicinity of mitochondria (Fig. 1.7). The pathway from the spiracle to the cells can show many modifications of the basic pattern. The spiracles are commonly provided with a valve-like mechanism that can regulate the convective inflow of air from the environment. The tracheae usually show some thin-walled dilatations in their initial parts; these sacs can in fact be ventilated, for example by the pumping movements of the abdomen that one may observe in wasps or bees. The actual tracheae that are branching into the body are formed by a rigid incollapsible chitin spiral that allows them to remain patent. O_2 flow through these channels is essentially by diffusion through the air, although some slight convection could be produced by accordion-like shortening and length-

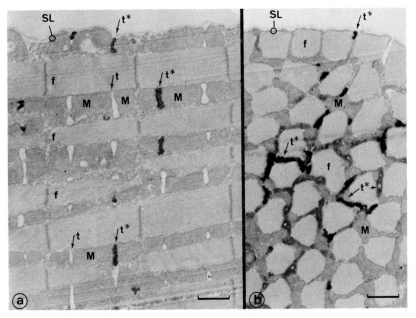

Fig. 1.7 Longitudinal (a) and transverse (b) sections of flight muscle of an insect demonstrate the close relation between tracheoles (t) and mitochondria (M). Some of the tracheoles (t*) were filled with oil from outside in a vacuum in order to demonstrate that they are filled with air. Note that the tracheoles are connected to the cell membrane or sarcolemma (SL) and course as a network between the myofibrils (f). Scale markers: 1 μm. (From Wigglesworth and Lee, 1982.)

ening of the tracheae caused by contraction of the muscles. Diffusion of O_2 through air is about 300,000 times faster than through water so that the insects' tracheal system can indeed assure adequate O_2 supply to the cells. But it depends essentially on being filled with air. Thus, even in aquatic insects the tracheal system is air-filled; they take O_2 either from an air-bubble that they maintain around their abdomen and periodically replenish at the water surface, or through a gas exchanger membrane that separates the tracheal system from the water. It is likely that the respiratory system of insects evolved in air as an adaptation to terrestrial life, whereas aquatic insects have adapted to their wet environment secondarily.

For most other higher animals the reverse is probably the case: the respiratory system evolved during aquatic life and was secondarily adapted to air breathing. When the size of aquatic animals began to increase, they were faced with a two-fold major problem: O_2 is poorly soluble in water and it diffuses very slowly through aqueous solutions, as compared with air. This called for two combined adaptations: an O_2 carrier had to be introduced that could take up large amounts of O_2, and this carrier had to be circulated between the cells and a specialized external gas exchanger that could load O_2 onto the carrier; this corresponds to the basic design of the pathway we developed in Figure 1.5.

A variety of O_2 carriers have evolved, but all share one common feature: they are metal-containing proteins that are colored so that they are often called respiratory pigments. One such molecule is *hemocyanin* which contains copper and is found in molluscs and some arthropods, such as crabs, dissolved in blood plasma as small molecular aggregates. The most common carrier is, however, *hemoglobin*, a protein that contains an iron-porphyrin ring; as we shall discuss later in detail, hemoglobin can bind up to four molecules of O_2 for each hemoglobin molecule. In some animals hemoglobin is found in solution in the plasma, but in nearly all vertebrates it is carried at high concentration in specialized cells, the *erythrocytes* or red blood cells. In 100 ml of human blood one finds 16 g of hemoglobin and this allows 20 ml of O_2 to be bound, as compared to no more than 0.2 ml O_2 that can be dissolved in the same volume of blood plasma. Hemoglobin thus increases the O_2 capacity of the blood by 100 times, and as a result the O_2 content of blood is the same as that of air, namely 20 ml O_2 per 100 ml of air or blood, a rather interesting phenomenon. This actually means that the O_2 content of blood capillaries in mammals is the same as that of the air-filled tracheae in insects. It is furthermore interesting to note that hemoglobin is phylogenetically a rather ancient molecule. We find it in many primitive or even unicellular organisms, such as protozoa or yeast, as a cytoplasmic pigment that can increase the cell's O_2 capacity and thus establish intracellular O_2 stores; moreover, it improves O_2 diffusion through the cell by what has been called facilitated diffusion, as we shall further discuss below with respect to mammalian muscle fibers which also contain a hemoglobin-like O_2 carrier.

It is, of course, important that such O_2 carriers do not bind O_2 too tightly. As we shall see in chapter 6, the O_2 binding properties of hemoglobin are such as to permit easy release of O_2 into the tissues as well as an efficient O_2 uptake in the external gas exchangers (lungs or gills). In principle this is due to the fact that the number of O_2 molecules bound to each hemoglobin molecule is a function of the prevailing P_{O_2}. Thus, if blood is exposed to a P_{O_2} of over 100 torr, as it prevails in ambient air, the hemoglobin becomes nearly saturated with four O_2 per hemoglobin molecule; but in the tissues the P_{O_2} is perhaps of the order of 40 torr and at this tension hemoglobin can hold no more than two O_2 molecules; the others are released. And thus, with circulation of the blood back and forth between the external gas exchanger and the tissues, a net flow of O_2 from ambient air to the cells via blood results as a function of P_{O_2} differences (Fig. 1.5).

Evolution of External Gas Exchangers

O_2 FLOW THROUGH EXTERNAL GAS EXCHANGERS

The external gas exchangers that have evolved in higher organisms — fish gills, bird lungs, and alveolar lungs of amphibia, reptiles, and mammals — have some basic features in common, irrespective of the different principles that determine their functioning in detail. For one, it is now commonly accepted that the flow of O_2 across the barrier separating blood from air or water occurs entirely by diffusion. Hence, it depends on the existence of a P_{O_2} gradient from the external medium to the blood which acts as the driving force for O_2 flow. This notion has not always been undisputed; for a long time, earlier in this century, a group of renowned respiratory physiologists believed that the air–blood barrier of the lung might be equipped with some kind of pump that could actively "secrete" O_2 into the blood. Such theories were essentially based on some physiological data sets which indicated that the P_{O_2} of blood may be higher than that of alveolar air; O_2 uptake would then have to occur "uphill," and this would require active pumping to overcome the diffusive back-flow of O_2 from blood to air. But even in those days the physiological data were not conclusive, partly owing—we now know—to inadequate measuring techniques, although the measurements were done as well as it was then possible. Indeed, we shall discuss later some of the formidable problems that are encountered when one wants to measure P_{O_2} gradients that are very small and are located in the depths of a large organ where one cannot penetrate with measuring probes, so that one essentially depends on deductions from indirect measurements.

The evidence available today suggests that the flow of O_2 from the external compartment into the blood can be simply described as a diffusive process which depends on the difference in partial O_2 pressures and on the conductance of the barrier separating the blood from air or water. We shall see that this conductance depends essentially on a large surface of contact between blood and air (or water) and on the great thinness of the tissue barrier that separates the blood from the external medium. This conductance is, indeed, large enough to allow all the O_2 flow that is needed to occur by diffusion.

MEETING DIFFERENT DEMANDS

Before we can go on to consider the basic designs used to build external gas exchangers we need to remember that respiration is but one of the many vital functions that an organism must maintain. Some of these functions will require design features that may have a negative effect on others, such as the following: In multicellular organisms it is essential that the cells are exposed to well-regulated environmental conditions; the fluids surrounding the cells must be maintained in a given narrow pH range, at a prescribed osmotic pressure, and sometimes in a given temperature range. To maintain this milieu intérieur, as it was termed by Claude Bernard, the organism must shield itself against the environment by an integument that prevents a loss or gain of water, or of ions and solutes — or, better still, that allows the ion, solute, or water exchange between the environment and the intercellular fluids to be regulated. Clearly, the structure of this integument will be very different depending on whether the animal lives in water or in air and whether the body temperature must be kept constant or not. But one thing is common to all higher organisms: the integument is made of several layers of cells that can serve as active shields of many kinds, and, as a consequence, it is fairly thick; furthermore, for reasons of economy, the surface over which the body is exposed to the often adverse environment must be kept as small as possible.

This introduces some problems when an external gas exchanger must be built. In such an organ we want to have blood come into extensive and very close contact with environmental water or air, so that O_2 and CO_2 can be rapidly exchanged by diffusion. The rate of gaseous diffusion across a barrier increases as the surface of contact becomes larger but decreases as the barrier becomes thicker. Thus gas exchange requires that a very thin barrier be established which confronts the blood and the environmental O_2 store over a very large surface. Clearly, these design conditions for a gas exchanger are contrary to those of the integument. They can only be achieved if the body finds additional ways of preventing water loss, ion imbalance, heat loss, and so on in that part of the body's surface that is used as a gas exchanger. Gas exchange through the skin is inadequate except in some very small organisms and can serve only as an auxiliary respiratory organ, as, for example, in amphibia. When special gas exchangers are built, a part of the body's surface is singled out for that specific purpose, given a large surface and a thin barrier. This surface is either evaginated (turned outward), resulting in the formation of gills used for respiration in water, or invaginated (turned inward), forming a lung used for breathing air.

RESPIRATION IN WATER: GILLS

Tadpoles develop a simple system of gills in the form of branched appendages. As the blood flows through the capillary network beneath the thin integument, it picks up O_2 and the P_{O_2} rises until it approximates that in the water at the gill surface (Fig. 1.8). It is

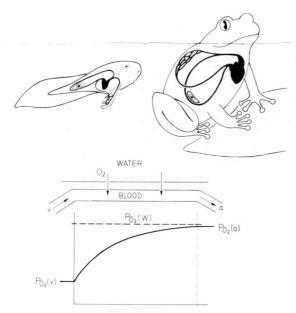

Fig. 1.8 Gas exchange through skin is used in the simple external gills of tadpoles and, to a limited extent, in adult amphibia. The P_{O_2} of blood flowing through capillaries between the veins and arteries becomes equilibrated with that in the water.

evidently essential that the water at the gill surface is continually exchanged, lest it be soon depleted of O_2. In the tadpole, as in some other lower aquatic forms, this is simply achieved by swimming through the water. This process is not very efficient and is only adequate in animals that have low O_2 requirements. Note that in adult frogs a similar mechanism of respiration through the skin is retained (Fig. 1.8), but it serves mostly as a means of eliminating CO_2 or as an auxiliary respiratory organ when the frog is submerged in water.

The design and functioning of *fish gills* is somewhat different. Here the respiratory surfaces are removed into a gill chamber that is covered by a lid, the operculum (Fig. 1.9). This chamber communicates with the buccal cavity through a set of slits which are separated by the branchial or gill arches so that water can be pumped from the buccal cavity through the gills. A large respiratory surface is established by the formation on these arches of a large number of long

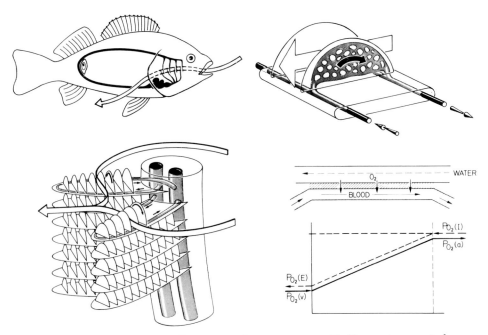

Fig. 1.9 In the fish the gills are complex structures with filaments mounted in paired rows on the gill arches; gas exchange occurs at the surface of numerous thin lamellae which are mounted on the filaments. Flow of water between the lamellae is in the opposite direction to blood flow. This counter-current exchanger allows the P_{O_2} in arterial blood to approach that in inspired water.

filaments which carry on their surface a dense set of parallel lamellae (Fig. 1.10). Arches and filaments are supporting structures which contain the proximal and distal limb of the branchial arteries, be-tween which capillary networks are formed that occupy the lamel-lae. Gas exchange takes place in the lamellae (Fig. 1.9). Now it is interesting to note that the water flows through the slits between the lamellae in a direction from front to rear, whereas the blood flows through the capillaries in the opposite direction. This so-called countercurrent system has tremendous advantages for gas exchange. As the venous blood of low P_{O_2} enters the lamella it is first exposed to outflowing water which has lost some of its O_2, but as it flows through the lamella the P_{O_2} of the water to which it is exposed gradually increases to that in the environmental water (Fig. 1.9). Thus the

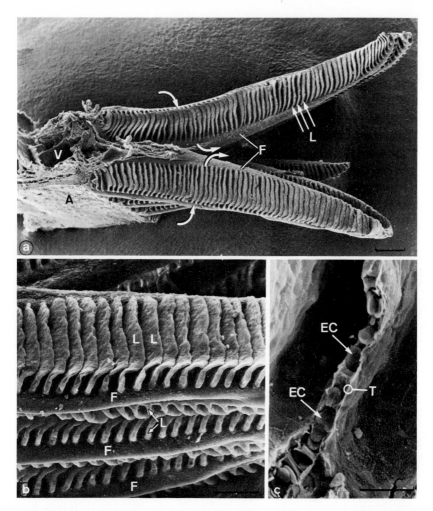

Fig. 1.10 Scanning electron micrographs of fish gills. (a) A pair of filaments (F) is seen to arise from a gill arch (A) with a large vessel (V) seen on its cross-section; the arrows indicate the direction of water flow between the lamellae (L). (b) Side view of three filaments (F) reveals that regularly spaced lamellae are mounted on both sides. (c) A broken lamella reveals erythrocytes (EC) in the capillaries and the thin tissue barrier (T) separating blood and water. Scale markers: (a) 200 μm; (b) 100 μm; (c) 20 μm.

blood leaving the gills can reach the same P_{O_2} as that prevailing in the environment. Note that if water and blood flowed through the gills in the same direction (cocurrent flow), as it was assumed in the model of Figure 1.4, this would not be possible; the outflowing blood and water would be equilibrated at some mid-value between the P_{O_2} of venous blood and that of environmental water. The countercurrent design thus greatly increases the efficiency of gills as gas exchangers so that the low O_2 content of water can be better exploited.

RESPIRATION IN AIR: LUNGS

Evaginated gills are not suitable for breathing in air, particularly since surface tension would make it very difficult to keep them separated; they would tend to stick together so that the surface available for gas exchange is very much reduced. Air breathing therefore requires the gas exchangers to be housed in invaginated pouches with the capillaries contained in thin walls that can be kept extended by tension (Fig. 1.11).

Such internal gas exchangers have not evolved from the skin, as was the case with gills, but rather from the gut where the integument is thinner a priori, being designed to allow the uptake of nutrients, and thus offers a distinct advantage for gas exchange. Removing the respiratory surfaces into an interior compartment has further obvious advantages for protection of the milieu intérieur from adverse effects of the environment: in air breathing the greatest danger is water loss by evaporation from the large surface and this can be minimized by controlling the air humidity in the lung, so that the barrier separating air and blood can be made very thin.

Primitive lungs of this kind occur in snails, for example. If fishes depend on air breathing, they too will develop lungs from outpouchings of the dorsolateral wall of the foregut, in addition to the gills they need for water breathing. This is the case in some African or South American lungfish that must survive when the river beds in which they live dry out in the dry season. In these fishes part of the blood that leaves the single-chambered heart from the aorta is diverted into the lung for gas exchange with air that is "swallowed" into the air spaces.

The lungs which are the evolutionary antecedents of the gas exchanger of terrestrial vertebrates are formed in amphibia and in reptiles from ventral invaginations of the foregut into the chest

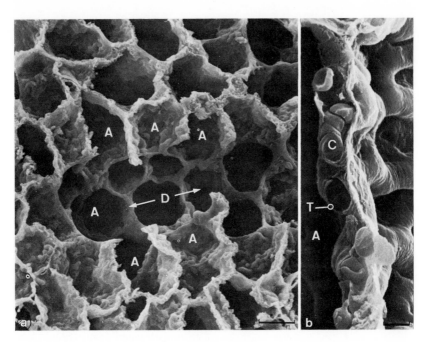

Fig. 1.11 (a) In alveolar lungs the gas exchange surface is enlarged by many pouches or alveoli (A) attached to airway ducts (D). (b) The walls between alveoli contain a dense network of blood capillaries (C), separated from air (A) by thin tissue barrier (T). Scale markers: (a) 50 μm; (b) 5 μm.

cavity. This is combined with a gradual separation of the blood circulation into two loops, one which carries the blood through the lung for oxygenation and one which directs the blood through the tissues for O_2 delivery.

The principal design feature of these lungs is that their gas exchange surface is made large by forming multiple walls that subdivide the air space and contain dense capillary networks (Fig. 1.11). The large number of air chambers resulting from this partitioning all communicate with the outside air through a system of usually branched tubes. These air chambers or alveoli are ventilated either by pushing air in from the buccal cavity, as in amphibia, or by sucking air in through the bellows action of the chest wall, as in mammals, and then breathing it out again. In either case, the air in the lung is renewed periodically by cyclic inspiration and expiration, and we must expect the P_{O_2} in the air chambers to be somewhat lower than in environmental air owing to the continuous extraction of O_2 by the blood that flows through the chamber walls (Fig. 1.12). In these *alveolar lungs* all air chambers are apparently ventilated as a pool and the P_{O_2} near the gas exchange surface is considered homogeneous because O_2 diffusion through air is so rapid as to instantaneously even out local differences due to O_2 extraction by the blood. Thus, in principle, the blood flowing through the capillaries becomes equilibrated to alveolar P_{O_2} which is lower than environmental P_{O_2} (Fig. 1.12) and at most as high, usually lower, than that of the air exhaled from the lung. Alveolar lungs, therefore, are less efficient than gills because they cannot cause the blood P_{O_2} to rise close to environmental P_{O_2}. Indeed, we shall see that the arterial blood P_{O_2} achieved in human lungs is only about 100 torr as compared to a P_{O_2} of 150 torr in ambient air at sea level.

Birds have evolved a more efficient lung by separating ventilation and gas exchange structures (Fig. 1.13). The *bird lung* is a small, rigid structure that is traversed by a parallel set of fine air tubes, called parabronchi, whose rather complex surface contains a maze of air capillaries that are interlaced with blood capillaries to form a large area for gas exchange across a very thin barrier (Fig. 1.14). These parabronchi are ventilated by a continuous stream of air from large abdominal air sacs that are periodically filled with fresh air; the outflowing air is collected into a separate set of anterior air sacs (Fig.

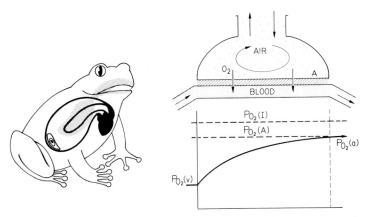

Fig. 1.12 In alveolar lungs as they occur in amphibia or mammals, gas exchange takes place between blood flowing by and air contained in an alveolar pool that is ventilated through the airways. Blood P_{O_2} becomes equilibrated to alveolar P_{O_2} which is, however, lower than that in inspired air.

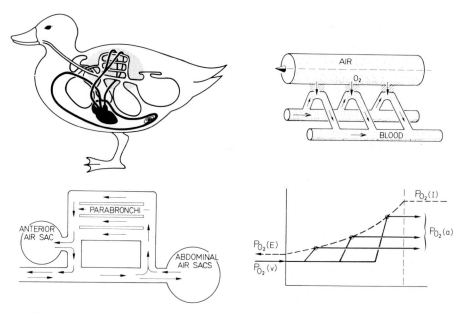

Fig. 1.13 In the bird lung, air flows from rear to front through parabronchi, with abdominal air sacs serving as bellows. The gas exchanger is arranged along the parabronchi and is perfused with blood according to a cross-current system. Arterial P_{O_2} may be higher than that in expired air.

1.13). Thus, the air entering the parabronchi is kept at a P_{O_2} equivalent to that in ambient air, and it will gradually fall along the parabronchial path as O_2 is being extracted by the capillaries that cross this pathway as parallel loops (Fig. 1.13). As a consequence, the blood leaving each capillary loop will have a different P_{O_2}, depending on its location along the parabronchial path, but the P_{O_2} of the mixed blood leaving the lung will be higher than the P_{O_2} of the air leaving the parabronchi to be eventually exhaled. It is thus apparent that the bird lung is more efficient than alveolar lungs in the sense that it can better exploit the O_2 content of the air passing through the lung. This may become a critical advantage for birds when they fly at high altitude and must get enough O_2 out of very thin air. Indeed, many birds can fly over the Himalayas, whereas man needs to breathe supplemental O_2 when going to these altitudes or when flying in an airplane.

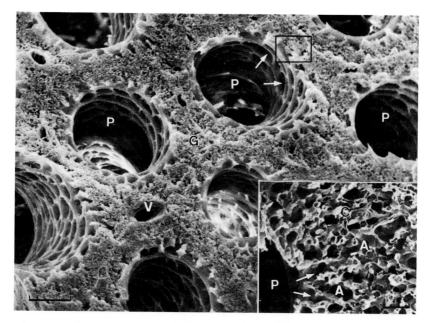

Fig. 1.14 The cross-section of a bird lung shows cylindrical parabronchi (P). Their wall is marked by bundles of smooth muscle that surround atria (arrows). Blood vessels (V) are embedded in the gas exchange tissue (G) between the parabronchi. The inset is a higher magnification of an area similar to that marked by a square; it shows that the gas exchange tissue between the parabronchi is a dense meshwork of blood capillaries (C) and air capillaries (A), the latter arising from atria in the parabronchial wall (arrows). Scale markers: 200 μm; (inset) 20 μm. (Scanning electron micrographs courtesy H. R. Duncker, Giessen, published in modified form in Duncker, 1978.)

Looking at the System as a Whole: Philosophy of the Approach

In the following chapters we shall be concerned with the design and the functioning of the mammalian respiratory system, whose characteristic properties can be summarized as follows: The external gas exchanger is an alveolar lung which is ventilated with air through a branched system of airways by means of the bellows action of the chest wall and diaphragm. Oxygen is transported between the lung and the tissues by a circulation in two serial loops, one leading through the lung, the other through the tissues, and each driven by a separate pump, the right and the left sides of the heart respectively. In the tissues an internal gas exchanger is set up by bringing the blood close to the cells where O_2 is being consumed.

In this system, O_2 flow is maintained because of two fundamental properties:

(1) *The structural design* sets up a sequence of closely linked compartments. It establishes a system of airway tubes for ventilation of the gas exchanger and a system of blood vessels for orderly circular blood flow. It also establishes close contact between air and blood and between blood and cells for efficient gas exchange. The subcellular structure organizes the relation between mitochondria and the blood capillaries that bring in O_2, and between mitochondria and the cellular elements that require ATP to perform the cells' functions.

(2) *Functional events* establish and maintain the driving forces that are needed to effect an O_2 flow. In the mitochondria, complex biochemical mechanisms perform the various steps of oxidative phosphorylation which control the O_2 needs of the organism. The heart maintains blood flow, and the muscles of the chest wall and diaphragm ventilate the lung. Most importantly, the proper match between these functions maintains adequate P_{O_2} gradients which direct the O_2 flow through the system.

The performance of the respiratory system hence depends both on structural and on functional properties which cannot be separated. If we want to consider the system as a whole we must face the problem of structure–function correlation. But in approaching it we meet with a procedural or even conceptual difficulty: professionalism in science has led to a compartmentalization of biology into various disciplines which look at the phenomena of life with different eyes and different prejudices. Function is the domain of the physiologist, structure that of the morphologist, and they operate with often vastly disparate concepts and approaches. To put it drastically, the physiologist will interpret his measurements of vital functions on the basis of models which get rid of as many structural complications as possible; it will often be "good enough" to consider the lung simply as an air bubble in contact with blood: as long as we can measure how much air flows into the bubble, how much blood passes along it, and how much O_2 is exchanged, we need not worry about how the two are brought into contact. Problems arise when such simple models, amenable to simple mathematical manipulations, are taken to be reality, for they are clearly artificial contraptions that ignore a lot of pertinent features of the system.

The morphologist, on the other hand, is often perplexed by the complexity of the structural systems he is looking at, a complexity that increases with the progressive resolving power of his microscopes. There are many different cells, membranes, vesicles, and other structures along the pathway that O_2 has presumably to follow. Are they important? The morphologist will say yes, and he is right; the physiologist will say no, and he is right too. The point is this: to set up and maintain a gas exchanger between air and blood requires a large spectrum of different functions, from the synthesis of fibers on which blood capillaries are suspended to membrane barriers that prevent blood fluids from leaking into the air spaces; but most of these functions affect the actual process of gas exchange only indirectly.

The scientific approach to structure–function correlation will have to strike a balance between these two biases by setting up models that account for a sufficiently realistic amount of structural information while still allowing functional data to be interpreted with reasonable simplicity. Most importantly, however, we have to acknowledge that any model of this kind is a highly abstracted picture of reality and can serve only a very limited purpose. We must be prepared to reject or modify it whenever we come up with essential information that is not compatible with the model, or not accounted for by it.

There is one other major difference between the traditional approaches chosen by morphology and physiology. Whereas the physiologist will, in general, attempt to single out phenomena which he can measure, the morphologist will look at structure as a whole and be content with precise, often meticulous descriptions, supported by generous pictorial evidence, although it is well possible to work out quantitative descriptions of structure as well. There is definite merit in each of these approaches, but when we tackle a specific problem of structure–function correlation both morphological and physiological data must be produced in comparable or compatible form. Although much fundamental insight can be gained by purely descriptive analysis of certain phenomena, in the end statements about correlation between structure and function will have to be supported by solid quantitative data which can be introduced jointly into appropriate models. Quantitative morphology or morphometry is, hence, an essential part of such studies. However, it must be stressed that nothing can be measured that is not precisely known, so that a thorough descriptive study of both the structural properties and the functional expressions of a system must precede measurement. Models are, indeed, based primarily on such descriptions and should be valid irrespective of the quantitative parameters that specify the magnitude of some of the model's components and features. We shall come up with several examples of this kind.

Summary

Oxygen plays a key role in the energy metabolism of living organisms. When carbohydrates are burned, O_2 is consumed and CO_2 and water are produced. The O_2 store in air is maintained because plants and algae regenerate carbohydrates and O_2 from CO_2 and H_2O using the energy of solar radiation, thus reversing the process. In oxidation, energy is liberated as electrons are transferred from an electron donor to an electron acceptor of higher electron affinity; O_2 is the ideal terminal electron acceptor because of its very high electron affinity. The energy liberated in this process is captured in small portions in high-energy phosphate bonds, mostly in the form of adenosine triphosphate, ATP. This transfer of energy is coupled to oxidation by means of enzyme systems contained in mitochondria, cell organelles which have presumably evolved from bacteria.

In the eukaryotic cell, sites of ATP generation (mitochondria) are separated from sites of ATP utilization. As organisms became larger by assembling many cells of different function, mechanisms for ensuring an adequate O_2 supply to the mitochondria had to evolve. They depend on O_2 diffusion and on convective O_2 transport. Diffusion is driven by P_{O_2} gradients and is affected by the conductance of the system, whereas convective transport depends on the flow rate of the carrier (air or blood, for example) and on its O_2 carrying capacity. In all higher organisms the transfer of O_2 from the air to the cells involves a series of transfer steps: convection of air (or water) into the external gas exchanger (lungs or gills); diffusion of O_2 into the blood; convective flow of blood to the tissues; diffusion of O_2 to the cells and mitochondria. The over-all driving force is a P_{O_2} cascade from the air to the cells.

Insects use air to carry O_2 to the mitochondria through a system of tracheae which penetrate into the cells. In all other organisms blood is used as an intermediate carrier; it contains a respiratory pigment, mostly hemoglobin, which increases the O_2 capacity 100 times as compared to water and binds O_2 loosely enough to discharge it to the cells as a function of lower P_{O_2}.

The external gas exchangers of vertebrates transfer O_2 to the blood by diffusion, driven by the higher P_{O_2} in the external medium. Respiration in water (fishes) occurs in gills, a system of filaments of large surface mounted on gill arches in the gill chamber. Water flows from front to back over the respiratory surface and blood flows in the opposite direction. This countercurrent system allows a high gas exchange efficiency as the blood leaving the gills can be equilibrated to the P_{O_2} in ambient water. Respiration in air required the evolution of lungs which can be kept expanded by tension and allow control of water and heat loss. Alveolar lungs, as they occur in amphibia, reptiles, and mammals, are ventilated and perfused as a pool; the P_{O_2} of arterial blood is lower than ambient P_{O_2}. In bird lungs ventilation of the gas exchanger occurs from air sacs and blood perfuses the gas exchanger in a cross-current pattern which allows better O_2 extraction of air, making the bird lung a more efficient gas exchanger than the alveolar lung.

The performance of the mammalian respiratory system — from the lung through the blood to the cells and mitochondria — is determined by both functional and structural properties which cannot be separated but need to be studied conjointly in an integrated approach.

Further Reading

Broda, E. 1978. The Evolution of Bioenergetic Processes. Oxford: Pergamon.

Hughes, G. M. 1963. Comparative Physiology of Vertebrate Respiration. Cambridge: Harvard University Press.

Hughes, G. M., and M. Morgan. 1973. The structure of fish gills in relation to their respiratory function. Biological Review 48:419–475.

Johansen, K. 1968. Air-breathing fishes. Scientific American 219:102–111.

Kleiber, M. 1961. The Fire of Life: An Introduction to Animal Energetics. New York: Wiley.

Margulis, L. 1981. Symbiosis in Cell Evolution. San Francisco: Freeman.

Piiper, J., and P. Scheid. 1977. Comparative physiology of respiration: functional analysis of gas exchange organs in vertebrates. *International Review of Physiology* 14:219–253.

Rahn, H., A. Ar, and C. V. Paganelli. 1979. How bird eggs breathe? *Scientific American* 240:46–55.

Scheid, P. 1979. Mechanisms of gas exchange in bird lungs. *Reviews of Physiology, Biochemistry and Pharmacology* 86:137–186.

Schmidt-Nielsen, K. 1972. *How Animals Work.* Cambridge: Cambridge University Press.

Wigglesworth, V. B. 1972. *The Principles of Insect Physiology.* 7th ed. London: Chapman & Hall.

References

Bentley, P. J., and J. W. Shield. 1973. Respiration of some urodele and anuran amphibia. II. In air, role of the skin and lungs. *Comparative Biochemistry and Physiology* 46A:29–38.

* Bernard, C. 1859. *Leçons sur les Propriétés Physiologiques et les Altérations Physiologiques des Liquides de l'Organisme.* Paris: Baillière.

Bouverot, P., and P. Dejours. 1971. Pathway of respired gas in the air-sacs–lung apparatus of fowl and ducks. *Respiration Physiology* 13:330–342.

Dejours, P. 1981. *Principles of Comparative Respiratory Physiology.* 2nd ed. Amsterdam: Elsevier North-Holland.

Duncker, H. R. 1972. Structure of avian lungs. *Respiration Physiology* 14:44–63.

———1978. Development of the avian respiratory and circulatory systems. In *Respiratory Function in Birds, Adult and Embryonic,* ed. J. Piiper. Berlin-Heidelberg: Springer, pp. 260–273.

Hughes, G. M., ed. 1976. *Respiration of Amphibious Vertebrates.* London: Academic.

Piiper, J., ed. 1978. *Respiratory Function in Birds, Adult and Embryonic.* Berlin-Heidelberg: Springer.

Piiper, J., and P. Scheid. 1975. Gas transport efficiency of gills, lungs and skin: theory and experimental data. *Respiration Physiology* 23:209–211.

Rahn, H., K. B. Rahn, B. J. Howell, C. Gans, and S. M. Tenney. 1971. Air breathing of the garfish (*Lepisosteus osseus*). *Respiration Physiology* 11:285–307.

Scheid, P., and J. Piiper. 1972. Cross-current gas exchange in avian lungs: effects of reversed parabronchial air flow in ducks. *Respiration Physiology* 16:304–312.

Schmidt-Nielsen, K. 1979. *Animal Physiology.* 2nd ed. Cambridge: Cambridge University Press.

Weibel, E. R., and C. R. Taylor, eds. 1981. Design of the mammalian respiratory system. *Respiration Physiology* 44:1–164.

Wigglesworth, V. B., and W. M. Lee. 1982. The supply of oxygen to the flight muscle of insects: a theory of tracheole physiology. *Tissue and Cell* 14:501–518.

Wigglesworth, V. B. 1972. *The Principles of Insect Physiology.* 7th ed. London: Chapman & Hall.

Wood, S. C., and C. Lenfant, eds. 1979. *Evolution of Respiratory Processes: A Comparative Approach.* New York: Dekker.

2

THE BODY'S NEED FOR OXYGEN

ALL CELL FUNCTIONS can be performed only if they are supplied with a certain amount of energy which they draw from high-energy phosphate bonds, as was mentioned in chapter 1. Moreover, this energy must be immediately available at the moment the function takes place. In order to ensure this, the cell stores a small amount of high-energy phosphates in the immediate surroundings of its functional units — enzymes, contractile proteins, and the like.

The main source of *immediate energy* is adenosine triphosphate, ATP, whose third phosphate group is attached with a bond that carries a lot of potential energy (Fig. 2.1). When this third phosphate group is split off, the energy liberated from the bond can be donated, for example, to reactants in a chemical reaction catalyzed by an enzyme or to the bonds between contractile proteins in muscle (see chapter 5) — that is, it can be used to do "biological work." The chemical result of this process is adenosine diphosphate, ADP, a compound of lower potential energy; it is recharged by what is called *phosphorylation,* but this evidently requires energy transfer from some other source, eventually from metabolic breakdown of food-stuffs (Fig. 2.1). It is interesting to note that this metabolic process is controlled by the level of ADP in the cell; when "biological work" requires the breakdown of ATP, resulting in an increase of ADP in the cell, phosphorylation increases. This process is relatively slow, however, so that a store of high-energy phosphates is essential to ensure adequate fueling of processes that require energy.

This is particularly important in muscle cells which must be

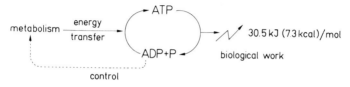

Fig. 2.1 High-energy phosphates play a key role in the transfer of energy in cells.

capable of performing sudden contractions and thus utilize energy from ATP very rapidly. However, muscle cells contain, at any one moment, only enough ATP to fuel maximal contractions for about 3 seconds. Because ATP cannot be supplied from the blood or from other cells, it must be regenerated within the cell, a process which requires energy. In muscle cells the energy required is drawn from another high-energy organic phosphate, creatine phosphate, CP, as it releases its phosphate group (Fig. 2.2). It turns out that muscle cells contain about 3–5 times more CP than ATP, so that creatine phosphate is considered to be a high-energy phosphate "reservoir" or store, which is, in turn, regenerated from ATP formed in the mitochondria. This system for storing high-energy phosphate has a number of advantages: for one, CP diffuses through the cell more easily than ATP and can thus reach the sites where energy is most needed; furthermore, it helps to finely regulate the concentration of ADP which, in turn, controls cell metabolism (see chapter 13).

The energy immediately available to muscle cells in the ATP-CP

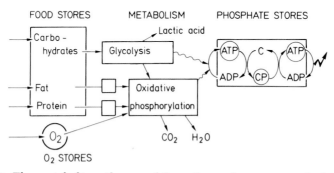

Fig. 2.2 The metabolic pathways of the cell transfer energy to the high-energy phosphate stores and draw on the food and O_2 stores; these need to be replenished from outside the cell.

stores is enough to fuel the work required for a 6-second sprint, a 1-minute walk, or a weight lift. Beyond that, work can only be maintained if energy is liberated from the breakdown of foodstuffs which are also stored within the cell (Fig. 2.2). This occurs along two metabolic pathways: anaerobic glycolysis and oxidative phosphorylation.

On a short-term basis, energy for phosphorylating ADP to ATP can be rapidly derived from the breakdown of glucose or glycogen through the process called glycolysis. As we shall see in chapter 4, this ends in the formation of lactic acid which must be eliminated from cells because it disturbs their acid–base balance. It first is discharged into the blood where one observes the concentration of lactate to increase; it is then disposed of in various ways which are, however, relatively slow. This pathway for gaining energy from foodstuffs does not depend on the availability of O_2; but its usefulness is limited in time and intensity because of the detrimental effects of its waste product, lactic acid.

Long-term energy supply must be secured through oxidative phosphorylation, which produces "clean" energy because its breakdown products, CO_2 and water, are easily eliminated. It is also most efficient with respect to foodstuffs: whereas from 1 mol glucose only 2 mol ATP can be gained by glycolysis, oxidative phosphorylation generates 36 mol ATP. Furthermore, the substrates for oxidative phosphorylation can also be drawn from fats and proteins through some intermediate metabolic steps (Fig. 2.2). But unlike glycolysis, oxidative phosphorylation is unconditionally dependent on a continuous supply of O_2. Although the cells, particularly some muscle cells, contain a certain amount of O_2 bound to intracellular O_2 stores (mostly to muscle hemoglobin or myoglobin, an iron pigment which causes muscle to be red), the amount of O_2 stored in the cells in this way does not last for very long. It must be replenished from environmental O_2 if energy production through oxidative phosphorylation is to continue.

In summary, when cells take up work they will first draw the energy required from their high-energy phosphate stores (ATP and CP); the rise in ADP concentration resulting from the breakdown of ATP will then trigger a metabolic chain reaction that first releases "fast" ATP from glycolysis and then proceeds to long-term ATP production by oxidative phosphorylation. It is only in this last phase that the energy needs of the cell become quantitatively reflected in the amount of O_2 consumed.

That this entails a certain delay is perhaps best seen in the case of physical exercise, where the energetic demands derive essentially from muscle work: when they are active, muscles have high energy requirements, and furthermore they make up about 40% of total body mass. Suppose now a subject whose O_2 consumption at rest is about 200 ml·min^{-1}. At point A on the time scale of Figure 2.3 we ask the subject to start running at a moderate speed which he is capable of maintaining over a certain time. The work output of his muscles instantaneously rises to the level required to run at the given speed, and then stays constant for, say, 12 minutes or longer. If we now measure O_2 consumption, we note that it rises slowly to reach a steady-state level after about 3–4 minutes (point B). If we assume that the steady-state level corresponds to the O_2 flow rate required for oxidative phosphorylation to "pay" the metabolic cost of running at that speed, then it is evident that the O_2 inflow during the first four minutes was insufficient to cover this cost. In the initial part of exercise there was an O_2 *deficit*, which means that the difference between the energy needed to do the work required (broken line in Fig. 2.3) and that provided by the O_2 uptake must be paid from other sources. It is now interesting to note that when exercise is suddenly stopped at point C, O_2 uptake falls rather slowly over a period of several minutes. What happens is that the body is apparently paying off a metabolic debt incurred in the course of exercise, in this case mostly during the initial parts of the run. The O_2 debt is the area under the $\dot{V}_{O_2}$ curve in Figure 2.3 from point C to that time when resting levels of O_2 consumption are reached again. The O_2 debt is

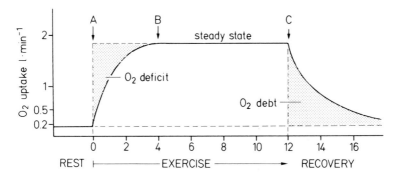

Fig. 2.3 O_2 consumption takes a few minutes to reach the steady-state level imposed by the energetic demands of exercise. The O_2 deficit in terms of energy balance at the start of exercise is reflected in a somewhat larger O_2 debt during recovery.

always a bit larger than the O_2 deficit, as if the loan had to be paid off with sizable interest.

How can we explain this difference, which was first described by A. V. Hill in 1924? If we refer back to Figure 2.2 we can see that, at the onset of exercise, the muscle cell will first draw on its high-energy phosphate stores to cover its immediate energy needs. As the ADP levels rise, metabolic events are triggered and will now begin to replenish the phosphate stores. This will at first occur through the rapid pathway of glycolysis, which furnishes ATP directly but also provides the substrates for oxidative phosphorylation in the mitochondria through the Krebs cycle and respiratory chain. Since oxidative phosphorylation seems to be somewhat slow in taking off, some of the chemical end products of glycolysis are spilled off into the blood as lactic acid. When oxidative phosphorylation begins, it will at first derive the required O_2 from the cell's O_2 stores; when these become somewhat depleted, the P_{O_2} gradient between the cell and the blood in capillaries is increased and more O_2 can now flow into the cell. This is then followed by adjustments in the complex system which supplies O_2 to the cells. Blood flow becomes increased by stepping up the heart rate, and the venous blood which leaves the muscles has a lower P_{O_2} owing to a greater O_2 extraction by the cells. The lung is perfused with blood at a higher flow rate and receives blood of lower P_{O_2}; more O_2 is taken up by the blood in the lung, and ventilation increases to meet this demand. The O_2 deficit is explained by the fact that this complex functional system requires some time to adjust to a new steady-state level of covering energetic needs through oxidative phosphorylation; but remember that long-term work can only be performed when this is achieved. On the other hand, this process sets up a number of gradients which help the flow of energy through the system: oxidative phosphorylation will adjust its level of activity to the ATP needs of the phosphate stores, gauged to the level of ADP available for rephosphorylation; and O_2 inflow from the blood will be determined by the level of depletion of the O_2 stores, and so on.

Once the energy demands on the system cease at the end of the exercise, oxidative phosphorylation will proceed until the phosphate stores are restored to the pre-exercise level; and, finally, O_2 inflow into the cells must proceed at a higher level until the partly depleted O_2 stores are filled up again. This reversal of the O_2 deficit that occurred at the beginning of exercise is part of the O_2 debt paid in the initial part of the recovery period, but there is clearly more to it. First, the heart rate does not fall to resting levels immediately, nor does ventilation, evidently because one still needs to bring in more O_2. Second, other physiological conditions must also be brought back to pre-exercise levels: body temperature rises somewhat during exercise and we need increased blood flow and perspiration to cool off; food stores in the cells must be replenished from the liver or from the diet, and so forth. All this explains why the O_2 debt is larger than the O_2 deficit. The original concept of A. V. Hill was that lactic acid formed at the onset and during exercise must be resynthesized into glucose in the liver and that this explained O_2 debt. While this may have to occur to some extent after very heavy, exhaustive exercise, it does not seem to play a major role in moderate exercise; it is now well established that lactic acid is directly utilized as a substrate for oxidative phosphorylation in some cells, particularly in the heart and the liver, but also in skeletal muscle.

I should finally mention that this system of energy flow to the sites where biological work is done appears to be rather well regulated to the actual energy needs. Figure 2.4 shows an experiment where a subject is made to run at constant speed up hills of increasing grade.

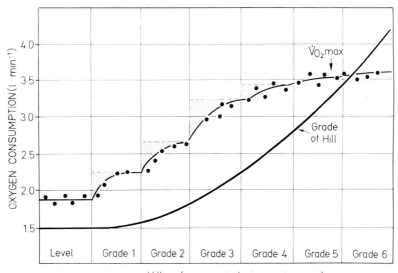

Fig. 2.4 In man, increasing the work load of running up a "hill" by increasing the grade causes a step-wise increase of O_2 consumption, each time with an O_2 deficit (stippled area), until $\dot{V}_{O_2}$max is reached. (After McArdle, Katch and Katch, 1981.)

At each grade a steady-state level of O_2 uptake is reached after a period of O_2 deficit, and this level is proportional to the work output required. This graph also shows that, at a certain point, the system has reached its limit and O_2 uptake can no more increase in spite of a higher imposed work load; we shall come back to this shortly.

In summary, we note that the O_2 needs of the body reflect rather closely the energetic needs of its cells because, on a long-term basis, the energetic cost of biological work must be paid by oxidative phosphorylation. The other mechanisms are available to the cells only for the short term and must eventually be repaid by oxidative phosphorylation in one way or another. We have demonstrated this with the example of muscle work because here the various events become so strikingly apparent; it is safe to say, however, that the same basic principles of liberating energy for biological work apply to all cells and their activities. The overall metabolic rate of the organism is therefore reflected in its rate of O_2 consumption, at least under steady-state conditions.

Levels of O_2 Consumption

The metabolic rate of an organism is not a fixed value but is modulated by various factors; accordingly, O_2 consumption will also be variable. In the preceding section we have seen that O_2 consumption is well regulated to energetic needs. As we do physical work of any kind we must breathe harder and our heart beats at a higher pace, reflecting the increased need for O_2. But there are other determinants of metabolic rate, such as temperature and body size. When we are exposed to cold without adequate clothing, we need more O_2 to compensate for the heat loss; on the other hand, we breathe more intensely when we are febrile. Lastly, small animals breathe more rapidly than large ones because their metabolic rate is higher.

Looking first at temperature effects, we must clearly distinguish body temperature from ambient temperature, because they will affect organisms differently. What one calls "cold-blooded" animals or *poikilotherms* are animals that will allow their body temperature to adjust to ambient temperature; "warm-blooded" animals or *homeotherms* will maintain a constant body temperature irrespective of the temperature in their surrounding, and they will achieve this by modulating their heat loss and their heat production.

The metabolic effect of *central body temperature* follows the rule that an increase in temperature is accompanied by an increase in metabolic rate; remember that, in fact, the rate of all chemical processes increases with temperature. One describes this temperature effect by a factor Q_{10} which indicates the rate increase due to a temperature increase by 10° C:

$$Q_{10} = \dot{V}_{O_2}(T + 10)/\dot{V}_{O_2}(T). \qquad (2.1)$$

This factor can be calculated from estimates of $\dot{V}_{O_2}$ at any two temperatures T_1 and T_2 by

$$Q_{10} = [\dot{V}_{O_2}(T_2)/\dot{V}_{O_2}(T_1)]^{10/(T_2-T_1)} \qquad (2.2)$$

or

$$\log Q_{10} = \frac{10}{T_2 - T_1} \cdot [\log \dot{V}_{O_2}(T_2) - \log \dot{V}_{O_2}(T_1)]. \qquad (2.3)$$

It turns out that for most animals Q_{10} has a constant value between 2 and 3 within the range of temperatures that are normally tolerated; this range is smaller in homeotherms than in poikilotherms. Note that if a mammal hibernates, it will drop its body temperature by some 20° C or more and can thus reduce its minimal metabolic rate by about a factor of 5 to 10.

When considering the effect of *ambient temperature* we now must distinguish between poikilotherms and homeotherms. In poikilotherms the body temperature becomes adapted to the ambient temperature; thus a fish or a frog living in cold water will have a reduced metabolic rate, and this reduction is described by equation 2.3, that is, it depends on Q_{10}. Homeotherms, however, will have to adapt their metabolic heat production to maintain their body temperature within the narrow tolerated range, and will therefore show a "reversed" change in metabolic rate: it will increase as ambient temperature falls and decrease as it rises, as shown in Figure 2.5. But there is a lower limit for resting metabolic rate, so that above what is called the lower critical temperature, metabolic rate remains constant. At much higher ambient temperatures above the higher critical temperature, $\dot{V}_{O_2}$ will rise again, because body temperature increases. The range in which temperature has no effect on metabolic rate is called

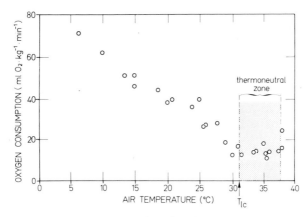

Fig. 2.5 O_2 consumption is inversely related to air temperature in a small mammal (pigmy possum) until a lower critical temperature (T_{lc}) is reached where the thermoneutral zone begins. (After Bartholomew and Hudson, 1962.)

the *thermoneutral zone*. This is the range which one can expect to measure the lowest metabolic rates in resting animals.

The effect of *body size* on the metabolic rate of animals is a most interesting phenomenon which we shall use as an experimental tool throughout this book. In principle, smaller animals require, per unit body mass, a higher metabolic rate than larger animals (Table 2.1). This is shown in Figure 2.6 (top) for mammals, where we see that a shrew weighing some 5 g consumes about 100 times more O_2 per gram body mass than an elephant weighing 4 tons. It turns out that the *specific metabolic rate* of mammals, $\dot{V}_{O_2}/M_b$, decreases as a power function of body mass, M_b

$$\dot{V}_{O_2}/M_b = a \cdot M_b^{-0.25}. \tag{2.4}$$

Figure 2.6 (bottom) shows that such a power function, which is called an *allometric function*, becomes a linear regression when the data are plotted on double-logarithmic scales. Alternatively, we can look at the *total metabolic rate* of the animal which we then find to increase with body mass to the power 0.75:

$$\dot{V}_{O_2} = a \cdot M_b^{0.75}. \tag{2.5}$$

Figure 2.7 shows the allometric plots of O_2 consumption rates for a wide variety of organisms, from unicellular organisms and poikilo-

TABLE 2.1. MAXIMAL O_2 CONSUMPTION IN MAMMALS RELATED TO BODY MASS (M_b).

Species	M_b (kg)	$\dot{V}_{O_2}max$ (ml·sec^{-1})	$\dot{V}_{O_2}max/M_b$ (ml·sec^{-1}·kg^{-1})
Pygmy mouse	0.0072	0.0314	4.36
Chipmunk	0.0902	0.358	3.97
White rat	0.205	0.330	1.61
Rat kangaroo	1.10	3.24	2.95
Banded mongoose	1.15	2.33	2.00
Spring hare	3.00	4.85	1.62
Suni	3.50	5.62	1.60
Grant's gazelle	11.2	10.0	0.89
Dog	21.0	55.4	2.64
Goat	21.1	18.3	0.86
Lion	30.0	30.0	1.00
Man	70.0	40.3	0.58
Wildebeest	98.0	72.6	0.75
Horse	105.0	169.0	1.61
Eland	217.0	131.0	0.60
Cow	254.0	125.0	0.49

Data from Seeherman et al. (1981) and Taylor et al. (1981).

therms to homeotherms, birds, and mammals. In each of the major groups, the data points fall onto linear regression lines with a slope of 0.75 which corresponds to the exponent in the power function of equation 2.5.

This universal relation between body size and metabolic rate is not easy to explain. It was first thought to be related to body surface and thus directly related to heat loss, because body surface increases with body mass to the power $\frac{2}{3} = 0.67$. In general terms, one can say that it would be impossible to build mammals of largely different body size which have the same weight-specific metabolic rate because of heat exchange problems through their skin: a steer with the metabolic rate of a mouse could not get rid of the heat produced in the depths of its body, whereas a mouse with the steer's metabolic rate could not keep warm. However, this "surface law" cannot be the whole story,

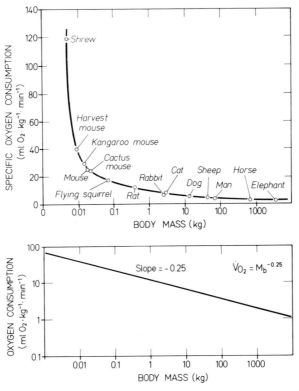

Fig. 2.6 Specific O_2 consumption in mammals increases steadily as body mass becomes smaller (top). The nonlinear function is expressed by a power function with slope -0.25 (bottom). (From Schmidt-Nielsen, 1979.)

because the slope of 0.75 found for metabolic rate is significantly different from 0.67 (Fig. 2.7). It may well be that other factors play an eminent role in determining these rates; among these the concept of "biological time" is of special interest, which says that small animals live "more quickly" than large ones.

What we have discussed so far are effects on what one usually calls the *standard resting metabolic rate*, that is, some kind of minimum O_2 requirement of the organism needed to fuel the basic functions that are never turned off. Some of these functions are: the necessity to pump ions through cell membranes in order to maintain the correct ionic balance; basic synthetic functions to maintain cells and tissues; conduction of electric impulses in the nervous system; secretory functions in the digestive tract, lung, or skin; urine formation in the

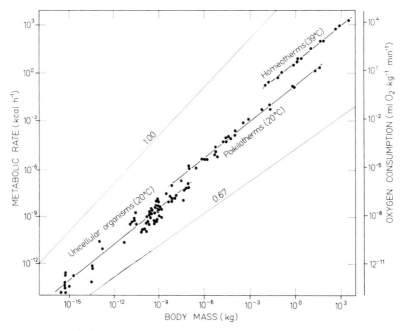

Fig. 2.7 Metabolic rate and O_2 consumption are power functions of body mass with slope 0.75 in all animals, from unicellular organisms to homeotherms. (After Hemmingsen, 1960.)

kidney; and, of course, the energetic costs of keeping the circulation and respiration going. The metabolic rate increases immediately and substantially as soon as muscles are being used to move about or do work; as we have seen above, this causes O_2 consumption to increase in proportion to the work done. It has been shown that, in a well-trained man, O_2 consumption can be increased by about 10 to 15 times above standard resting metabolism by running, for example. There seems to be an upper limit, however, above which $\dot{V}_{O_2}$ cannot be increased any further, although the body may be required to further increase its work output (Fig. 2.4). This upper limit is called *aerobic capacity* or *maximal O_2 consumption*, $\dot{V}_{O_2}$max.

Estimating the Limits of O_2 Consumption

It is evident that the limit of O_2 consumption is an important parameter when we attempt to characterize the respiratory system: it describes the maximal flow rate for O_2 that the system allows. To set this into relation with various structural and functional characteristics of the system will be one of my main endeavors in most of this book, because the power of a functional system is best described by its limits. How can we estimate the overall functional limit or capacity of the respiratory system?

We have seen in the preceding section that there are two ways by which we can make an organism, specifically a homeotherm, increase its metabolic rate: by exposure to a cold environment and by physical work.

Exposure to cold increases O_2 consumption in about linear proportion to temperature (Fig. 2.5), because the animals need to generate heat to keep their body temperature constant. About 60% of the energy freed by oxidative catabolism of substrates is lost as heat; so increasing the rate at which glucose and fat are metabolized generates heat. This is a normal process used to regulate body temperature; mainly small animals and newborn humans have a tissue specialized for that purpose: brown adipose tissue which is particularly rich in mitochondria. When the body is exposed to abnormally low temperatures, muscles may also participate in generating heat; when this occurs suddenly, the animal may shiver, as we shiver when we feel cold. One interesting question is whether this process leads to an excess production of ATP or whether phosphorylation is uncoupled from electron transfer. It should be mentioned that not much is gained in this instance by glycolysis, because this liberates little heat, as we shall see.

One can exploit this feature to estimate some limit of O_2 consumption, a method that has been used extensively with small mammals. If ambient temperature is lowered toward $O°$ C, O_2 consumption may reach the five-fold of the resting value obtained in the thermoneutral zone (Fig. 2.5). The problem with this approach is that it is difficult to know whether limiting conditions of O_2 consumption have been reached. One usually measures central body temperature and measures O_2 flow at the ambient temperature at which body temperature begins to fall. The metabolic rate measured at this temperature is called *summit O_2 consumption*, $\dot{V}_{O_2}$sum. It has been shown to amount to about 80% of maximal $\dot{V}_{O_2}$ induced by exercise.

The most reliable method for estimating the limits to O_2 consumption is to measure the increase in $\dot{V}_{O_2}$ as the animal is induced to *increasing levels of muscular exercise*, such as by running on a treadmill or swimming. A system as we have used it for much of the work to be described is to let the animal — it can of course, also be a human being — run on a treadmill at controlled speed and to measure O_2 consumption continuously (see chapter 3).

With this method one finds O_2 consumption to increase linearly with running speed up to a certain level, above which it remains constant, as shown in Figure 2.8; a dog running up an incline of 14°, for example, will reach running speeds up to 5 m·sec^{-1} (or 18 km per hour), but its O_2 consumption reaches the maximal level at about 3.5 m·sec^{-1}. Similar values are obtained for other species. Thus we could conclude that the plateau observed in this curve corresponds to *maximal O_2 consumption*, which we have designated $\dot{V}_{O_2}$max. Indeed, this is justified for the following reason. If we take small blood samples at the various speeds and measure the rate at which the lactate concentration in blood plasma increases, we find that this

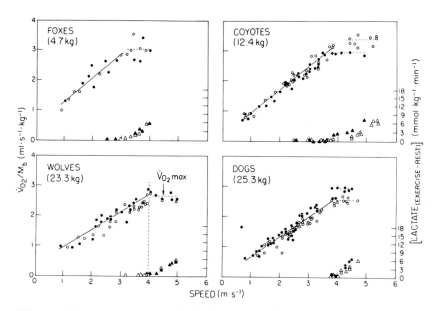

Fig. 2.8 O_2 consumption per kg body mass (circles) increases linearly with running speed in four species of canids running on a treadmill inclined at 14°. When $\dot{V}_{O_2}$max is reached, additional energy required to run faster is produced by glycolysis, resulting in an increase of lactate delivery into the blood (triangles). The full and open symbols refer to two individual animals from each species. (Data from C. R. Taylor, published in Weibel et al., 1983.)

rate goes up at the speed at which $\dot{V}_{O_2}$ reaches the plateau. This is clearly a sign that the muscles now use glycolysis to generate the extra ATP required to run at still higher speeds. And the lactate concentration in plasma increases in proportion to the additional energy required. In Figure 2.8 we have adjusted the scale for lactate increase to be proportional to that of $\dot{V}_{O_2}$ in terms of "energetic equivalents" or ATP produced. (We shall see later that 0.67 mol lactate formed from glycogen breakdown or 0.16 mol O_2 consumed correspond to 1 mol ATP generated.)

We conclude from these observations that muscles have a higher capacity to do work than they can cover by oxidative phosphoryl-ation because the O_2 that can be delivered to the mitochondria in the muscle cells is somehow limited. We shall therefore consider as *maximal O_2 consumption* that value of $\dot{V}_{O_2}$ obtained during strenuous muscular exercise of such intensity that glycolysis must be involved to provide supplemental ATP.

It is evident, however, that exercise levels which require supplemental energy from increased levels of glycolysis cannot be maintained for a very long time because they lead to an accumulation of lactate in the blood and in the tissues, causing severe imbalance in the ionic environment of the cells. Accordingly, the performance levels where $\dot{V}_{O_2}$max is just about reached can be considered the limit of long-term or endurance exercise. This further strengthens the significance of $\dot{V}_{O_2}$max for estimating the limits of energetics in the body.

A last point to be discussed is how $\dot{V}_{O_2}$max is related to the other levels of O_2 consumption, particularly to standard resting metabolic rate, and how it varies among animals. It turns out that O_2 consumption can be increased about 10-fold from resting to maximal in all mammals so far investigated, but there is considerable variation. In particular, there are large differences in the level of $\dot{V}_{O_2}$max reached between different species, and even between different individuals in one species. In Figure 2.8 one can note that the two dogs whose data are shown in the lower right-hand panel increase O_2 consumption along the same regression line as speed increases; but one of them reaches a $\dot{V}_{O_2}$max level which is 15% higher, so that one of them has a higher aerobic capacity than the other. In humans one finds that well-trained athletes have an aerobic capacity which is up to 50% higher than in untrained individuals. On the other hand, Table 2.1 shows that the $\dot{V}_{O_2}$max of dogs is about three times higher than that of

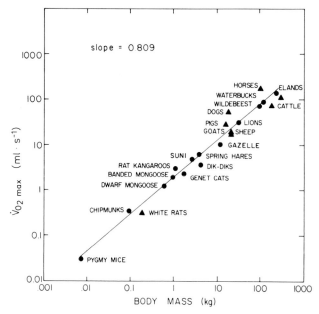

Fig. 2.9 Average values of $\dot{V}_{O_2}$max of 21 mammalian species increase with body mass to the power 0.81. (From Taylor et al., 1981.)

goats of the same body mass, and the $\dot{V}_{O_2}$ of the horse twice that of the wildebeest. Such differences are highly relevant for our purpose because they allow us to look for relations between the limits to O_2 flow and design properties of the respiratory system.

Such differences within size classes are, however, small compared to the differences in metabolic rate as a function of body mass. Thus we find that mass-specific $\dot{V}_{O_2}$max ($\dot{V}_{O_2}$max/M_b) is about ten times greater in the pygmy mouse than in cattle (Table 2.1). Considering the allometry of $\dot{V}_{O_2}$max, we find that it increases in proportion to the 0.8 power of body mass (Fig. 2.9), thus with an allometric regression similar to that found for resting metabolism (Fig. 2.7). This again we shall exploit in seeking relations between limiting O_2 flow rates and design features of the respiratory system.

Summary

The energy required by cells is drawn from high-energy phosphates —mostly ATP—of which a small amount is stored in the cells for immediate use. Muscle cells contain enough ATP to fuel a 6-second sprint or a weight-lift. Beyond that new ATP must be made by phosphorylation of ADP. This is rapidly achieved anaerobically through glycolysis, but it is wasteful with substrates and leads to the formation of lactate which has detrimental effects. Long-term energy supply must be secured through oxidative phosphorylation in mitochondria, whose waste products CO_2 and H_2O are harmless because they are easily eliminated. When, in exercise, muscles begin to work, they first draw on their high-energy phosphate stores, then use glycolysis to make ATP before oxidative phosphorylation becomes fully operative; O_2 consumption reaches its full level only after a few minutes, a delay called the O_2 deficit. At the end of the exercise oxidative phosphorylation continues for some time, a phenomenon called the O_2 debt. Oxidative phosphorylation and O_2 consumption are tightly regulated to the cells' need in ATP, so that total O_2 consumption reflects the total energetic needs of the body.

The metabolic rate and hence the O_2 consumption of the body are modulated by various factors, besides their dependence on energetic needs arising from work. The effects of ambient temperature are different. In poikilotherms (cold-blooded animals) central body temperature is adjusted to ambient temperature and the metabolic rate falls as temperature falls; the same occurs, with degrees, in a hibernating mammal. In homeotherms (warm-blooded animals) central body temperature must be kept constant; as ambient temperature falls metabolic rate increases to compensate for the higher heat loss.

Body size affects metabolic rate, with small animals having a higher metabolic rate per unit of body mass than large animals, in proportion to $M_b^{-0.25}$. Accordingly total metabolic rate increases with $M_b^{0.75}$, a relation which holds for all living creatures, from unicellular organisms to mammals.

The limit of O_2 consumption (aerobic capacity, maximal O_2 consumption) is an important characteristic of the respiratory system: it describes the maximal O_2 flow rate the system allows. It is estimated either by cold exposure or by intensive exercise. Cold exposure yields metabolic rates which increase linearly with falling temperature. Running on a treadmill causes the metabolic rate to increase linearly with speed. Maximal O_2 consumption is achieved in running, whereas by cold exposure only about 80% of this level is reached. If the body is asked to work in excess of what can be covered by oxidative phosphorylation at the aerobic capacity, the muscle cells will revert to anaerobic glycolysis to make the additional ATP required, resulting in an increase of lactate concentration in the blood and in a fall of pH (acidosis).

Further Reading

Åstrand, P.-O., and K. Rodahl. 1977. *Textbook of Work Physiology.* New York: McGraw-Hill.

Brody, S. 1968. *Bioenergetics and Growth.* Princeton: Reinhold-Van Nostrand. New York: Hafner.

Lehninger, A. L. 1982. *Principles of Biochemistry.* New York: Worth, chapters 13 and 14.

Margaria, R. 1976. *Biomechanics and Energetics of Muscular Exercise.* London: Oxford University Press.

McArdle, W. D., F. I. Katch, and V. L. Katch. 1981. *Exercise Physiology.* Philadelphia: Lea & Febiger.

Taylor, C. R., and N. C. Heglund. 1982. Energetics and mechanics of terrestrial locomotion. *Annual Review of Physiology* 44:97–107.

References

* Adolph, E. F. 1949. Quantitative relations in the physical constitution of mammals. *Science* 109:579–585.

Bartholomew, G. A., and J. W. Hudson. 1962. Hibernation, estivation, temperature regulation, evaporative water loss, and heart rate of the pigmy possum, *Cercaertus nanus. Physiological Zoölogy* 35:94–107.

Dejours, P. 1981. *Principles of Comparative Respiratory Physiology.* 2nd ed. Amsterdam: Elsevier North-Holland.

Di Prampero, P. E., and R. Margaria. 1968. Relationship between O_2 consumption, high energy phosphates and the kinetics of the O_2 debt in exercise. *Pflügers Archiv* 304:11–19.

Hemmingsen, A. M. 1960. Energy metabolism as related to body size and respiratory surfaces, and its evolution. In *Reports of the Steno Memorial Hospital,* vol. 9, pt. 2. Copenhagen: Steno Memorial Hospital, pp. 1–110.

* Hill, A. V., C. N. H. Long, and H. Lupton. 1924. Muscular exercise, lactic acid and the supply and utilization of oxygen. *Proceedings of the Royal Society of London (Biology)* 97:84–95.

Margaria, R., P. Cerretelli, P. Aghemo, and G. Sassi. 1963. Energy cost of running. *Journal of Applied Physiology* 18:367–370.

* Margaria, R., H. T. Edwards, and D. B. Dill. 1933. The possible mechanism of contracting and paying the oxygen debt and the role of lactic acid in muscular contraction. *American Journal of Physiology* 106:689–715.

McArdle, W. D., F. I. Katch, and V. L. Katch. 1981. *Exercise Physiology.* Philadelphia: Lea & Febiger.

Pasquis, P., A. Lacaisse, and P. Dejours. 1970. Maximal oxygen uptake in four species of small mammals. *Respiration Physiology* 9:298–309.

Schmidt-Nielsen, K. 1972. Locomotion: energy cost of swimming, flying and running. *Science* 177:222–228.

—— 1979. *Animal Physiology.* 2nd ed. Cambridge: Cambridge University press.

Seeherman, H. J., C. R. Taylor, G. M. O. Maloiy, and R. B. Armstrong. 1981. Design of the mammalian respiratory system. II. Measuring maximum aerobic capacity. *Respiration Physiology* 44:11–23.

Taylor, C. R. 1973. Energy cost of animal locomotion. In *Comparative Physiology,* ed. L. Bolis, K. Schmidt-Nielsen, and S. H. P. Maddrell. Amsterdam: North-Holland, pp. 23–42.

Taylor, C. R., N. C. Heglund, and G. M. O. Maloiy. 1982. Energetics and mechanics of terrestrial locomotion. I. Metabolic energy consumption as a function of speed and body size in birds and mammals. *Journal of Experimental Biology* 97:1–21.

Taylor, C. R., N. C. Heglund, T. A. McMahon, and T. R. Looney. 1980. Energetic cost of generating muscular force during running: a comparison of large and small animals. *Journal of Experimental Biology* 86:9–18.

Taylor, C. R., G. M. O. Maloiy, E. R. Weibel, V. A. Langman, J. M. Z. Kamau, H. J. Seeherman, and N. C. Heglund. 1981. Design of the mammalian respiratory system. III. Scaling maximum aerobic capacity to body mass: wild and domestic mammals. *Respiration Physiology* 44:25–37.

Taylor, C. R., K. Schmidt-Nielsen, and J. L. Raab. 1970. Scaling of energetic cost of running to body size in mammals. *American Journal of Physiology* 219:1104–1107.

Weibel, E. R., C. R. Taylor, P. Gehr, H. Hoppeler, O. Mathieu, and G. M. O. Maloiy. 1981. Design of the mammalian respiratory system. IX. Functional and structural limits for oxygen flow. *Respiration Physiology* 44:151–164.

Weibel, E. R., C. R. Taylor, J. J. O'Neil, D. E. Leith, P. Gehr, H. Hoppeler, V. Langman, and R. V. Baudinette. 1983. Maximal oxygen consumption and pulmonary diffusing capacity: a direct comparison of physiologic and morphometric measurements in canids. *Respiration Physiology* 54.

3

LINKING STRUCTURE AND FUNCTION: MODEL, MEANS, AND TOOLS

IN REVIEWING EVOLUTION in chapter 1 we have noticed that all higher organisms secure an adequate O_2 supply to their cells through a respiratory system that can essentially be subdivided into three compartments (Figs. 3.1 and 1.5): (A) the respiratory medium, air or water, that enters the external gas exchanger; (B) blood that serves as O_2 carrier; and (C) the cells that house the furnaces where O_2 is consumed. These compartments are arranged in series, and we have seen that a flow of O_2 becomes established either by bulk flow of the carriers within the compartments or by exchange of O_2 between the compartments at their interfaces. This principle of organization holds also for the mammalian respiratory system which, in essence, differs from that of other forms only in the design of the lung and circulation.

The flow of O_2 through this system is clearly determined by the rate at which O_2 disappears into the mitochondria in the process of making ATP in order to fuel cell functions. Thus a runner, who may consume in his muscles 3 liters of O_2 per minute to fuel a fast and steady run, will have to collect O_2 from the air at the same rate. In the lung he will need to transfer O_2 to his erythrocytes at the rate of $3 \, l \cdot min^{-1}$; blood flow will have to carry them to the tissues where they can discharge O_2 at the rate of $3 \, l \cdot min^{-1}$, the rate at which the mitochondria use O_2 to make ATP by oxidative phosphorylation. And we have seen in chapter 2 that cell metabolism is well-regulated to energetic needs so that the muscle cells will only consume as

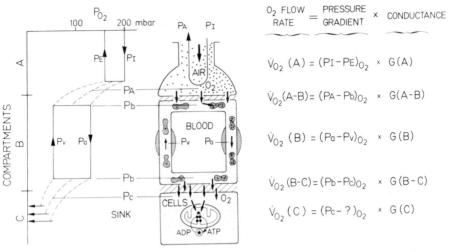

$$\frac{O_2\ FLOW}{RATE} = \frac{PRESSURE}{GRADIENT} \times CONDUCTANCE$$

$$\dot{V}_{O_2}(A) = (PI - PE)_{O_2} \times G(A)$$

$$\dot{V}_{O_2}(A\text{-}B) = (PA - Pb)_{O_2} \times G(A\text{-}B)$$

$$\dot{V}_{O_2}(B) = (Pa - Pv)_{O_2} \times G(B)$$

$$\dot{V}_{O_2}(B\text{-}C) = (Pb - Pc)_{O_2} \times G(B\text{-}C)$$

$$\dot{V}_{O_2}(C) = (Pc - ?)_{O_2} \times G(C)$$

Fig. 3.1 Model of the respiratory system of mammals in the form of a cascade (compare Fig. 1.5). The O_2 flow rate through each of the sequential steps is the product of a pressure difference and a conductance. In a steady state the flow rates through all steps must be equal. (After Taylor and Weibel, 1981.)

much O_2 as needed to replenish the phosphate stores in response to ATP consumption.

From this we derive one basic condition for the functioning of the repiratory system: the flow rates of O_2 through each link of the chain must be equal and matched to the rate at which O_2 disappears in the mitochondria, so that

$$\dot{V}_{O_2}(A) = \dot{V}_{O_2}(A\text{-}B) = \dot{V}_{O_2}(B) = \dot{V}_{O_2}(B\text{-}C) = \dot{V}_{O_2}(C) \tag{3.1}$$

accounts for steady-state conditions.

The flow rate of O_2 through any of the elements of the respiratory system can conveniently be expressed by the product of a conductance, G, with the difference between the O_2 partial pressures at the entrance (in) and at the exit (ex) of the element:

$$\dot{V}_{O_2} = G \cdot [P_{O_2}(in) - P_{O_2}(ex)]. \tag{3.2}$$

Note that this is Ohm's law, well-known from the physics of electricity, which relates the current J to the tension ΔU between the poles of a conductor and its resistance R, which is simply the reciprocal of the conductance (Fig. 3.2a). This same formula also holds for the flow of fluid through a tube where now the driving force is the hydrostatic pressure difference, ΔP, between inflow and outflow side of the tube (Fig. 3.2b). And we have seen in chapter 1 that diffusion of a solute across a barrier is driven by the difference in concentration or partial pressure of the solute on both sides of the barrier (Figs. 1.1 and 3.2c). Equation 3.2 is therefore of very general applicability. It is most useful for our purpose because it expresses O_2 flow rate as a function of two variables which separate the effect of O_2 from that of the system: O_2 affects O_2 flow rate through the partial pressure difference, whereas the conductance G contains all the design parameters of the respiratory system that influence $\dot{V}_{O_2}$.

This now allows us to set up a complete physiological model for the mammalian respiratory system, as it is shown in Figure 3.1. The structural framework is, evidently, the chain of compartments—air, blood, and cells—that interact in the lung and in the tissue. The basic functional "driving force" for O_2 flow through this system is a cascade of O_2 partial pressures which gradually decrease from the P_{O_2} in ambient air of about 150 torr (200 mbar) to very low values in the region of the mitochondrial O_2 sink.

If we look at the scheme in detail, we notice that the P_{O_2} cascade is not a simple step function. It is more complicated because the P_{O_2}

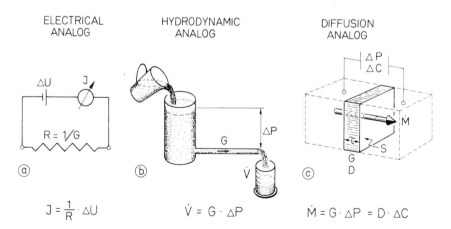

ELECTRICAL ANALOG	HYDRODYNAMIC ANALOG	DIFFUSION ANALOG

$$J = \frac{1}{R} \cdot \Delta U \qquad \dot{V} = G \cdot \Delta P \qquad \dot{M} = G \cdot \Delta P = D \cdot \Delta C$$

Fig. 3.2 In either an electrical, a hydrodynamic, or a diffusion analog model the flow rate is the product of a conductance with a driving force in the form of a tension gradient across the conductor.

gradient is not the only, perhaps not even the actual, driving force for O_2 flow within the compartments A and B, where O_2 is carried by bulk flow of air and blood, respectively. In compartment A, the P_{O_2} difference is that between inspired and expired air and hence depends essentially on the extraction of O_2 that occurs in the lung, but also on the rate at which the lung is ventilated with fresh air. Similarly, in compartment B the P_{O_2} difference between arterial and venous blood is the result of O_2 extraction in the tissue, of O_2 inflow in the lung, and of blood flow. Even with respect to the gas exchangers in lung and tissue, the P_{O_2} differences are not simple to define. In describing the external gas exchangers in chapter 1 (Figs. 1.8 to 1.13) we have noticed that these gradients are quite different for the different designs, and that they may show local differences as well. And finally, the P_{O_2} prevailing in the region of the O_2 sink is ill-defined: it appears that mitochondria can perform oxidative phosphorylation within a wide range of P_{O_2}, possibly down to very low values.

In spite of these apparent difficulties it is convenient for our purposes to retain the P_{O_2} cascade as a unifying basic parameter determining O_2 flow through the system, mainly because O_2 solution in water, O_2 diffusion, and O_2 binding to carriers such as blood can be easily defined in relation to P_{O_2} as a common parameter.

How Does Structure Affect O_2 Flow?

A further convenience of the model of Figure 3.1 with the P_{O_2} cascade as driving force is that the O_2 flow rate is affected by structural design features through the conductance G of equation 3.2. The structural parameters which must be considered in defining G at the various levels of the system will be different, depending on whether O_2 flow is by diffusion, bulk flow of a carrier, or consumption in the sink.

CONDUCTANCE FOR DIFFUSIVE O_2 EXCHANGE

Diffusive exchange between two compartments occurs across a barrier made of material that usually is different from that constituting the two compartments. Thus the gas-exchange barrier in the lung is made of tissue and separates air and blood (Fig. 3.3). Three properties affect the diffusion conductance of such a barrier: the area, S, over

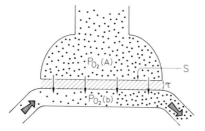

Fig. 3.3 Model for O_2 flow by diffusion from alveolar air (A) to capillary blood (b) which depends on the P_{O_2} difference and on the surface (S) and thickness (τ) of the barrier.

which the barrier establishes contact between the compartments, the thickness of the barrier, τ, and its material properties which are expressed by a permeability coefficient K. Fick's law says that

$$\dot{V}_{O_2}(\text{A-B}) = K_x \cdot \frac{S}{\tau} \cdot [P_{O_2}(A) - P_{O_2}(B)]. \tag{3.3}$$

By comparing with equation 3.2, we see that the conductance

$$G(\text{A-B}) = K_x \cdot \frac{S}{\tau} \tag{3.4}$$

is directly proportional to the barrier surface area and inversely proportional to its thickness, the two basic parameters of barrier design. We shall see later on that we must be somewhat more specific about the precise meaning of "surface" and "thickness" with respect to real structures, because, on the one hand, the two surfaces of the barrier may be of different area, and, on the other hand, the barrier thickness may show important local variations. But we shall defer this until we set up detailed models that describe gas exchange in the lung or in the tissues.

The coefficient K_x is called Krogh's permeability or diffusion constant and needs some explanation. It is, in fact, the product of two material properties: the diffusion coefficient, D_{O_2}, for O_2 and the solubility β_{O_2} of O_2 in this material:

$$K_x = D_{O_2} \cdot \beta_{O_2}. \tag{3.5}$$

The diffusion coefficient D_{O_2} indicates the quantity of O_2 that moves in the unit time through a unit cross-sectional area of the barrier under a *concentration* gradient ΔC_{O_2} over the unit length of diffusion distance; it has the dimension $cm^2 \cdot sec^{-1}$. Thus, in fact, diffusion across the barrier depends on concentration differences and can be written as

$$\dot{V}_{O_2}(A\text{-}B) = D_{O_2} \cdot \frac{S}{\tau} [C_{O_2}(A) - C_{O_2}(B)]. \qquad (3.6)$$

The solubility coefficient β_{O_2}, on the other hand, establishes the relation between concentration and partial pressure, in that

$$\beta_{O_2} = \Delta C_{O_2} / \Delta P_{O_2} \qquad (3.7)$$

indicates the quantity of O_2 that becomes dissolved in the unit barrier volume if the partial pressure is raised by one unit; it has the dimension $mol \cdot cm^{-3} \cdot torr^{-1}$, or, if expressed in volume of O_2 at STPD,* ml O_2 (STPD) $\cdot cm^{-3} \cdot torr^{-1}$. The Krogh permeability coefficient therefore establishes the relation between O_2 flow and *partial pressure* gradient and has the dimension $mol \cdot cm^{-1} \cdot sec^{-1} \cdot torr^{-1}$ or ml O_2 (STPD) $\cdot cm^{-1} \cdot sec^{-1} \cdot torr^{-1}$.

The permeability coefficient is quite different for different materials, as shown in Table 3.1, because both diffusion coefficient and solubility vary with the material and with temperature. An increase in temperature increases the diffusion coefficient of O_2 in aqueous media but decreases its solubility, so that one finds K_{O_2} to increase by less than 1% for a temperature rise by 1° C.

In working out the effect of structural design on O_2 flow rate due to diffusion between compartments, we will therefore have to find the

---

* The amount of a gas of a given species — such as O_2 — is a quantity of substance, best expressed in mol, one mol containing $6.02 \cdot 10^{23}$ molecules (Avogadro's number). If the amount of gas is expressed as a volume, then the conditions must be specified because the volume of a given amount of gas varies with temperature and pressure (laws of Boyle-Mariotte and Gay-Lussac). STPD means Standard Temperature Pressure Dry where T = 0° C and P = 760 torr. A given amount of a gas assumes a well-defined volume at STPD; thus, 1 mol O_2 has a volume of 22.39 l STPD. Other conditions useful in physiology are BTPS, which means body temperature, ambient pressure, saturated with water vapor at body temperature, which corresponds to the state of the gas in the lung; and ATPS, where the gas is at ambient temperature and pressure and saturated with water pressure at ambient temperature.

TABLE 3.1. DIFFUSION, SOLUBILITY, AND PERMEABILITY COEFFICIENTS FOR O_2 IN VARIOUS MATERIALS.

Material	D_{O_2} ($cm^2 \cdot sec^{-1}$)	β_{O_2} ($nmol \cdot ml^{-1} \cdot torr$)	K_{O_2} ($nmol \cdot cm^{-1} \cdot sec^{-1} \cdot torr^{-1}$)
Air, 20° C	0.20	55	11
Water, 20° C	$25 \cdot 10^{-6}$	1.82	$45 \cdot 10^{-6}$
37° C	$33 \cdot 10^{-6}$	1.41	$46 \cdot 10^{-6}$
Connective tissue, 37° C	$10 \cdot 10^{-6}$	1.4	$14 \cdot 10^{-6}$
Muscle	$12 \cdot 10^{-6}$	1.4	$16 \cdot 10^{-6}$
Chitin	—	—	$1.3 \cdot 10^{-6}$

Data from Altman and Dittmer (1971), table 14.

permeability coefficient that characterizes the barrier material and estimate the critical barrier dimensions, namely its cross-sectional area and its effective thickness.

CONDUCTANCE FOR O_2 TRANSPORT BY BULK FLOW OF A CARRIER

The transport of O_2 by means of a carrier which is moved in bulk will depend on two factors: on the flow rate of the carrier and on the quantity of O_2 it can carry in a unit volume, that is, on the concentration of O_2 in the carrier, C_{O_2}. Thus blood which flows at a rate $\dot{Q}_B$ will carry along an O_2 flow

$$\dot{V}_{O_2}(B) = \dot{Q}_B \cdot C_{O_2}. \tag{3.8}$$

With respect to the respiratory system we are, however, mostly interested in the delivery of O_2 by blood to the tissues and will therefore want to know the net O_2 flow rate supported by blood flow, that is, the difference between the O_2 flow rate reaching the tissue with arterial blood and that which leaves the tissue in venous blood (Fig. 3.4), so that we seek

$$\dot{V}_{O_2}(B) = \dot{Q}_B \cdot C_{O_2}(arterial) - \dot{Q}_B \cdot C_{O_2}(venous)$$
$$= \dot{Q}_B \cdot [C_{O_2}(a) - C_{O_2}(v)]. \tag{3.9}$$

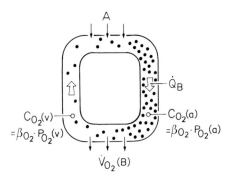

Fig. 3.4 O_2 delivery by the blood, $\dot{V}_{O_2}(B)$, depends on blood flow $(\dot{Q}_B)$ and on the difference in O_2 content (C_{O_2}) between arterial (a) and venous (v) blood.

Now, in equation 3.7 we have introduced a "solubility" or capacitance coefficient β_{O_2} which relates C_{O_2} to P_{O_2}; accordingly we can write equation 3.9 as

$$\dot{V}_{O_2}(B) = \dot{Q}_B \cdot \beta_{O_2}(B) \cdot [P_{O_2}(a) - P_{O_2}(v)] \qquad (3.10)$$

and we immediately find that the conductance for O_2 by bulk flow of a carrier

$$G(B) = \dot{Q}_B \cdot \beta_{O_2}(B) \qquad (3.11)$$

is the product of carrier flow rate and capacitance of the carrier for O_2. Note that this will apply as well to O_2 transport by the blood through the circulation (compartment B, Fig. 3.1), as by air flow in the pulmonary airways (compartment A). It is most interesting to note in this context that the O_2 capacity of blood is about the same as that of air because hemoglobin is a potent O_2 carrier, as mentioned in chapter 1; accordingly, the blood flow rate and the ventilation rate are of similar magnitude.

It is not as easy to indicate, in a general way, the effect that structural design may have on the conductances for O_2 flow by bulk transport. But even here we shall find such effects. For example, the capacity of blood to bind O_2 will depend on the number of red blood cells it contains in the unit volume. Furthermore, the dimensions of the tubes which guide the blood into the tissues, or the air into the pulmonary gas exchange region, will affect the bulk flow rate, particularly the distribution of flow to the many small units that participate in gas exchange in the lung or in the tissue.

CONDUCTANCE FOR O_2 FLOW INTO THE SINK

What is, finally, the all-important conductance that determines the O_2 flow rate into the mitochondrial O_2 sink and thus actually determines all the flow rates through the entire respiratory system? We shall be considering this question in some detail in chapter 5, but I would still like to set up a basic relation at this time.

Let us consider two points: (1) On passage through the respiratory chain of the mitochondria, molecular O_2 disappears in water, so that we can postulate that the P_{O_2} in the "depth of the sink" is zero. Thus it appears that the O_2 flow into the sink should be described by

$$\dot{V}_{O_2}(C) = G(C) \cdot [P_{O_2}(C) - 0] \qquad (3.12)$$

where $P_{O_2}(C)$ is the O_2 partial pressure in the cytoplasm of the cells. (2) The consumption of O_2 in the respiratory chain is quantitatively coupled to the generation of ATP, so that the molar flow of O_2 into the mitochondria is proportional to the flow of ATP out of the mitochondria:

$$\dot{M}_{O_2}(C) = k \cdot \dot{M}_{ATP} \qquad (3.13)$$

where $k = \frac{1}{6}$, as we shall see. Now, biochemical processes which are catalyzed by enzyme systems, such as oxidative phosphorylation, operate at a certain critical rate, so that the total rate of ATP production is going to depend on the total number of enzyme units available in the cell. And because these enzyme units are packed into a specialized organelle, the mitochondrion, we can expect the conductance of the sink to be proportional to the number of respiratory chains and to the mass of mitochondria available in the cells (Fig. 3.5):

$$G(C) \propto N(\text{resp. chain}) \propto V(\text{mitochondria}). \qquad (3.14)$$

To be more specific, what we must consider as "mitochondrial mass" in relation to the respiratory system is the *total* mass of all mitochondria in all cells active at a certain time.

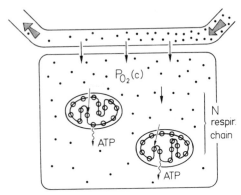

Fig. 3.5 The flow of O_2 to the mitochondrial sink depends not only on the P_{O_2} in the cell but also on the energetic demands of the cell, reflected by the number of respiratory chain units present.

It is thus evident that the structural design of the cell, specifically the quantity of mitochondria it contains, will be an important determinant of O_2 flow through the respiratory system.

Are Animals Built Reasonably?

We have seen in the preceding section, as well as in chapter 1, that the design of the respiratory system has multiple important effects on its functional performance. The design of the external gas exchanger determines the degree of O_2 extraction from the environment, as evidenced by comparing fish gills, bird lungs, and mammalian lungs. The design of blood vasculature determines the distribution of blood to various organs, and the number of red cells the quantity of O_2 that can be carried. We have also seen that the number of mitochondria should be an important determinant of the O_2 needs of the organism. And, finally, the conductance for O_2 diffusion from air to blood depends on a thin barrier of very large surface that keeps air and blood apart. How important are such design parameters? Are they adjusted to functional needs? In other words, are animals built reasonably?

At this point I must confess to a deep-rooted prejudice which, in fact, I would like to set out testing in much of the subsequent discussions. The prejudice relates to a firm belief that animals — and man — are built reasonably. Thus there should be no waste, or as little waste as possible. Clearly, if we only make the lung large enough, it would be capable of any O_2 flow rate we may fancy to demand. But we do not really need flow rates in excess of what our muscles can possibly consume, for example the 3 liters per minute mentioned above. Any surface area in excess of that required to support this flow rate would be wasteful. Similarly, our muscles do not have to contain more mitochondria than are needed to produce ATP at the rate required by the contractile matter to perform work, for example during running; any excess would again be wasteful.

Now there are good reasons to believe that the organism may try to minimize such structures to the level required. First, because all components of the body have a natural tendency to deteriorate, they must be continuously renewed, and this is costly in terms of resources and energy. Second, it is well known that the body will reduce certain of its components when they are not used; remember the wasting of muscles when a leg is immobilized in a plaster cast, to mention only one example.

For animals to be built reasonably we would therefore expect the design and dimensions of the respiratory system to be matched to functional requirements. There should be just enough, but no more, alveolar surface in the lung, just enough, but no more, mitochondrial mass in the muscle to support the largest energy needs of the body.

THE PRINCIPLE OF SYMMORPHOSIS

Clearly, this postulate specifies for the special case of the respiratory system the main elements of a rather general principle of regulated economical construction which should apply to all levels of biological organization, from the cells and their organelles to organs and functional systems, and finally to the organism. The principle uses as a gauge the functional needs. Since all elements of a functional system are basically sized with respect to the same gauge, they should all be well balanced to each other. We have proposed to call this principle *symmorphosis*, defining it as a state of structural design commensurate to functional needs resulting from regulated morphogenesis. The formation of structural elements (morphogenesis) that occurs during growth, and during maintenance of structures in the grown-up organism, should be regulated to satisfy but not exceed the requirements of the functional system.

The term "functional needs" is a bit loose, and purposely so.

Indeed, the functional needs may not always be quite simple to define because, in a functional system as complex as the one we are considering there is important interaction and cross-influence from one part to the other. We shall see later on that various ancillary cell functions are needed to maintain a large surface between air and blood in the lung, for example. It is also likely that the body cannot optimally exploit all parts of the respiratory system all the time. For such reasons the design of the respiratory system must allow for some safety factors, or inherent redundancies. The principle of symmorphosis still holds if inherent redundancies are part of the design, that is, imposed by functional needs.

A principle of this kind is too general for testing because, in fact, it describes a biological process that we cannot directly observe. What we see are the results of symmorphosis after it has happened. So we must now deduce from this principle a set of hypotheses that predict how the structural properties of the respiratory system should be related to its functional performance if the principle of symmorphosis holds. We can then set out studying animal organisms with well specified aims in mind. Step by step we can then see whether our observations agree with the predictions or not. This should, in the end, allow us to draw some conclusions on whether the principle of symmorphosis holds in general or within certain limits, that is, whether and to what extent animals are built reasonably.

THREE HYPOTHESES FOR TESTING

Let us now formulate a few general hypotheses which we shall further specify in subsequent chapters as we look at the various stages in the pathway for O_2.

> *Hypothesis 1: The structural design is a rate-limiting factor for O_2 flow at each level of the respiratory system.* This hypothesis tells us that we must choose as the functional parameter for our correlations the *maximal O_2 flow rate* that the system can accommodate. We will therefore have to estimate the maximal O_2 consumption that an animal can achieve and ask the question why and how it is limited, in particular by structural design features.

> *Hypothesis 2: The structural design is adaptable*, at least within certain limits. This means that the body can increase the size of

its respiratory structures if a higher need for O_2 flow is imposed, or decrease it if the demand is reduced.

Hypothesis 3: The structural design is optimized, that is, there is just enough structure at each level to support the maximal O_2 flow rate, perhaps allowing for a certain safety factor. Optimization means striking a balance between cost and benefit, the benefit obviously being O_2 flow; the cost derives from the necessity to involve numerous metabolic functions — such as protein synthesis and cell proliferation — in building and maintaining the structural elements of the respiratory system. The smaller the number of such elements the lower the energetic and metabolic cost of their maintenance, just as a smaller house is cheaper to build, heat, and maintain. But evidently a smaller house can accommodate fewer people, and, similarly, a smaller gas exchanger has a lower capacity for O_2 flow rate.

THE EXPERIMENTAL APPROACH

These hypotheses could evidently be tested if we were able to measure precisely the P_{O_2} gradients and all the factors affecting the conductances at each step of the general model of Figure 3.1, in order to estimate the maximal O_2 flow rate by means of a good physical model. Unfortunately this is not easily possible because most of the models we can use are gross abstractions from a rather complex reality, models which focus on a limited number of variables at the neglect of many others. Remember that a model is a convenient artifice that may help us understand a small facet of a large and intricate machinery.

The group of hypotheses just formulated predicts, however, that within certain limits the structural design of the respiratory system is malleable to match the functional needs of an organism. We can therefore proceed to testing them by comparing organisms that differ sufficiently in terms of their O_2 flow requirements. Nature has given us two ways to approach this task, and a third approach may be derived from man's ability to modify nature to a limited extent.

Comparing animals of different levels of activity.   It is quite evident that a shepherd dog keeping his flock of sheep together is consuming energy at a much higher rate than the sheep as he races back and forth, encircling the flock, and also more than the shepherd who looks on. Shepherd dogs and sheep are of about the same size, but the dog consumes two to three times the amount of O_2 that the sheep does (Table 2.1). On the basis of our hypothesis we would therefore expect the dog to have 2–3 times more mitochondria and a lung 2–3 times larger than the sheep's.

One can find in all size classes pairs of animals that differ in a similar way with respect to the activity level imposed by their behavioral pattern. Horses are clearly more active than cows; their O_2 consumption is also 2–3 times higher. Wild hares are much more active than cage rabbits. White rats are lazier than chipmunks or ground squirrels, or than wild rats. The Swiss laboratory mice are very slow moving compared to the Japanese waltzing mice kept as pets because they amuse us by their continuous dancing around, sometimes in wild swirls.

Therefore the first approach we shall use is to simply compare the structural design of the various parts of the respiratory system in such pairs of mammals of similar size but different O_2 needs. If the size of respiratory structures, measured by any parameter but mostly by an appropriate conductance, G, is proportional to O_2 consumption, we should find it proportionally larger in an animal of higher O_2 needs, as shown graphically in Figure 3.6.

Comparing animals of different size: allometry.   The difference in O_2 needs due to behavioral differences is rather small when compared to that found between large and small animals. Since the pioneering work of Kleiber (1932) it has been known that the meta-

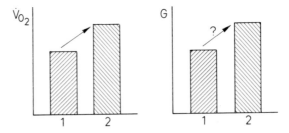

Fig. 3.6 The hypothesis of structure–function correlation can be tested, first, by comparing two groups of animals (1 and 2) and asking whether the conductances (G) in the respiratory system (Fig. 3.1) are proportional to O_2 consumption of the organism.

bolic rate of mammals—and, in fact, of all organisms—increases with the $\frac{3}{4}$ power of body mass (Figs. 2.7 and 2.9). As a consequence of this, a mouse weighing 20 grams consumes about 12 times more O_2 per unit body mass than a cow of 500 kg, although, in terms of behavior, both classify as slow, lazy beasts.

The approach in this case is to see how the different structural and functional parameters of the respiratory system change as a function of body mass. The analytical tool is that of *allometry*, or of studying the *scaling* of structures and functions relative to body mass, as introduced by Huxley (1932) and Bertalanffy (1951). In allometry one determines the *power function* that describes the change in the magnitude of any functional or structural parameter Y as body mass, M_b, changes:

$$Y = a \cdot M_b{}^b. \tag{3.15}$$

The exponent b is called the *scaling factor* and is, for our purpose, the critical parameter of allometric relations. As already mentioned, Kleiber (1932, 1961) has found that standard resting O_2 consumption of mammals changes with body mass as

$$\dot{V}_{O_2}\text{std} = a \cdot M_b^{3/4}. \tag{3.16}$$

If the size of the respiratory structures is matched to functional needs—as predicted by our hypotheses—then we would expect them to change with body mass in proportion to O_2 needs, that is, their scaling factors to be equal, or at least similar to that for O_2 consumption. We therefore shall base this analysis on a comparison of the scaling factors b.

Analytically this is made possible because a power function such as equation 3.15 can be transformed into a linear equation by taking the logarithm:

$$\log Y = b \cdot \log M_b + \log a. \tag{3.17}$$

Graphically this means plotting the data on double-logarithmic coordinates. The meaning of this transformation is shown in Figure 3.7. The degree of nonlinearity of the curve measured by the exponent b is reflected in the slope of the log transformation: if $b = 1$ the line is at 45° to the log x and log y axes, but if $b < 1$ it is flatter. The

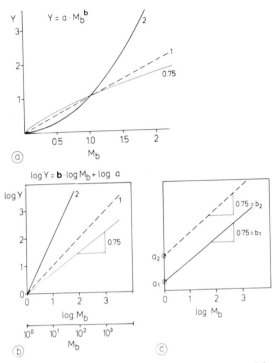

Fig. 3.7 Structure–function correlation can also be tested by comparing species across a large range of body sizes. This is best done by allometry, that is, linearizing the power functions (a) through logarithmic transformation (b). The approach (c) is to compare the exponents b of the power functions, but also the intercepts a with $\log M_b = 0$.

parameter a does not affect the slope but determines the position of the line function, that is, its intercept with the ordinate at $\log x = 0$. Thus we would expect two parameters that scale identically to be represented by parallel lines on a double log plot (Fig. 3.7c), the essence of the allometric approach.

I should mention that we are using allometry in this context simply as a tool for comparing animals of vastly different body mass. We shall not use it in a strictly analytical sense, attempting to unravel laws of biological similitude; this would require a different framework which is still rather theoretical and abstract in many ways. I hope that eventually the two approaches will come together.

Modifying O_2 needs.   The most direct way to test the third hypothesis — that the respiratory system should be adaptable to altered functional needs — is to impose on some individuals a behavioral pattern that modifies their O_2 needs. If we engage in a systematic training program for running, rowing, cross-country skiing, or any other endurance sport we will increase our O_2 needs as our work performance improves. This training effect is well known. The question for us is whether the increased maximal O_2 flow rate is, at least partly, due to adaptive increases of the structures supporting the respiratory system.

To impose training programs of this kind on animals offers the possibility for well-controlled studies on the degree to which the various elements of the respiratory system are malleable to match the functional needs for O_2 flow. It also allows us to examine the question whether symmorphosis is operative during the animal's growth period only, or whether it is wholly or partly retained in the grown-up. Such questions are rather important not only for understanding some biological principles but also for practical medical problems. For example, if an adult has lost a substantial part of his lung, is he capable of enlarging the gas exchanger of his remaining lung? If not, at what age does this capacity to adapt cease? The problems with this experimental approach are manifold, however. On the one hand, they are rather costly in terms of time and manpower and require considerable experimental skill, as well as a good knowledge of animal behavior if such experiments are to be done humanely and, if possible, even in a way that animals enjoy what they are asked to do. On the other hand, the adaptive response one can induce in this way is usually relatively modest, resulting in an increase of O_2 needs rarely exceeding 50%. It is therefore essential to design tightly controlled experiments and to use precise methods of measurement, lest inconclusive results are obtained; and this could not justify the use of experimental animals, nor of the scarce material resources available for research.

THE DOUBLE STRATEGY

In trying to establish relations between the size of respiratory structures and maximal O_2 flow through the system we shall, as far as possible, follow a double strategy in examining how these parameters vary with O_2 consumption (1) independently of body mass by using the comparative approach, and (2) as a function of body mass by the allometric approach described above. We will, in fact, not accept any correlation as valid, as established fact, unless the two

approaches result in compatible results. If this does not happen—
and you shall see that this will occur—we shall not question the
validity of the data, provided we can have confidence in the methods
used, but rather the validity of the models which we used to interpret
them. Models, I have said it before, are artificial abstractions and we
can easily go wrong by neglecting some factors that may be more
important than our prejudices make us believe.

The third approach listed above, that of experimentally modifying
O_2 needs, we shall use in a way as a special variant of the first
approach, since in fact we are artificially creating by our experiment
two groups of animals of differing O_2 needs and same body mass
which belong, in addition, to the same species, or may even be
littermates.

The Tools

To approach our problem of structure–function correlation in the
respiratory system we must obtain two basically different sets of
measurements: we must estimate the functional performance of the
system by measuring O_2 uptake, and we must obtain quantitative
data on the construction of the various conductances. In other words,
we must borrow our tools from both physiology and morphometry.

ESTIMATING O_2 CONSUMPTION

Under steady-state conditions O_2 consumption by the body is totally
reflected in O_2 uptake through the lung. We can therefore estimate
total body O_2 consumption at the mouth (and nose) by measuring the
amount of O_2 extracted from air per unit time.

Breathing is a cyclical process: we inspire a certain amount of air,
allow it to interact with the blood that flows through the lung, and
then expire. In the lung, the blood takes up a certain amount of O_2
and releases CO_2; because the amount of CO_2 given off approximately corresponds to the amount of O_2 taken up, the volume of air
expired is the same as that inspired. So in order to measure O_2 uptake
per minute, $\dot{V}_{O_2}$, all we have to do is to measure the amount of air we
breathe in and out per minute, and the difference in O_2 content
between inspired and expired air. We can write

$$\dot{V}_{O_2} = [\dot{V}_I \cdot C_{O_2}(I)] - [\dot{V}_E \cdot C_{O_2}(E)]$$
$$= \dot{V}_E \cdot [C_{O_2}(I) - C_{O_2}(E)] \tag{3.18}$$

where $C_{O_2}(I)$ and $C_{O_2}(E)$ are the O_2 concentrations, and $\dot{V}_I$ and $\dot{V}_E$ the ventilation rates, that is, volume per minute, of inspired and expired air, respectively. Since we assume $\dot{V}_I = \dot{V}_E$ the O_2 uptake is directly proportional to the O_2 concentration difference between inspired and expired air, so that we only need to measure three quantities $\dot{V}_E$, $C_{O_2}(I)$, and $C_{O_2}(E)$.

In practice this becomes complicated by the fact that the O_2 concentrations vary with the temperature, the barometric pressure, and the humidity of air, so that one needs to introduce some corrections that account for these factors. The two standardized conditions to which one refers any quantities describing air are:

STPD: standard temperature (0° C), pressure (760 torr), dry (water pressure 0 torr);

BTPS: body temperature (37° C in man), ambient pressure, saturated with water at body temperature (resulting in a water pressure of 47 torr in man).

The BTPS conditions are those which reign in the lung, but these are not important for the present purpose because the measurements we must consider are done outside the body. It will, however, be important to relate all the data to STPD conditions for them to be meaningful. The concentration of O_2 in air, for example, clearly depends on the gas conditions. It is defined as

$$C_{O_2} = M_{O_2}/V \tag{3.19}$$

where M_{O_2} is the molar quantity of O_2 and V is the containing volume; thus C_{O_2} will change if the air volume changes, for example, due to temperature differences.

The concentration of O_2 is not easy to measure, but we can get around this by considering its dependence on O_2 partial pressure. For that purpose we have introduced in equation 3.7 the useful capacitance coefficient β which expresses the increase in concentration that occurs when the partial pressure is increased by one unit. Equation 3.18 then becomes

$$\dot{V}_{O_2} = \dot{V}_E \cdot \beta_{O_2}[P_{O_2}(I) - P_{O_2}(E)].$$ (3.20)

The value of β_{O_2} in air depends on temperature; it amounts to 58.7 μmol $O_2 \cdot L^{-1} \cdot torr^{-1}$ at $0°$ C, that is, with respect to STPD, and to 51.7 at $37°$ C. This relation has further simplified our task because the P_{O_2} of inspired air is well known. The fractional concentration of O_2 in ambient air is everywhere 0.2095 (20.95%), and therefore $P_{O_2}(I)$ is simply obtained from barometric pressure, P_B, by

$$P_{O_2}(I) = 0.2095 \cdot P_B$$ (3.21)

and amounts to 159 torr in dry air at sea level with $P_B = 760$ torr.

We can now devise three methods by which we can measure $\dot{V}_{O_2}$ (Fig. 3.8):

(1) *Collecting expired air* in a spirometer over a given time period (Fig. 3.8a), we estimate $\dot{V}_E$. On a sample of the collected air we estimate $P_{O_2}(E)$ with an O_2 analyzer, and by equation 3.20 O_2 consumption is directly calculated.

(2) The *open circuit method* allows us to further simplify the measurements by measuring the O_2 that is being extracted from an open circuit by an individual breathing into a mask (Fig. 3.8b) or in a chamber (Fig. 3.8d) through which we draw ambient air at a known rate, $\dot{V}_{mask}$, which is larger than $\dot{V}_E$. We then need to measure P_{O_2} in a dry sample of the outflowing air, which is reduced with respect to that flowing in by the amount of O_2 that is being removed due to respiration. It is easily seen that we now estimate $\dot{V}_{O_2}$ by

$$\dot{V}_{O_2} = \dot{V}_{mask} \cdot \beta_{O_2}[P_{O_2}(IN) - P_{O_2}(OUT)]$$ (3.22)

which is simply a modification of equation 3.20.

(3) The *closed chamber method* also allows us to measure $\dot{V}_{O_2}$ directly by a volumetric method if the individual breathes from and into a closed chamber (Fig. 3.8c). All we need to do is to absorb the CO_2 that is being expired, by a suitable method, for example by KOH; the chamber gas volume then becomes reduced by the volume of O_2 that is taken up in the lungs, and this can be measured by connecting the chamber to a spirometer. The problem with this method is that O_2 becomes depleted in the chamber atmosphere; it therefore works only for short

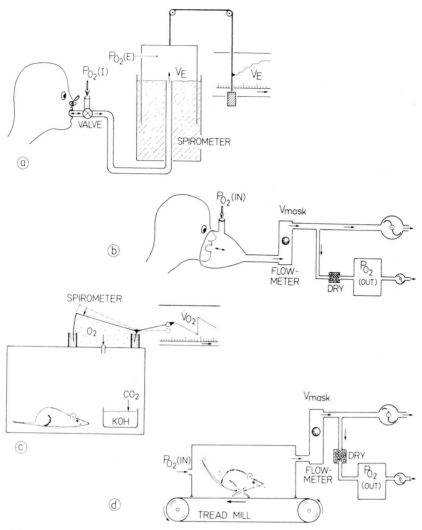

Fig. 3.8 Four methods for measuring O_2 consumption in man and in animals.

periods of time, or if pure O_2 is fed in from the spirometer, rather than air. It is also necessary to monitor the temperature, P_{O_2}, and P_{CO_2} in the chamber.

We have so far assumed that the quantity of CO_2 given off through the lung is the same as that of O_2 taken up; this means that the respiratory quotient, R, the ratio of CO_2 flux to O_2 flux,

$$R = \dot{V}_{CO_2}/\dot{V}_{O_2} \hspace{4cm} (3.23)$$

is assumed to be equal to 1. But this is not necessarily so; it rather depends on the substrates used in oxidative phosphorylation. In chapter 4 we shall have a closer look at this; for the present purpose the following remarks must suffice. When we burn glucose, we consume 6 mol O_2 for every mol glucose and produce 6 mol CO_2; thus, in this case, $R = 1$. Burning 1 mol fatty acids uses a volume of O_2 that is greater than the volume of CO_2 produced, so that $R = 0.7$; the catabolism of amino acids yields intermediate values. Since we normally generate ATP from a mixture of substrates, the respiratory quotient will be smaller than 1. This will, however, have a small effect on the air flow rates during inspiration and expiration because the part of the ventilated air volume affected by R is small: about $\frac{1}{4}$ of the O_2 inspired, which amounts to 20.95% of the air volume, is taken up and replaced by CO_2; thus, if $R = 0.8$, we would expect $\dot{V}_E$ to be about 1% smaller than $\dot{V}_I$, and this is negligible because it is of the same order as the measuring error. Also we should notice that differences in R may affect the results obtained with method 1 but have no effect on methods 2 and 3.

When we look at individual parts of the system, for example at the muscles of the leg only (Fig. 3.9), we must take a different approach. In this case, we can consider O_2 consumption in these muscles to be reflected in the rate of O_2 extraction from the blood supplying these muscles. If we revert to equation 3.9 we note that we can estimate $\dot{V}_{O_2}$ in muscle group X through a slightly modified formula:

$$\dot{V}_{O_2}(X) = \dot{Q}_B(X) \cdot [C_{O_2}(a) - C_{O_2}(v)]. \hspace{2cm} (3.24)$$

To do this, we evidently need to estimate blood flow through the group of muscles under consideration, $\dot{Q}_B(X)$. We furthermore need to take small blood samples from arterial blood and from venous blood flowing out of compartment X and estimate their O_2 content. This method is commonly called the Fick principle after the German physician A. Fick who not only formulated the laws of diffusion through a barrier (equation 3.3) but also proposed, in 1870, the above equation for estimating blood flow from a measurement of O_2 uptake and O_2 content in in-flowing and out-flowing blood. This method is widely used to estimate total cardiac output by measuring O_2 consumption through the lung and O_2 content in arterial and mixed

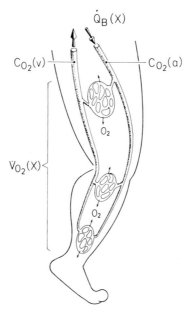

Fig. 3.9 O_2 consumption by a part (X) of the body, for example one leg, depends on the blood flow through that part, $\dot{Q}_B(X)$, and on the difference in O_2 content between arterial and venous blood entering or leaving that part.

venous blood. In our case we use it differently by considering $\dot{V}_{O_2}(X)$ to be the unknown variable. But we can still use the Fick principle to estimate $\dot{Q}_B(X)$ if, instead of O_2, we use some other independent tracer y which we can add to the in-flowing blood. We can then estimate $\dot{Q}_B(X)$ by measuring the rate of loss of y into the tissue, $\dot{V}_y(X)$, and the content of y in the arterial and venous blood. The tracer can be a radioactive gas, or it can be a small amount of heat which dissipates while the blood passes through the tissue. Under experimental conditions one may often impose a known blood flow onto the system, so that we only need to estimate the O_2 content in arterial and venous blood to calculate $\dot{V}_{O_2}(X)$.

LOOKING INTO TISSUES AND CELLS

The foregoing discussions have revealed that an analysis of structure–function correlation can only be carried out if the structural data are obtained in quantitative terms: we need to estimate the volume of mitochondria in cells, the surface area of the air–blood barrier in the lung, its thickness, and so on. The approach is hence that of quantitative morphology, or morphometry.

But here we meet with a methodological problem, because all the structures we are interested in are *internal* components of organs, tissues, and cells, and they need to be "opened to the eye," made amenable to the study with a microscope of adequate resolving power. To be more specific, mitochondria and their membranes can only be seen in the electron microscope at magnifications of the order of $10,000\times$ to $100,000\times$, and even the lung surface can only be properly resolved at magnifications of several thousand times.

The problems to be overcome are two-fold. The first is that we can rarely approach a morphological question by direct observation of living tissue. We therefore must prepare tissues in such a way that they become accessible to microscopic observation, that is, the tissue must be fixed, embedded in some suitable material, and cut or sliced into very thin sections, methods that are, in fact, well worked out today. But if the results obtained are to be biologically meaningful, it is mandatory that we choose methods which preserve the structure of the living tissue as faithfully as possible. I can make no general recommendations with regard to specific methods to use, because this will depend so much on the tissue to be studied, on the physiological state that is to be preserved, and on the specific question asked. Very often fixation by vascular perfusion under well-controlled conditions comes closest to preserving the natural physiological state at the time of fixation; its main disadvantage lies in the fact that it removes the blood from the tissue. Methods that depend on rapid freezing appear very attractive, but they are suitable only under very particular circumstances; most of the time the process of freezing is not rapid enough to prevent severe damage to cells. There is only one rule: the methods of tissue preparation must be controlled, and this requires that the same result be obtained by at least two different methods, and that the result must evidently be reproducible. In other words, methods of tissue preparation can be accepted as producing faithful images of tissue structure if the results they produce are consistent. There is another, more general rule, namely that the diligent choice of good methods is an essential part of designing a scientific investigation and is therefore one of the primary responsibilities of the investigator; it is part of what makes a good scientist.

The second methodological problem results from the fact that such studies need to be done on very thin sections of the tissue, obtained by microtomes. The process of sectioning destroys the all-important three-dimensional nature of the structure; we see only a distorted picture, one essentially reduced to a two-dimensional image with no clues as to its spatial nature. The traces left by the spatial structural elements on a random plane that traverses them are, indeed, rudimentary: an object that has a certain volume appears as a planar patch, whereas its surface appears as a linear trace around the patch, and a thin fiber is seen as a fine dot. Another problem is this: we cannot be sure that the size of such a profile on section faithfully represents the size of the spatial particle from which it has been cut; indeed, it usually does not because a random section very rarely passes right through its major or characteristic cross-section. A small profile can therefore just as well represent a central section of a small as a peripheral section of large particle. How is it then possible to do any reliable, meaningful measurements on sections?

The fundamental problems underlying this difficulty have been solved by *stereology* and sound practical measuring methods have been developed. The theory of stereology has its roots in geometrical probability theory, so that stereological methods are statistical in nature. I have hinted above that microtome sections hit the structural elements at random. A large element therefore has a greater chance of being hit than a small one. Also an element that occurs in greater number may result in more profiles than one which is rare. With respect to a sphere of given size one can furthermore determine theoretically the probability that a circular profile of a certain size, or rather size class, is obtained. These few statements, which can be intuitively accepted, must suffice for the present. To expand further on the mathematical theory that forms the basis of stereology would be beyond the scope of this book; I have dealt with it elsewhere in great detail.

Although the mathematical basis of stereology is not trivial, the most important measuring methods derived from this theory are astonishingly simple and easy to apply. I would only like to explain the method for measuring volumes and surfaces which can, indeed, help us answer some of the most important questions of structure–function correlation. Let us, for that purpose, look at a model structure (Fig. 3.10) — it could be, for example, a cell — which we label X, containing mitochondria, labeled Y. We can now characterize the mitochondrial content of this cell — something we may want to

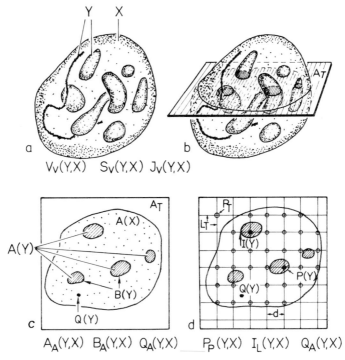

Fig. 3.10 The morphometric descriptors of a cell, for example, or of any structure (a) can be derived by stereological methods from measurements obtained on random sections of the structure (b-d).

know in order to estimate the cell's capacity to make ATP — as the fractional cell volume occupied by mitochondria, which would be

$$V(Y)/V(X) = V_V(Y,X). \tag{3.25}$$

In stereology, this is called the mitochondrial volume density, symbolized by V_V with the identifier of the phase in parentheses (Fig. 3.10a). We may perhaps also be interested in the surface area, $S(Y)$, over which these mitochondria are in contact with the cytoplasm; a characteristic and meaningful parameter might be the surface contained in the unit volume of the cell

$$S(Y)/V(X) = S_V(Y,X) \tag{3.26}$$

which one calls their "surface density" in the cell, symbolized by S_V in analogy to the volume density.

Let us now cut this cell with a random plane (Fig. 3.10b). In the microscope we will then see a profile of the cell — more or less large, depending on where the section hits the cell — which contains some profiles of mitochondria (Fig. 3.10c). One of the fundamental principles of stereology now states that the fraction of the cell profile area occupied by profiles of the mitochondria is, on the average, equal to the volume density of the mitochondria in the cell, or expressed in an equation:

$$A(Y)/A(X) = A_A(Y,X) = V_V(Y,X). \tag{3.27}$$

Note that the mitochondrial area $A(Y)$ is the sum of the area of all mitochondrial profiles on the section. Note also that I have said "on the average," which means that $A_A(Y,X)$ is no more than an estimator of $V_V(Y,X)$ whose statistical quality evidently depends on the number of cell profiles measured; as a rule, such estimates must always be based on several independent measurements that are averaged.

The mitochondrial profiles seen on section are bounded by a linear trace which, in fact, is the "profile" of the mitochondrial surface. A second fundamental stereological principle states that the total length of these boundary traces, $B(Y)$, contained in the cell profile area, $A(X)$, is proportional to the surface density:

$$B(Y)/A(X) = B_A(Y,X) = \frac{\pi}{4} S_V(Y,X). \tag{3.28}$$

Here again, of course, B_A is but an estimator of S_V, whose statistical quality depends on the number of measurements made.

So in principle one could now simply measure — for example, by planimetry — the profile area of the cell, $A(X)$, that of the mitochondria, $A(Y)$, and their combined boundary length, $B(Y)$, and thus estimate both the volume and surface density of mitochondria in the cell. But such measurements are rather laborious, unless one possesses an expensive computerized image analyzer. Stereology, however, offers some very simple and easy point-counting methods as alternatives that do the same job very inexpensively and most efficiently. One places, for example, a square grid of lines onto the section, or, mostly, on the micrographs (Fig. 3.10d). The cross-sections of these lines constitute "test points," P_T, which hit the mitochondria, or not, and hit the cell, or not. One finds that the relative number of such points which fall on mitochondrial profiles estimates the volume density of mitochondria:

$$P(Y)/P(X) = P_P(Y,X) = A_A(Y,X) = V_V(Y,X). \qquad (3.29)$$

One can actually try to prove this estimation principle for oneself by considering that each point represents an area d^2, where d is the spacing of the lines in the grid.

There is a similarly simple point-counting method for estimating the surface density. We see in Figure 3.10d that some of the test lines of the grid intersect the profile boundaries of the mitochondria. If we designate the number of these intersections with I(Y) we have

$$I(Y)/L(X) = I_L(Y,X) = \frac{2}{\pi} B_A(Y,X) = \frac{1}{2} S_V(Y,X) \qquad (3.30)$$

where L(X) is the test line length contained in the cell profile. This principle is not so simple to demonstrate because questions of orientation between the test lines and the surface must be considered.

We now see that these stereological principles give rise to two very simple methods for measuring the volume and surface density of many tissue components:

$$V_V(Y,X) = \hat{P}_P(Y,X) \qquad (3.31)$$

$$S_V(Y,X) = 2 \cdot \hat{I}_L(Y,X) \qquad (3.32)$$

where the "hat" over the point counts means that these are averages from many samples. These measurements can be obtained with virtually no equipment; a simple grid, pencil, and pad suffice, but evidently one can greatly facilitate the task by using any small computing facility — desktop calculators often do the job very well. But there are two points I want to stress: (1) the parameters V_V and S_V are *estimated* by these relations and not measured, so that P_P and I_L must be averages of several counts; and (2) stereological parameters are always expressed with respect to some *reference*: in our example we have used the cell volume as a reference, but when we estimate the alveolar surface area the lung volume will serve as reference.

Both these remarks indicate that proper sampling of the tissue to be examined is most important. We are usually not interested in the make-up of one particular cell but rather of a typical or average cell, so that one needs to look at many cell profiles, taken, for example, from all parts of the muscle.

Stereological methods have a number of limitations that preclude their application to certain special problems. Because they depend on random sampling they are not suitable, for example, for evaluating the progression of dimensions in hierarchical structures such as trees, the branching airways of the lung, or larger blood vessels. Here one will have to find other nonrandom measuring methods. The methods are also subject to a number of biases; for example, at high magnifications the thickness of the "section"—which is actually more like a slice—may introduce some systematic errors. But I shall not pursue this any further. With proper precautions, stereological methods offer excellent tools for estimating most morphometric parameters that we will be interested in.

Summary

The respiratory system can be described as having three compartments in series: (A) the respiratory medium (air or water), (B) the blood as O_2 carrier, and (C) the cells as O_2 consumers. In (A) and (B) O_2 is transported by convection of the medium, in (C) molecular O_2 disappears. At the interfaces (A – B) and (B – C) O_2 is exchanged by diffusion. Under steady-state conditions convective O_2 flow rate through each of the compartments of this model and diffusive flow rates between them must all be equal to the O_2 flow rate into the mitochondrial sink. By describing these flow rates as a product of a conductance and a P_{O_2} difference, structural and functional parameters of O_2 flow can be separated. The conductances for diffusive O_2 flow depend on the surface area of contact between air and blood in the lung, or between blood and cells in the tissue, as well as on the diffusion distances, for example, the air–blood tissue barrier in the lung. The conductance for convective O_2 flow is determined by the flow rate of the carrier (air or blood) and its O_2 capacitance which in the blood depends on the number of red blood cells. The O_2 flow rate into the sink is proportional to the rate of ATP consumption and is determined by the number of respiratory chain units available in the mitochondria.

The central question is whether the design of the respiratory system is matched to functional needs, whether animals are built reasonably. The principle of symmorphosis postulates that the structural design of a system (or of the body) is commensurate to functional needs as a result of regulated morphogenesis both during growth and during maintenance of structures in the grown-up. To explore the validity of this principle we shall attempt to test three hypotheses which derive from it: (1) the structural design is a rate-limiting factor for O_2 flow at each level of the respiratory system; (2) the structural design is adaptable to altered functional needs; and (3) the structural design is optimized. To this end we shall compare animals of different energetic and O_2 needs using primarily two experiments of nature: (a) animals of similar size but different O_2 needs because of different levels of activity; and (b) animals of different body size, since O_2 consumption is proportional to $M_b^{0.75}$ and hence is relatively much greater in small than in large animals. In this latter instance allometry should show whether the size of structures that determine O_2 flow is matched to functional needs. A third approach is to modify O_2 needs by imposing higher levels of activity in experimental training programs, both on man and on animals.

The tools used to perform these studies are two-fold. We need to estimate O_2 consumption by physiological methods while animals perform work by running on a treadmill; at the level of cells, corresponding biochemical studies are needed. The structural design of the various parts of the system must be evaluated by morphometric methods; stereology offers the tools to reliably estimate volumes, surfaces, lengths, and distances.

Further Reading

Kleiber, M. 1961. *The Fire of Life: An Introduction to Animal Energetics.* New York: Wiley.

Weibel, E. R. 1979. Oxygen demand and the size of respiratory structures in mammals. In *Evolution of Respiratory Processes,* ed. S. C. Wood and C. Lenfant. New York: Dekker, pp. 289–346.

——— 1979/80. *Stereological Methods.* Vol. 1: *Practical Methods for Biological Morphometry.* Vol. 2: *Theoretical Foundations.* London: Academic.

Weibel, E. R., and C. R. Taylor. 1981. Design of the mammalian respiratory system. *Respiration Physiology* 44:1–164.

West, J. B. 1974. *Respiration Physiology: The Essentials.* Baltimore: Williams & Wilkins.

References

Altman, P. L., and D. S. Dittmer. 1971. *Biological Handbooks: Respiration and Circulation.* Bethesda: Federation of American Societies for Experimental Biology.

Bachofen, H., A. Ammann, and E. R. Weibel. 1982. Perfusion fixation of lungs for structure–function analysis: credits and limitations. *Journal of Applied Physiology* 53:528–533.

Bertalanffy, L. von. 1951. *Theoretische Biologie. II. Stoffwechsel, Wachstum.* 2nd ed. Bern: Francke.

Dejours, P. 1981. *Principles of Comparative Respiratory Physiology.* 2nd ed. Amsterdam: Elsevier North-Holland.

* Fick, A. 1870. *Ueber die Messung des Blutquantums in den Herzventrikeln.* Sitzungsbericht 16. Würzburg: Physikalisch Medizinische Gesellschaft.

* Huxley, J. S. 1932. *Problems of Relative Growth.* London: Methuen.

* Kleiber, M. 1932. Body size and metabolism. *Hilgardia* 6:315–353.

McMahon, T. A. 1973. Size and shape in biology. *Science* 179:1201–1204.

Rahn, H. 1967. Gas transport from the external environment to the cell. In *Development of the Lung,* ed. A. V. S. de Reuck and R. Porter. Ciba Foundation Symposium. London: Churchill, pp. 3–23.

Schmidt-Nielsen, K. 1975. Scaling in biology: the consequences of size. *Journal of Experimental Zoology* 194:287–308.

Stahl, W. R. 1967. Scaling of respiratory variables in mammals. *Journal of Applied Physiology* 22:453–460.

Taylor, C. R., and E. R. Weibel. 1981. Design of the mammalian respiratory system. I. Problem and strategy. *Respiration Physiology* 44:1–10.

Weibel, E. R., W. Limacher, and H. Bachofen. 1982. Electron microscopy of rapidly frozen lungs: evaluation on the basis of standard criteria. *Journal of Applied Physiology* 53:516–527.

4

CELL RESPIRATION

IN THE NEXT TWO CHAPTERS we shall have a closer look at the mechanisms by which cells can get biologically useful energy through the combustion of foodstuffs, sugars, fats, and proteins. The part of the O_2 pathway we shall be considering is its terminal segment, that which begins when O_2 enters the cell (Fig. 4.1). What we shall examine in the present chapter is what the cell has to do to break down the substrates by sets of enzymes which are either in the cytoplasm or in the mitochondria, and how O_2 intervenes in the very last step. In the next chapter we shall have a closer look at mitochondria as the sites for oxidative phosphorylation. Thus, while the present chapter deals essentially with biochemistry and cell physiology, the next chapter will approach the question of structure–function correlation at this level of the system.

Gaining Energy from Combustion

In the first two chapters I have repeatedly stated that cells can gain energy by combustion of foodstuffs using O_2 in the process. Let us look at a simple example, the combustion of glucose, which in the presence of sufficient O_2 can be broken up completely into carbon dioxide and water molecules:

$$C_6H_{12}O_6 + 6O_2 \longrightarrow 6CO_2 + 6H_2O.$$

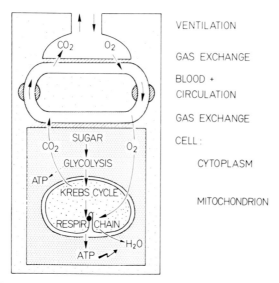

Fig. 4.1 Cell metabolism liberates energy through a sequence of biochemical steps that take place either in the cytoplasm or in mitochondria. O_2 inflow and CO_2 discharge are important for that part taking place in mitochondria.

For each mol of glucose, which is about 180 grams, this process liberates energy to the amount of 2870 kJ or 686 kcal (1 kcal = 4.186 kJoule). This is quite a bit of energy, for it is enough to heat nearly 7 liters of ice water to the boiling point. The main logistic problem that the cells must solve is how to gradually extract this energy in little portions which can then be used to drive the cell's many functions. This is achieved by controlled breakdown of the foodstuff molecules through a series of enzymes that are built into the cell according to a well-ordered plan.

In our context it is furthermore important to note that the combustion of 1 mol glucose consumes 6 mol O_2, which is the amount of O_2 contained in 130 liters of pure O_2 gas or in 650 liters of air. Thus the metabolic need for O_2 is quite large, and this would seem to make energy metabolism primarily dependent on the availability of O_2. While this is a reasonable postulate for most contemporary organisms, this has not always been the case. Indeed, much recent evidence indicates that life originated in the absence of O_2 and that our O_2-rich environment is, in fact, the result of living organisms populating the earth. And yet even early forms of life had to obtain

energy through "combustion" of foodstuffs and thus had to evolve
mechanisms which allowed "oxidation" without the presence of
molecular O_2. These mechanisms are still used in all our cells and
constitute one of the main devices for extracting energy in small
units.

In order to understand this we must first ask what occurs in the
process of oxidation that liberates energy stored in the foodstuff
molecules. When the glucose molecule breaks up, it sheds off hydrogen which is then captured by molecular O_2 to make water. This
process, called oxidation, involves the transfer of two hydrogen ions
or protons ($2H^+$) together with two electrons ($2e^-$) to what is called an
electron or proton acceptor which becomes reduced. Thus *oxidation*
of an electron (or proton) *donor* is coupled with *reduction* of an
electron (or proton) *acceptor*. Such processes are called *oxidation-
reduction reactions* or "redox" reactions. Energy becomes liberated
because the acceptor has a higher affinity for electrons than the
donor, which means that the transferred electrons lose part of their
energy, donating it to the environment, for example in the form of
heat.

Molecular O_2 is the perfect electron acceptor because its affinity for
H^+ and its associated electrons is so high that it results in very tight
binding of the hydrogen ion in the water molecule, thus allowing the
largest amount of free energy to be liberated. But there are many
alternative electron acceptors which bind H^+ less tightly and thus
allow smaller portions of the electrons' energy to be liberated in one
step. Such electron acceptors allow oxidation of foodstuffs to occur
even if molecular O_2 is not available. Clearly, it was essential for
primitive cells to find such molecules during the early period of
biological evolution when there was no or very little molecular O_2 in
the atmosphere. Several such H^+ acceptors are still found and used
extensively in present-day organisms. One such widely used molecule is the pyridine nucleotide NAD (nicotinamide adenine dinucleotide), which can be reduced to NADH as shown in Figure 4.2. Its
"backbone" is a nucleotide, that is, the same type of chemical of
which the genetic material DNA (deoxyribonucleic acid) is made, in
terms of biological evolution probably the most ancient compound
made. In this case, the nucleotide is not used as a carrier of genetic
information but as a carrier for protons and electrons.

The process of oxidation-reduction of NAD is very important and
fundamental, and we need to dwell on it for a moment because it
helps us to understand what is happening in oxidation-reduction

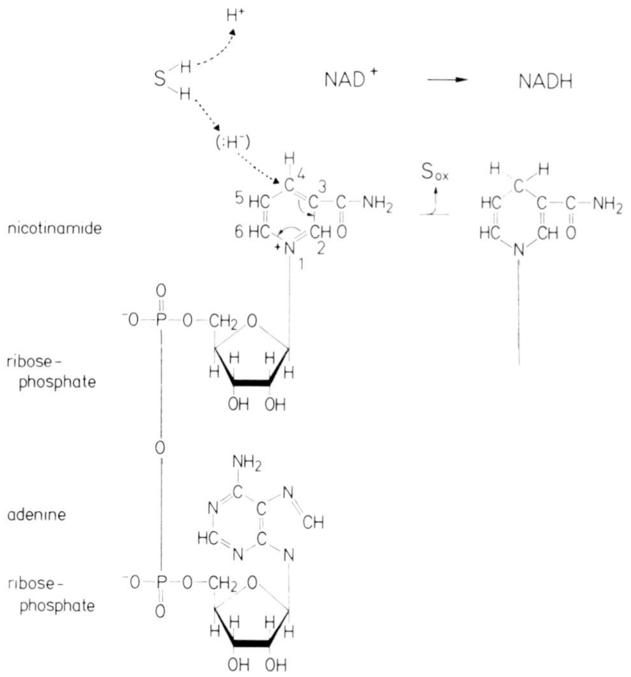

Fig. 4.2 Substrate oxidation results in reduction of nicotinamide adenine dinucleotide (NAD) as electron carrier.

reactions as they are used to extract energy from the combustion of foodstuffs. NAD^+, the oxidized form of NAD, contains a positive charge at the nicotinamide ring (Fig. 4.2). In order to reduce NAD^+ to NADH, two electrons must be donated from a foodstuff molecule or substrate, $S\text{-}H_2$ in Figure 4.2. This is achieved by dehydrogenation of the substrate, which liberates two hydrogens (two protons, H^+ and two electrons), called *reducing equivalents*. One of the hydrogens is transferred to the 4-position of the nicotinamide ring in form of a hydride ion $(:H^-)$ (Fig. 4.2), that is, it carries the two electrons along, which ultimately leads to a reduction at positions 1 and 4. The other hydrogen is lost to the medium as a H^+ ion. So in principle this reaction can be written as

$$S\text{-}H_2 + NAD^+ \longrightarrow S_{ox} + NADH + H^+.$$

When we say, in the following discussion, that NADH is a carrier of hydrogen, we actually always mean $(NADH + H^+)$ because we shall see that NADH carries a H^+ ion along when it enters the respiratory chain to be reoxidized to NAD^+.

It is evident that oxidation of substrates by this system can only proceed if the acceptor is present in adequate quantity, so NAD^+ needs to be resupplied at the rate at which it is reduced to NADH. However, it is thermodynamically impossible to secure an adequate supply by continuous synthesis of NAD, as this would consume more energy than is made available by the process of combustion that NAD serves. Thus NAD^+ needs to be regenerated by oxidizing NADH, that is, by transferring its hydrogen to another H^+ acceptor, called terminal electron acceptor. The *cofactors* NAD^+ and NADH therefore serve as a link in a chain of H^+ and electron transfer from the foodstuff molecule to the terminal electron acceptor, a key feature being the cyclical manner in which the cofactor is oxidized and reduced, as shown in Figure 4.3.

In this process, the *terminal H^+ acceptor* X can be molecular O_2, in which case we talk about oxidative or *aerobic* metabolism, and we shall see later that this is the most efficient mechanism. However, there are alternatives which become active under *anaerobic* conditions when the supply of molecular O_2 is not sufficient. In such cases, the terminal electron acceptor is an organic molecule which has a higher electron affinity than the cofactors; in glycolysis, the main anaerobic process for getting energy in higher organisms, the terminal electron acceptor is pyruvate, which becomes reduced to lactate, as we shall see. Anaerobic metabolism, which is called *fermentation*, is quite inefficient in that much less energy can be gained per mol of foodstuff than by aerobic metabolism; but it is still useful if O_2 is not available at an adequate flow rate. It becomes important even in

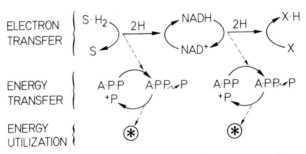

Fig. 4.3 Sequence of electron and energy transfer.

higher organisms when they require energy at a rate in excess of that which can be covered by the flow of O_2 from outside air to the cells.

The oxidation-reduction reactions shown in Figure 4.3 liberate a certain amount of free energy when hydrogen (protons and electrons) passes from an oxidizing to a reducing agent — that is, from a molecule with lower to one with higher electron affinity — since this causes the electrons to lose some energy. The problem now is to trap a substantial part of that energy in useful form — as chemical energy that can be transferred to a multitude of chemical and physical processes that allow the cell to function and stay alive. The solution to this problem — one of the most significant steps in early biological evolution — which predominates in present-day organisms is to load this energy into *high-energy phosphate bonds* of organic phosphates. The primary fuel of this kind is the nucleoside phosphate *adenosine triphosphate (ATP)*, shown in Figure 4.4, which is generated by adding a third inorganic phosphate group to ADP (adenosine diphosphate), making use of the energy liberated by H^+ transfer (Fig. 4.3). The energy stored in ATP is considerable, for upon hydrolysis of ATP to ADP + P about 30 kJ/mol are liberated and can be utilized to drive biological processes of many kinds. Thus the "energy acceptor" ADP is again regenerated in a cyclical manner, and this at a rate which corresponds to the energy requirements of the cell. We have seen in

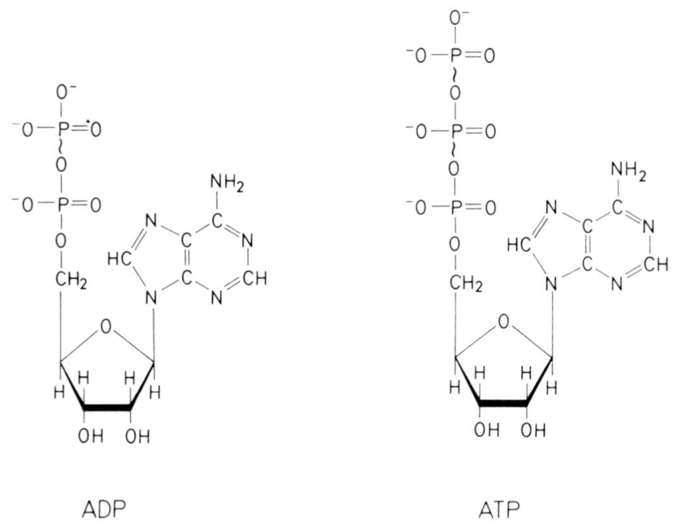

Fig. 4.4 Chemical structure of ADP and ATP.

chapter 2 that, indeed, the level of ADP in the cell is the main regulator of the metabolic machinery leading to phosphorylation.

There is another energy carrier that is of interest in this context, namely coenzyme A, usually abbreviated CoA. As shown in Figure 4.5, this molecule can bind to small organic compounds with a high-energy thiolester bond, again making use of the energy liberated by H^+ transfer processes. The hydrolysis of the bond liberates energy of the same order of magnitude as the hydrolysis of ATP. The metabolism of many compounds depends upon activation by conversion to CoA derivates, as we shall see below.

The interesting feature of this process of harvesting energy from the "oxidation" of foodstuffs — in the presence or absence of molecular O_2 — is that they depend on a set of carriers that can be regener-

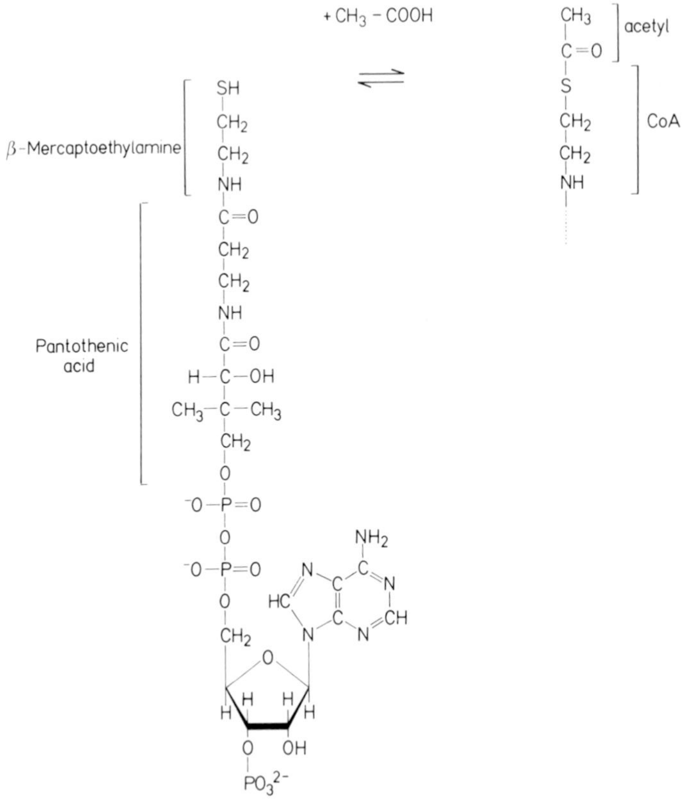

Fig. 4.5   Chemical structure of coenzyme A (CoA) and reversible binding of acetyl group for entrance into the Krebs cycle.

ated in a cyclical manner. NAD is a carrier for H$^+$, ADP a carrier for high-energy phosphate bonds, and CoA a carrier for organic compounds that must be introduced into metabolic pathways. And furthermore, most interestingly, these carriers have a similar chemical backbone made of ribonucleosides and are hence in a way akin with the carriers of genetic information. They are all very ancient elements of biological systems that occur in all present-day living organisms.

Metabolic Pathways of the Cell

The basic mechanisms for harvesting energy from the combustion of foodstuffs described in the following section must take place in an orderly and controlled fashion in the cell. The process does, in fact, not take place spontaneously but is controlled by a set of enzymes that serve as catalysts for the step-by-step degradation of foodstuffs in the process of which energy is being collected. The complete combustion of glucose to CO_2 and H_2O takes place through something like two dozen steps or more, involving a similar number of enzymes and resulting in the formation of a total of 36 molecules of ATP per molecule of glucose consumed. This pathway can be conveniently broken up into three major steps as shown in Figure 4.6:

(1) *Glycolysis*, an anaerobic fermentation process that results in the formation of two three-carbon molecules, pyruvate or lactate, and produces NADH as well as ATP;

(2) *Krebs cycle*, in which the pyruvate produced by glycolysis is further broken down to CO_2, and in which NADH is produced;

(3) *Respiratory chain*, where the hydrogen collected in NADH is transferred to molecular O_2 generating ATP from the energy liberated during transfer.

We shall see that glycolysis is, in essence, independent of the other steps whereas the Krebs cycle can only function if it receives its substrate from either glycolysis or the metabolism of fatty acids or proteins and if the NADH generated along the cycle can be efficiently reoxidized to NAD$^+$ in the respiratory chain. Thus glycolysis is an anaerobic fermentative process, whereas the Krebs cycle belongs to aerobic metabolism, although no O_2 is used in the cycle itself.

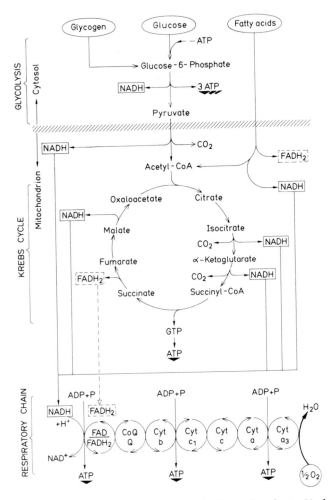

Fig. 4.6 The three stages of oxidative metabolism: glycolysis, Krebs tricar-boxylic acid cycle, and respiratory chain. (From Weibel, 1979.)

GLYCOLYSIS

The sequence of events of glycolysis, shown in Figure 4.7, begins with phosphorylation of glucose to glucose-6-phosphate, transforming a neutral sugar to a negatively charged one by addition of a phosphate group. If this initial priming step occurs with free glucose obtained from the blood, it requires hydrolysis of an ATP molecule to supply both the phosphate and the required binding energy; if, on the other hand, the glucose molecule is derived from glycogen in the cell,

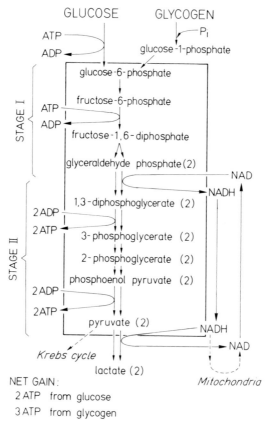

Fig. 4.7 The sequence of steps in anaerobic glycolysis which ends in the formation of lactate when pyruvate is used as electron acceptor for oxidizing NADH formed in the process. When NADH can be oxidized by mitochondria, pyruvate can enter the Krebs cycle.

no ATP is required as inorganic phosphate can be bound directly. After transformation to fructose-6-phosphate, another ATP molecule is required to attach a second phosphate group, and the resulting diphosphate is split into two molecules of glyceraldehyde-3-phosphate. This completes the first stage of glycolysis in which simple six-carbon sugars were collected and converted to pairs of three-carbon phosphates, a process which required an input of energy in the form of ATP.

In the second stage oxidoreduction and phosphorylation steps take place which generate ATP and in which the glyceraldehyde-3-

phosphate molecules are gradually converted to pyruvate. Note that both molecules derived from glucose follow identical steps. In a first step, and indeed the most important step of the glycolytic sequence, a second inorganic phosphate group is attached to form 1,3 diphosphoglycerate. The energy required for this is derived from a hydrogen transfer to NAD^+, resulting in the formation of NADH which will have to be reoxidized to NAD^+ at a later step. Now the 1,3 diphosphoglycerate can react enzymatically with ADP, transferring the phosphate group at position 1 to form ATP. Together with the preceding step, the energy of aldehyde oxidation has thus been conserved as the phosphate bond energy of ATP. In the three further steps of the glycolytic sequence the remaining phosphate group is first shifted from position 3 to 2 and then the molecule is dehydrated to phosphopyruvate; this molecule can now again react enzymatically with ADP and transfer its phosphate group so that the sequence ends with the production of another ATP molecule and pyruvate.

We now see that the glycolytic breakdown of glucose to pyruvate has used 2 mol ATP per mol glucose as a primer to get the sequence started, but has then produced 4 mol ATP in the second stage of the sequence. Thus glycolysis results in a net gain of 2 mol ATP per mol glucose that can be used to drive other energy-requiring cell functions. Note, however, that an additional mol of ATP is obtained if the glucose molecule that enters the sequence was obtained from glycogen.

The process has also resulted in the formation of NADH which needs to be reoxidized to NAD^+ because, as we have seen, the glycolytic sequence can only enter its second and most important stage if H^+ acceptors are available. The mechanisms for reoxidizing NADH are different under aerobic and anaerobic conditions. If O_2 is available, oxidation occurs in the respiratory chain, as described below. But since the mitochondrial membranes are impermeable to NADH, the latter is oxidized by transferring its reducing equivalents to FAD, the flavine adenine dinucleotide which, we shall see, is part of the respiratory chain; $FADH_2$ can enter the mitochondrion. Under anaerobic conditions, NADH is oxidized by donating its electrons to pyruvate, which thus becomes reduced to lactate; this reaction is catalyzed by the enzyme lactate dehydrogenase.

Thus, under anaerobic conditions, lactate is the end product of glycolysis, 2 mol lactate being released to the blood as waste for every mol of glucose consumed. This is rather important. We have seen in chapter 2 that organisms revert to glycolysis as the main mechanism for obtaining ATP if the flow rate of O_2 into the cells is insufficient to cover their energetic needs, as it occurs in very heavy work above $\dot{V}_{O_2}$max (Fig. 2.8). Under such circumstances one will observe the lactate concentration in the blood to rise. However, the organism can utilize lactate as a substrate for the Krebs cycle in some cells, particularly in heart muscle, liver, kidney, and also in skeletal muscle, so that it can get rid of some of the lactate generated by glycolysis in places where oxidative phosphorylation cannot cope with the demand. Finally, some of the lactate can also be used to resynthesize glucose in a process called gluconeogenesis, but this requires energy.

AEROBIC METABOLISM

In reference to Figure 4.6 I have mentioned that the pathway for aerobic metabolism can be divided into two parts, the Krebs cycle and the respiratory chain. The Krebs cycle essentially produces CO_2 and NADH, whereas in the respiratory chain O_2 is consumed and NAD^+ regenerated, since, in this case, molecular O_2 serves as terminal electron acceptor.

The *Krebs tricarboxylic acid cycle* is the common and universal pathway of oxidative catabolism of all foodstuff molecules in aerobic cells. The principle is this: a molecule of acetic acid (two carbons) enters the Krebs cycle by condensation with oxaloacetic acid to form citric acid (Fig. 4.6). Through a sequence of steps the two carbon atoms gained from acetic acid are removed as two CO_2 molecules by decarboxylation, and oxaloacetic acid is eventually regenerated, thus completing the cycle. The overall net reaction catalyzed by the cycle can be written as follows:

$$CH_3COOH + 2H_2O \longrightarrow 2CO_2 + 8H.$$

So, evidently, for each acetic acid entering the cycle we obtain not only two CO_2 molecules but also eight hydrogens, four of which are donated to NAD^+ to make four NADH by the process described above (Fig. 4.2). This dehydrogenation of acetic acid is indeed the essential part of the cycle because it is this process which permits the extraction of free energy from the acetic acid in a form that can subsequently be used to make ATP in the respiratory chain. It is seen from this brief account that the Krebs cycle depends on two critical steps:

(1) the introduction of acetic acid, and (2) the reoxidation of NADH so as to maintain an adequate supply of the electron acceptor NAD$^+$.

THE KREBS TRICARBOXYLIC ACID CYCLE

The backbone of the Krebs cycle is a four-carbon dicarboxylic acid, oxaloacetic acid (Fig. 4.8); the cycle begins by condensing this molecule with one molecule of acetic acid which is donated by acetyl CoA (Fig. 4.5), a reaction which is catalyzed by the enzyme citrate synthase and results in citric acid, a six-carbon tricarboxylic acid. The Krebs cycle constitutes a sequence of reactions by which citric acid is reconverted to oxaloacetic acid, releasing two molecules of CO_2 and a number of hydrogens in the process (Fig. 4.6).

After transformation of citric acid to isocitric acid, a coupled decarboxylation and dehydrogenation reaction (catalyzed by isocitrate dehydrogenase) releases one CO_2 molecule and one pair of hydrogens which are picked up in NADH; it results in the five carbon α-ketoglutaric acid. The next step, the oxidation of α-ketoglutarate to succinate, occurs in two steps. The first combines again a decar-

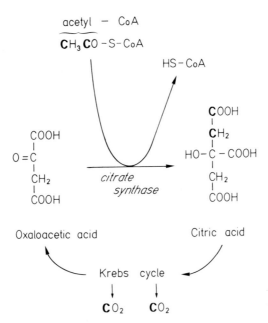

Fig. 4.8 The initial step in the Krebs cycle is the condensation of oxaloacetic acid with acetyl CoA to make the tricarboxylic acid citric acid.

boxylation and dehydrogenation, releasing CO_2 and 2H, but the resulting four-carbon molecule is now bound to CoA as succinyl CoA by means of a high-energy thiolester bond (compare Fig. 4.5); in a second step this bond is cleaved and the energy released causes the formation of GTP (guanosine triphosphate) using GDP and inorganic phosphate. Reversal of GTP to GDP causes the formation of an ATP molecule at this point (Fig. 4.6). Succinate is then oxidized by succinyl dehydrogenase to yield fumarate; the two hydrogens which are removed are, however, donated to a different electron acceptor, flavin adenine dinucleotide (FAD), which is covalently bound to the succinyl dehydrogenase and also forms part of the respiratory chain, as discussed below. It is of interest in this context that succinyl dehydrogenase is tightly bound to the inner mitochondrial membrane as is the respiratory chain. In the last two steps of the cycle H_2O is added to fumarate and the resulting malate is dehydrogenized to oxaloacetate, with the hydrogen trapped in NADH.

Three points are noteworthy: (1) The cycle has preserved its "backbone," the four-carbon dicarboxylic acid, which can again be condensed with acetic acid, and the cycle can begin another round. (2) The Krebs cycle does not consume any energy other than that which is contained in the acetyl CoA fed into the cycle. (3) The Krebs cycle is catalytic in two senses: every step is, of course, catalyzed by enzymes; but each intermediate has by itself a catalytic effect, since the addition of one molecule of any of the intermediates catalyzes the breakdown of many additional acetate molecules.

The existence of a cycle involving citric acid as an essential part of aerobic metabolism was postulated in 1937 by Krebs and Johnson on the basis of brilliant reasoning and ingenious though simple experiments; it was proven to exist as a universal mechanism that is found in bacteria and plant cells as well as in all cells of higher organisms. This process was first called the "citric acid cycle" and then the "tricarboxylic acid cycle." It is, however, perfectly justified to label it "Krebs cycle" in recognition of the classic, fundamental contributions of Hans Krebs (1900–1981).

ENTRANCE INTO THE KREBS CYCLE

Acetic acid is introduced into the Krebs cycle from a complex with coenzyme A called acetyl CoA (Fig. 4.5). If the foodstuff to be oxidized is a carbohydrate, or sugar, the process starts with pyruvate, the provisional end product of glycolysis (Fig. 4.7). If the pyruvate is oxidized in the presence of NAD^+ and CoA, the rather complex reaction, which is catalyzed by the pyruvate dehydrogenase system, results in acetyl CoA, NADH, and CO_2. The NADH will need to be reoxidized in the respiratory chain for the system to be continuously functioning. It is now important to note that glycolysis does not have to end in the wasteful production of lactate; in the presence of O_2 the pyruvate can be directed into the Krebs cycle through the intermediate step of acetyl CoA. At the end of the cycle the three-carbon molecule pyruvate will have been disassembled into three CO_2 molecules and will have generated five NADH molecules; since in CO_2 the carbon atom is completely oxidized, its energy is much lower than in pyruvate, and the energy released is first picked up by NADH for further use (Fig. 4.6).

The entrance of other foodstuffs into the cycle also occurs through the intermediary of acetyl CoA. Fatty acids are an important source of energy; they are available in the blood, or stored in the cells as lipid droplets. Fatty acids are broken up step by step into two-carbon fragments by a process called β-oxidation. The fatty acids are first activated by binding to CoA to make fatty acyl CoA esters which enter, indirectly, the mitochondrial matrix (Fig. 4.6). There, β-oxidation proceeds through four steps that are catalyzed by enzymes, resulting in the cleavage of a two-carbon fragment attached as acetic acid to CoA and leaving the fatty acyl CoA complex shortened by two carbons. The process then begins anew and cycles in the form of a spiral until the fatty acid chain is completely broken up. The acetyl CoAs formed in this process enter the Krebs tricarboxylic acid cycle to be further oxidized to CO_2 and H_2O.

The entrance of amino acids into the Krebs cycle is not uniform, and we shall not dwell on the mechanisms involved. Suffice it to say that about half the amino acids also enter the Krebs cycle via acetyl CoA which is made by different degradation pathways. The other amino acids enter the Krebs cycle at other points in that the intermediate that occurs in the Krebs cycle is formed from the amino acid, one example being the formation of α-ketoglutarate from arginine through glutamate, involving glutamate transaminase as a catalyst. The contribution of amino acid derivates to the energy gained in the Krebs cycle depends on their point of entry. For those that enter as acetyl CoA the result is evidently no different than for carbohydrates or fatty acids. Derivates that are intermediates of the tricarboxylic acid cycle and thus enter at other points contribute a reduced number of hydrogens for subsequent oxidation in the respiratory chain, but they will have an overall catalytic effect on the rate at which acetic acid can be metabolized in the cycle, as mentioned above, because they contribute additional "backbone."

THE RESPIRATORY CHAIN

We have seen in the preceding sections that the catabolism of substrates through glycolysis, fatty acid oxidation, and the Krebs cycle releases a considerable number of reducing equivalents which are carried away mostly as $NADH + H^+$. The energy captured in this way must now be transferred to the high-energy phosphate bond of ATP while the reducing equivalents must be delivered to the terminal electron acceptor, oxygen. This coupled process is called *oxidative phosphorylation*, and it is accomplished by letting the electron pairs, which are related to the reducing equivalents, flow down a chain of electron-carrier enzymes of successively lower energy level, called the respiratory chain (Fig. 4.6), until they finally reduce molecular oxygen to water. The free energy stored in NADH amounts to approximately 220 kJ/mol, but only about 30 kJ/mol are needed to attach the third phosphate group of ATP; the enzyme sequence in the respiratory chain allows a stepwise extraction of this energy so that three ATP molecules can be generated.

Before we can go on to describe the events in the respiratory chain we need to understand a few basic facts which will be described without any details; a deeper understanding can be obtained from standard texts on biochemistry. The first question is why do we talk about electron transport in the respiratory chain when "actually" a transfer of hydrogen to O_2 is meant? The point is that *oxidation-reduction (or redox) reactions* are those reactions in which electrons are transferred from an electron donor (or reducing agent) to an electron acceptor (or oxidizing agent); for comparison, protons (H^+) are being exchanged in acid–base reactions. Thus an oxidation-reduction reaction can be described as follows:

$$\text{Reductant} \qquad\qquad \text{Oxidant}$$

$$\text{electron donor} \rightleftharpoons e^- + \text{electron acceptor}.$$

The equilibrium of this relation results in an electrical potential because of the free electrons, which can be measured with respect to a standard reference electrode that can reversibly accept electrons; this potential is called the *standard reduction potential* and describes the tendency for reducing agents to lose electrons. Thus a more negative potential means a lower electron affinity, that is, a higher tendency to lose or "donate" electrons. The standard of reference is the reduction potential of the reaction

$$H_2 \rightleftharpoons 2H^+ + 2e^-$$

which is set at 0.0 volt at pH 0.0, and becomes -0.42 volt at pH 7.0, the reference pH used in relation to biochemical reactions. For comparison, the reaction

$$H_2O \rightleftharpoons \tfrac{1}{2}O_2 + 2H^+ + 2e^-$$

has a strongly positive standard reduction potential of $+0.815$ volt; thus water has a very low tendency to lose electrons since O_2 has a very high electron affinity.

Returning to the problem at hand, we remember that NADH trapped "reducing equivalents" donated from a substrate (Fig. 4.3). The NAD-NADH redox couple is linked to dehydrogenation of the substrate which liberates two hydrogens and two electrons; the redox reaction is

$$S\text{-}H_2 \longrightarrow S_{ox}$$
$$\Big\downarrow \text{dehydrogenase}$$
$$NADH + H^+ \rightleftharpoons NAD^+ + \overbrace{2H^+ + 2e^-}$$

which has a standard reduction potential of -0.32 volts. We have seen that one of the protons and both electrons are used to reduce NAD^+ to NADH, so that NADH is a carrier of two electrons that can be used for further redox reaction since they are relatively loosely bound, as evidenced by the highly negative reduction potential.

This description of oxidation-reduction reactions explains how the respiratory chain transfers electrons from NADH to molecular O_2, which can then bind H^+ ions to make water. This is achieved by arranging in series a set of redox couples (electron carriers) of increasing electron affinity, or decreasing reduction potential. Thus electrons flow down a cascade as they are donated and received between the links of the respiratory chain.

The electron carriers which make the respiratory chain (Fig. 4.6) are of three kinds whose properties we shall only briefly sketch:

The first member is a *flavin adenine dinucleotide*, FAD, which belongs to the same class as NAD and acts in a similar way: its isoalloxazine ring becomes reduced by accepting two electrons and binding two hydrogens so that the reduced form of FAD is designated $FADH_2$. The FAD-$FADH_2$ couple of the respiratory chain is bound to succinyl dehydrogenase and can receive electrons directly from this enzyme.

The second member is a benzoquinone derivative called *coenzyme Q* or *ubiquinone*, which can be reduced by accepting $2e^- + 2H^+$. It appears to serve as a shuttle between FAD and the subsequent cytochromes.

The following members are *cytochromes*, a group of iron-containing proteins that can transfer electrons. The iron is present in the form of a heme, that is, it is contained in a porphyrine ring (Fig. 4.9), just as in hemoglobin, for example. Electron transport by cytochromes is linked to the iron which can undergo cyclic or reversible valence changes between the oxidized form Fe(III) and the reduced form Fe(II) by accepting or releasing electrons. A number of different cytochromes, which differ by the nature of the protein

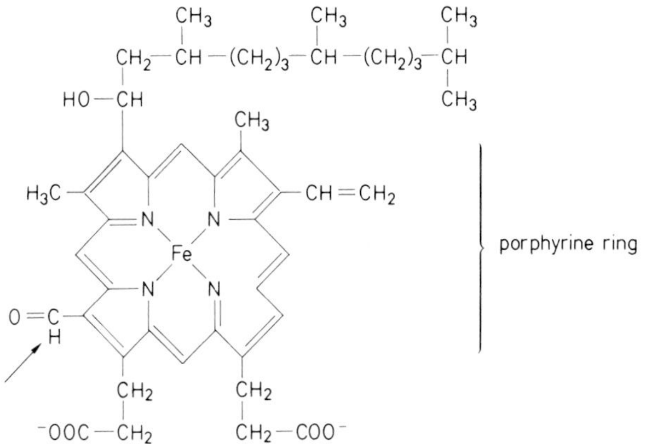

Fig. 4.9 Chemical structure of heme, as it occurs in cytochromes or in hemoglobin.

attached to the prosthetic group, have been identified in cells where they serve different functions. In the respiratory chain five cytochromes are found which are labeled Cyt b, Cyt c_1, Cyt c, Cyt a, Cyt a_3, in the sequence in which they transfer electrons (Fig. 4.6). The terminal cytochrome a_3, which can react with molecular O_2, is called *cytochrome oxidase*. Cytochromes a + a_3 seem to be present as a complex. It is interesting that the cytochromes occur in a fixed molar ratio in the respiratory chain, the current estimate being $b : c_1 : c : a : a_3 \cong 2 : 1 : 2 : 2 : 2$.

As mentioned before, the different members of the respiratory chain perform the electron transfer from NADH to molecular O_2 because they have a decreasing reduction potential, as shown in Figure 4.10. This goes along with a sequential decline in free energy which is proportional to the reduction potential: as a pair of electrons moves from one member to the next, a certain amount of free energy is lost. The total energy loss from NADH to O_2 amounts to -220 kJ. The formation of a high-energy phosphate bond in the reaction

$$ADP + P_i \rightleftharpoons ATP + H_2O$$

requires $+30$ kJ, so that the energy released in the respiratory chain is sufficient to make several ATP molecules from ADP and phos-

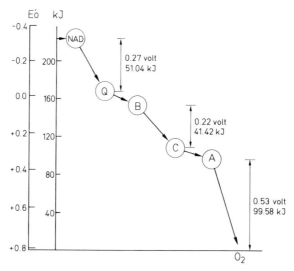

Fig. 4.10 As electrons move along the respiratory chain they lose some of their energy. In three steps this energy drop is large enough to drive the phosphorylation of one ADP to ATP. (After Lehninger, 1975.)

phate, provided a suitable coupling mechanism is available. Refer-ring to Figure 4.10 we see that three of the steps release an amount of free energy which is sufficiently large to allow this reaction to occur, and consequently each passage of an electron pair through the respi-ratory chain generates three molecules of ATP, as shown in Figure 4.6.

We would now need to consider the mechanism by which the synthesis of ATP is coupled to the stepwise energy loss along the respiratory chain. But I shall defer this to chapter 5 because it is intimately related to the structural arrangement of the respiratory chain in the inner mitochondrial membrane. Suffice it to say, at this point, that the energy gained at the three major steps of the respira-tory chain (Figs. 4.6 and 4.10) is transferred to an enzyme ATPase which is also bound to the inner mitochondrial membrane and can perform the synthesis of ATP from APD and phosphate.

The Cell's Energetic Balance Sheet

We have now seen that the cell is capable of transferring the free energy stored in foodstuff molecules, such as sugars and fatty acids, to the high-energy phosphate bonds of ATP. The process involves a multitude of small steps of dehydrogenation and decarboxylation catalyzed by enzymes in which intermediate hydrogen carriers are formed; phosphorylation of ATP occurs when these intermediates transfer their energy to the terminal hydrogen acceptor, oxygen. This process is brought to completion when the foodstuff molecule is degraded to CO_2 and H_2O, and this can happen only if O_2 is available. This is why energy metabolism is directly linked to respiration.

Let us now look once more at these processes in overview, and let us consider their efficiency. The questions are: how many ATP molecules are formed from one foodstuff molecule, how much O_2 is needed to allow completion of catabolism, and how much of the energy stored in the foodstuff molecule can be gathered in the ATP, that is, how efficient is this part of the system?

To understand this approach, let us first have a look at the last step in the chain of events, namely the energy transfer from NADH to ATP by coupled oxidative phosphorylation in the respiratory chain. The overall equation of this process

$$NADH + H^+ + 3ADP + 3P_i + \tfrac{1}{2}O_2 \longrightarrow NAD^+ + 4H_2O + 3ATP$$

has two components, one in which energy is lost, called the *exergonic* component,

$$NADH + H^+ + \tfrac{1}{2}O_2 \longrightarrow NAD^+ + H_2O,$$

and one in which energy is gained, the *endergonic* component,

$$3ADP + 3P_i \longrightarrow 3ATP + 3H_2O.$$

The change in standard free energy, called ΔG, that occurs in each of these component reactions is calculated from the difference in the free energy contained in the molecules on each side of the arrow. In the exergonic reaction the molecules on the left contain more energy than those on the right, so that ΔG is negative, amounting to -220 kJ. In the endergonic reaction it is positive; since phosphorylation of one mol ADP requires 30.5 kJ, we find $\Delta G = 3 \times 30.5 = 92$ kJ for the phosphorylation that is coupled to oxidation of one mol NADH. We thus see that $(\frac{92}{220}) \cdot 100 = 42\%$ of the energy released is trapped in ATP, the difference being lost as heat. The efficiency of this reaction is hence 42%. This is, in fact, quite good efficiency compared with manmade machines, but there is evidence that under steady-state conditions in intact mitochondria the efficiency may be considerably higher.

Let us now use the same approach to look at the energy balance sheet that results from the catabolism of foodstuffs, looking at the two main sources of energy, carbohydrates and fatty acids. Some basic data are reported in Table 4.1. The complete catabolism of *glucose* is described by

$$Glucose + 6O_2 + 36ADP + 36P_i \longrightarrow 6CO_2 + 42H_2O + 36ATP.$$

The exergonic component liberates $\Delta G = -2,870$ kJ, of which $\Delta G = +1,010$ kJ are recovered in the endergonic phosphorylation part, so that the efficiency is about 39%. The balance sheet for *fatty acids* depends on the chain length of the molecule; taking as example the 16-carbon palmitic acid, that enters the process as palmitoyl CoA, we have

$$Palmitoyl\ CoA + 23\ O_2 + 131ADP + 131P_i \longrightarrow$$
$$16CO_2 + 146H_2O + 131ATP.$$

TABLE 4.1 RESPIRATORY AND ENERGETIC DATA FOR GLUCOSE, PALMITIC ACID, AND THE AMINO ACID ALANINE, CONSIDERING BOTH AEROBIC AND ANAEROBIC BREAKDOWN OF GLUCOSE. NOTE THAT ENERGETIC EQUIVALENT OF O_2 IS VERY SIMILAR WITH ALL THREE SUBSTRATES.

Variable	Glucose $C_6H_{12}O_6$ Aerobic	Glucose $C_6H_{12}O_6$ Anaerobic	Palmitic acid $CH_3(CH_2)_{14}COOH$	Alanine $CH_3CH(NH_2)COOH$
Quantity of substance, M				
In mol	1	1	1	1
In g	180	180	256	89
O_2 consumed, M_{O_2}, in mol	6	—	23	3
CO_2 produced, M_{CO_2}, in mol	6	—	16	2.5
Respiratory quotient M_{CO_2}/M_{O_2}	1	—	0.7	0.83
Other products	H_2O	Lactate H_2O	H_2O	Urea H_2O
Energy produced ΔG (exergonic)				
In kJ/mol	2,871	136	9,794	1,318
ATP production				
In mol/mol	36	2	130	
Energy consumed (endergonic)				
In kJ/mol	1,100	61.1	3,972	
ATP efficiency	38%	40%	41%	
Energetic equivalent of O_2				
$\Delta G/M_{O_2}$, in kJ/mol O_2	478	—	426	439

From Dejours (1981).

This liberates $\Delta G = -9872$ kJ and recovers $\Delta G = +4001$ kJ, resulting in an efficiency of about 41%.

Thus — and this is now most important — whatever the foodstuff substrate, the efficiency of oxidative phosphorylation is about 40%, and *six molecules of ATP are generated for each molecule of O_2 consumed.* (In biochemistry one says that the P:O ratio of these reactions is 3.) For this reason the amount of O_2 consumed is a direct measurement of the energy made available to the cell in the form of ATP: respiration and energy metabolism are directly linked.

We have seen, however, that the cell has a way to make ATP from glucose in the absence of O_2, or when the O_2 supplied is insufficient. Glycolysis results in a net gain of two ATP for each glucose molecule split into two molecules of pyruvate, but this also produces one molecule of NADH which is oxidized, under anaerobic conditions, by reducing pyruvate to lactate by fermentation. *Anaerobic glycolysis,* described by

$$\text{Glucose} + 2\text{ADP} + 2\text{P}_i \longrightarrow 2 \text{ lactate} + 2\text{H}_2\text{O} + 2\text{ATP},$$

liberates -135.6 kJ and recovers $+61.1$ kJ and thus also has an efficiency of about 40%. However, it is wasteful with foodstuffs since it recovers only about 5% of the energy that glucose could generate by aerobic metabolism. The lactate released into the blood still contains quite a lot of free energy; the organism will, if possible, use lactate as a substrate for the Krebs cycle or to regenerate glucose, but this can be effective only under aerobic conditions. Thus, by using glycolysis, the cells incur an O_2 debt which must be paid off at a later stage, and, often, by different cells.

Although glycolysis is wasteful, the organism will revert to this pathway under two conditions:

(1) when ATP must be rapidly made, such as in short-term muscle work (weight lifting, for example), or at the beginning of an exercise load, as discussed in chapter 2;

(2) when oxidative phosphorylation cannot cope with the need for ATP or with the oxidation of NADH produced by glycolysis, as occurs when we reach the limit of aerobic energy production.

Summary

Cells get biologically useful energy through the combustion of food-stuffs (sugars, fats, proteins) using O_2 in the last step of the process. One mol glucose liberates 2,870 kJ (686 kcal) of energy and this uses 6 mol O_2. The problem is how to extract this energy in small portions in order that an important fraction can be captured in ATP. Oxidation involves the stepwise transfer of two hydrogen ions or protons (2 H^+) together with two electrons to an electron or proton acceptor which becomes reduced. Such reactions are called oxidation-reduction reactions. During breakdown of substrates (glucose, for example) protons are transferred to the cofactor NAD^+, reducing it to NADH. The system requires NAD^+ to be regenerated by proton and electron transfer to a terminal electron acceptor. Under aerobic conditions, molecular O_2 is the ideal terminal electron acceptor; under anaerobic conditions pyruvate plays this role, becoming reduced to lactate. The energy liberated by electron transfer is captured in the high-energy phosphate bond of ATP which requires 30 kJ per mol ATP formed.

These processes take place in an orderly fashion in the cells, controlled by a set of enzymes that are housed either in the cytoplasm or in the mitochondria. They can be broken up into three major steps: (1) glycolysis, an anaerobic fermentation process resulting in two molecules of pyruvate from each molecule of glucose and producing NADH and some ATP; (2) Krebs cycle, in which pyruvate is broken down to CO_2 and NADH is formed: (3) respiratory chain, where the H^+ collected in NADH is transferred to molecular O_2, generating ATP. The glycolytic fermentation of glucose produces 2 mol ATP per mol glucose, and some NADH which needs to be reoxidized; under anaerobic conditions this is achieved by reducing pyruvate to lactate. Under aerobic conditions, the NADH is oxidized in the mitochondria, and the pyruvate serves as a substrate for the Krebs cycle. The Krebs tricarboxylic acid cycle is the common and universal pathway of oxidative catabolism of all foodstuff molecules in aerobic cells. A molecule of acetic acid — derived from pyruvate, fatty acids, or some amino acids — enters the cycle by condensing with oxaloacetic acid to make citric acid. Through a sequence of enzyme-controlled steps the two carbon atoms gained from acetic acid are removed as two CO_2 molecules and oxaloacetic acid is eventually regenerated, thus completing the cycle. Eight H^+ are removed in the process, four of which are collected in NADH; this requires the presence of NAD^+ which must be regenerated by oxidation of NADH. This function is performed by the respiratory chain, a system of seven electron-carrier enzymes (flavin adenine dinucleotide, ubiquinone, cytochromes) which form an assembly within the inner mitochondrial membrane. As these enzymes transfer electrons eventually to molecular O_2 to make water, they build up a high-energy state which can be used to make ATP from ADP and inorganic phosphate, a complex process called oxidative phosphorylation.

Oxidative phosphorylation works with an efficiency of about 40%, that is, 40% of the energy contained in NADH is transferred to ATP. The complete catabolism of 1 mol glucose results in the formation of 36 mol ATP, with an efficiency of again 40%. The efficiency of oxidative catabolism of fatty acids is similar. Through glycolysis 1 mol glucose yields only 2 mol ATP, but this too occurs with an efficiency of 40% because the waste product, lactate, still carries a lot of energy; this process is ultimately inefficient, however, because it extracts only 5% of the energy contained in the substrate. Nevertheless, it is used by cells whenever they need to make ATP rapidly or when O_2 is in short supply.

Further Reading

Boyer, P. D., B. Chance, L. Ernster, P. Mitchell, E. Racker, and E. C. Slater. 1977. Oxidative phosphorylation and photophosphorylation. *Annual Review of Biochemistry* 46:955–1026.

Hochachka, P. W. 1980. *Living without Oxygen: Closed and Open Systems in Hypoxia Tolerance*. Cambridge: Harvard University Press.

Hochachka, P. W., and G. N. Somero. 1973. *Strategies of Biochemical Adaptation*. Philadelphia: Saunders.

Krebs, H. A. 1970. The history of the tricarboxylic cycle. *Perspectives in Biology and Medicine* 14:154–170.

Lee, C. P., G. Schatz, and L. Ernster, eds. 1979. *Membrane Bioenergetics*. Reading, Mass.: Addison Wesley.

Lehninger, A. L. 1982. *Principles of Biochemistry*. New York: Worth, chapters 13–19.

Racker, E. 1976. *A New Look at Mechanisms in Bioenergetics*. New York: Academic.

See also "Further Reading" in chapter 5.

References

Dejours, P. 1981. *Principles of Comparative Respiratory Physiology*. 2nd ed. Amsterdam: Elsevier North-Holland.

Hatefi, Y., A. G. Haavik, L. R. Fowler, and D. E. Griffiths. 1962. Studies on the electron transfer system. XLII. Reconstruction of the electron transfer system. *Journal of Biological Chemistry* 237:2661–2669.

* Keilin, D., and E. F. Hartree. 1939. Cytochrome and cytochrome oxidase. *Proceedings of the Royal Society of London (Biology)* 127:167–191.

* Kennedy, E. P., and A. L. Lehninger. 1949. Oxidation of fatty acids and tricarboxylic acid cycle intermediates by isolated rat liver mitochondria. *Journal of Biological Chemistry* 197:957–972.

* Krebs, H. A., and W. A. Johnson. 1937. The role of citric acid in intermediary metabolism in animal tissue. *Enzymologia* 4:418–422.

Lehninger, A. L. 1975. *Biochemistry*. 2nd ed. New York: Worth.

* Martius, C., and F. Knoop. 1937. Der physiologische Abbau der Citronensäure. *Zeitschrift Physiologische Chemie* 246:1–2.

Pullman, M. E., H. S. Penefsky, A. Datta, and E. Racker. 1960. Partial resolution of enzymes catalyzing oxidative phosphorylation. *Journal of Biological Chemistry* 235:3322–3330.

Weibel, E. R. 1979. Oxygen demand and the size of respiratory structures in mammals. In *Evolution of Respiratory Processes*, ed. S. C. Wood and C. Lenfant. New York: Dekker, pp. 289–346.

5

MITOCHONDRIA:
THE CELL'S FURNACES

MITOCHONDRIA WERE DISCOVERED by Richard Altmann in 1890 and described by Carl Benda in 1898 as "thread-like little bodies"; this is what the term "mitochondrion" means. Altmann had already pointed out that the functional role of this organelle is related to energy metabolism, and there is today no doubt that they are the sites of oxidative phosphorylation in the eukaryotic cell, housing the enzyme systems of the respiratory chain, Krebs cycle, and β-oxidation of fatty acids.

Although the mitochondria are often described as "particles," it is well established that most of them are indeed long thread-like structures which may branch or assume all sorts of bizarre shapes. It has been shown that some smaller cells such as yeasts or lymphocytes contain just two mitochondria which are rather long and tortuous so that a section will cut each mitochondrion several times; the cell then appears to contain many mitochondrial profiles. In muscle cells mitochondria form branched bands which encircle myofibrils in the form of a network.

Shortly after the introduction of the electron microscope into cell research, Fritjov Sjöstrand and George E. Palade independently discovered in 1953 that mitochondria were bounded by membranes which folded up to partially partition the interior. Today it is well established that the mitochondrion is bounded by a continuous *outer membrane*; a second *inner membrane* is apposed to the outer membrane but forms multiple infoldings, the *cristae* (Fig. 5.1). The inner membrane thus separates two spaces: a narrow *intermembrane space*

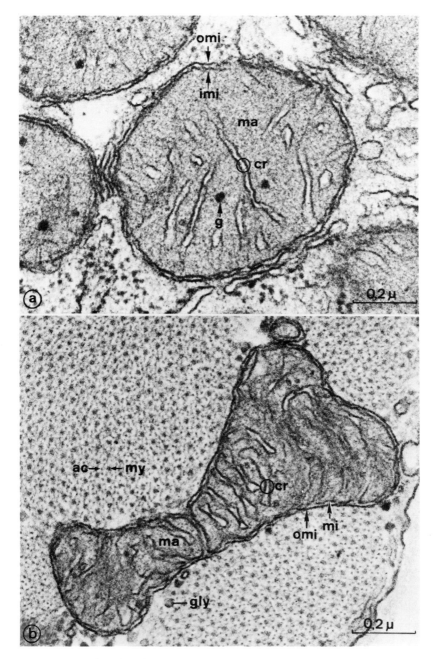

Fig. 5.1 Mitochondria from liver (a) and skeletal muscle (b) showing matrix (ma) with granule (g), outer (omi) and inner (imi) membrane, and cristae (cr). Note the higher density of cristae in muscle mitochondria. Cross-section of myofibrils in (b) shows regular arrangement of actin (ac) and myosin (my) filaments in A band, and glycogen granules (gly). (From Weibel, 1979.)

and the *mitochondrial matrix* (Fig. 5.2). We shall see that the separation of these two spaces by a membrane plays an important functional role. On electron micrographs the matrix appears relatively dense; it usually contains several dark granules which have been shown to contain divalent cations, mostly Ca^{++} and Mg^{++}, and appear to play a role in regulating mitochondrial function.

For a long time the question how the mitochondrial complement of a cell grows, particularly following cell division, was a matter of debate; the issue was *de novo* synthesis versus growth and division. Today the matter appears settled: mitochondria divide and grow. One decisive factor was the discovery that mitochondria contain a circular double strand of DNA, so that they possess their own genome which must be replicated in order to be preserved. By *de novo* synthesis this would be hard to accomplish. Mitochondria also contain their own population of ribosomes which differ somewhat from cytoplasmic ribosomes. Mitochondria are therefore able to synthesize some proteins autonomously. However, not all mitochondrial

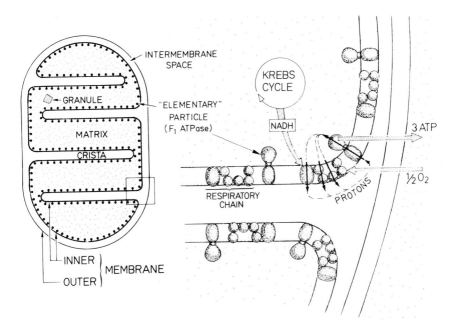

Fig. 5.2 Scheme of mitochondrial organization and of modular structure of inner mitochondrial membrane shows how these elements take part in the process of oxidative phosphorylation. (Modified from Weibel, 1979.)

proteins are coded for by mitochondrial DNA; an important part is made on cytoplasmic ribosomes bound to the endoplasmic reticulum, and are hence programmed from nuclear DNA. Indeed, there seems to be a quite active interchange of material between endoplasmic reticulum and mitochondria: besides some mitochondrial components originating in the endoplasmic reticulum, some of the ER enzymes derive part of their heme (the iron-containing prosthetic group) from mitochondria. Remember also the current hypothesis that mitochondria may have derived, during evolution of the eukaryotic cell, from aerobic bacteria which entered a symbiotic association with other prokaryotes; this can explain the fact that mitochondria are to some extent self-sufficient through their own genome — one which furthermore resembles that of bacteria.

Thus it appears that mitochondria form a comparatively "stable" organelle population of eukaryotic cells for which one finds a partial continuity through cell division, similar to that of the nucleus, the perinuclear membrane, or the cell membrane.

Putting Some Order into Cell Metabolism

We have seen in chapter 4 that the biochemical pathways leading to ATP production involve several major steps (Fig. 4.6). The substrates must first be broken down to acetyl CoA, which enters the Krebs cycle; reducing equivalents (NADH + H$^+$) derived from these steps are then oxidized in the respiratory chain, coupled with phosphorylation. All these steps are catalyzed by enzymes.

The construction of an efficient pathway of this kind calls for a certain spatial order which allows the different steps to be linked appropriately. For example, most of the dehydrogenases of the Krebs cycle are NAD-linked, that is, they function only if sufficient NAD$^+$ is present as immediate electron acceptor. These enzymes should therefore not be too far removed from the respiratory chain that transfers the electrons to the terminal electron acceptor, thus regenerating NAD$^+$ from NADH. One would also like to see all enzymes of the Krebs cycle housed in the same compartment to facilitate the sequential transfer of the breakdown products from one enzyme to the next. A further requirement is that the respiratory chain be linked with the ATPase that makes ATP. We shall see below that, according to current views, this necessitates their incorporation into a barrier between two compartments.

On the basis of these requirements we find the common pathways of oxidative phosphorylation, Krebs cycle and respiratory chain, to be contained totally within the mitochondria (Figs. 5.2 and 4.6). The oxidoreductases and cytochromes of the respiratory chain form spatially compact units that are built into the inner mitochondrial membrane and to which the ATPase is related; I shall expand on this below. The enzymes of the Krebs cycle are all contained in the mitochondrial matrix. They are thus contained in a compartment that is completely bounded by respiratory chains; in fact, because of the formation of cristae, the contact surface between inner membrane and matrix is so large that the distance from any Krebs cycle enzyme molecule to the nearest respiratory chain unit is no more than 10–20 nm, thus ensuring an easy exchange of NAD^+ and NADH between the enzyme and the respiratory chains. But there are some closer associations: we had seen that one Krebs cycle enzyme, succinyl dehydrogenase, is linked to the flavoprotein FAD as electron acceptor rather than to NAD; since FAD is part of the respiratory chain (Fig. 4.6), one finds succinyl dehydrogenase to be bound to the inner mitochondrial membrane, which ensures the required tight link between enzyme and electron acceptor.

The mitochondrial matrix also houses some additional enzyme systems, for example those which catalyze β-oxidation of fatty acids, or the pyruvate dehydrogenase system, which both result in the formation of acetyl CoA, the entrance currency for the Krebs cycle. The location of these enzymes in the mitochondrial matrix is again logical because they also generate NADH and depend on an adequate supply of NAD^+.

In summary, we can therefore say that the complex of mitochondrial matrix and cristae (or inner mitochondrial membrane) establishes a narrow space in which electrons gained by dehydrogenation of substrates can be efficiently transferred to O_2 through a sequence of well-controlled steps.

Glycolysis, is, in a way, independent of this mechanism because the NADH formed in its course can be reoxidized by reducing pyruvate, the product of glycolysis, to lactate. The enzymes that catalyze glycolysis are therefore situated in the unstructured part of the cytoplasm, that is, in the same compartment as glycogen, the main carbohydrate store of the cell.

The enzymes which catalyze the various steps that lead from

TABLE 5.1. DISTRIBUTION OF MARKER ENZYMES OF CELL METABOLISM TO STRUCTURAL UNITS.

Structural unit	Functional unit	Marker enzyme
Cytoplasmic matrix	Glycolysis	Hexokinase
Mitochondria		
Outer membrane	Entrance of Substrates	Monoaminoxidase
		Acyl CoA synthase
Intermembrane space		Adenyl kinase
Inner membrane	Respiratory chain	Cytochrome c
		Cytochrome oxidase
	Krebs cycle	Succinyl dehydrogenase (SDH)
	Phosphorylation	F_1 ATPase
Matrix	Krebs cycle	Citrate synthase
	Substrate oxidation	Lactate dehydrogenase (LDH)
		?(Acyl decarboxylase)

foodstuffs to ATP are therefore built into the cell according to a plan reflected by their association with well-defined structural units. A synopsis of this order is shown in Table 5.1, where I have listed a number of so-called marker enzymes in relation to the structural units in which they are located.

Most of these enzymes are housed within the mitochondria. The outer mitochondrial membrane is thus the basic structural element that separates them from the cytoplasm. This membrane is interesting in the sense that it is rather leaky and allows an easy passage of even large molecules such as sucrose. It also incorporates a number of enzymes whose main function appears to be to facilitate the entrance of substrates into the mitochondria in suitable form.

Oxidation–Phosphorylation Coupling Depends on Structure

In chapter 4 and Figure 4.10 we have seen that the passage of one reducing equivalent (NADH + H$^+$) through the electron-transport chain liberates, in three steps, a sufficient amount of energy to attach the third phosphate group in ATP; thus, one reducing equivalent causes three ATP to be made and $\frac{1}{2}O_2$ to be consumed. The process is apparently indirect because phosphorylation is not performed by the oxidoreductases of the respiratory chain but rather by a special enzyme called coupling factor or F_1-ATPase. How are the three quanta of energy gained from oxidation transferred to the ATPase?

This evidently fundamental question has been debated very intensely for several decades, and essentially three hypotheses have been advanced. The first is that of *chemical coupling*, in which a high-energy intermediate would be generated along the electron-transport chain; this compound would then transfer its energy to the ATPase. Such a high-energy compound has never been found. The second hypothesis considers *conformational coupling*. Some proteins of the system — for example, the ATPase itself — would store energy through a conformational shape change in a large number of weak bonds which are then "concentrated" into the high-energy phosphate bond. There is little more than suggestive evidence in support of this hypothesis.

The most widely — if not by now generally — accepted third hypothesis is that of *chemiosmotic* coupling proposed in 1961 by Peter Mitchell, a British biochemist whose ingenious work was honored with the Nobel Prize in 1978. In this hypothesis — now often called a theory — oxidation and phosphorylation are not coupled by a compound but rather by a *high-energy intermediate state* that involves the entire mitochondrion and is dependent on its structural integrity. This high-energy state is an electrochemical *gradient of protons* (H^+) across the inner mitochondrial membrane, that is, between the matrix and the intermembrane space; it serves as a coupling device if it is generated by the electron carriers and if the ATPase can use its energy to make ATP. Much of the evidence available indicates that this is the case.

What is this evidence? One important feature is that the inner mitochondrial membrane is a good H^+ barrier because its structural "backbone" is a bimolecular phospholipid barrier that does not let charged molecules or ions through. The proteins of the electron-transport chain are incorporated into this lipid bilayer in the form of four complexes of very different size. There is still some debate about how these complexes are precisely arranged, to which side of the membrane they are exposed, and where protons are translocated; a simplified version of the current "best guess" is shown in Figure 5.2.

The first complex is the largest (MW $\sim$ 500,000) and it is definitely in contact with the matrix side because this is where NADH + H$^+$ enters and interacts with what is called the NADH-linked dehydro-genase. Also the small FAD containing complex, linked to succinyl dehydrogenase, is on the matrix side. The third complex contains the cytochromes b and c$_1$ and is on the outer side, whereas the fourth complex, which is made of the cytochromes a and a$_3$ (cytochrome oxidase), spans the entire membrane.

It is now well established through a number of different experi-ments that the electron-transport chain can translocate protons vec-torially from the matrix to the intermembrane space, using the energy liberated by electron transfer (Fig. 4.10). There is still some debate about how this precisely happens; in Figure 5.3 one of the

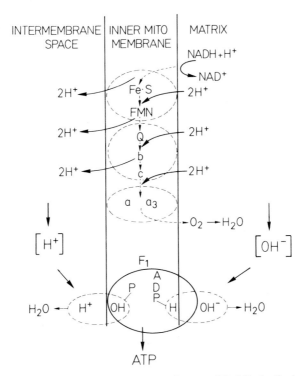

Fig. 5.3 According to the chemiosmotic theory of P. Mitchell, the electron flow along the respiratory chain (broken line, small arrows) causes three proton pairs to be shifted from the matrix into the intermembrane space. This model shows how the resulting pH gradient could be used to make ATP, although this is highly oversimplified.

possible sequences is illustrated in relation to the electron flow along the chain. The net result of this process is that the H^+ concentration increases in the intermembrane space and OH^- concentration in the matrix, and this builds up a strong "proton-motive force" or pH gradient across the inner mitochondrial membrane.

This force is now used by the F_1-ATPase to make ATP. How this really happens is still a matter of debate. One simple — probably much too simple — mechanism is again shown in Figure 5.3. In order to bind a phosphate group to ADP the phosphate must lose an OH^- group and ADP an H^+; if the OH^- is delivered toward the outside and the H^+ toward the matrix by virtue of the concentration gradients, H_2O is formed on both sides and the pH gradient is reduced. Many other more complex mechanisms have been proposed, but in the end they should all have the same effect: as ATP is formed the pH gradient is reduced. In fact, the coupling between H^+ translocation and ATP formation is so intense that one cannot measure any pH difference between the matrix and the intermembrane space: the protons translocated are immediately used.

The phosphorylation mechanism shown in Figure 5.3 is probably too simple because the element which carries out phosphorylation and is now called F_1-ATPase has a fairly complicated shape. It actually corresponds to the "elementary particles" of the inner mitochondrial membrane — sometimes also called "inner membrane spheres" — which have been shown by electron microscopy. These particles appear to be made of two major parts (Fig. 5.2); a base plate is incorporated into the membrane and carries by means of a slim stalk the spherical head piece which projects into the matrix. This element has been extensively studied and shown to be made of some twelve different subunits, which can intervene in various ways in transferring the energy of the proton gradient to the high-energy phosphate bond.

In summary, the theory of chemiosmotic coupling provides the simplest and most direct explanation of all available experimental evidence. For our purpose this concept is of further importance because it establishes an important relation between mitochondrial structure and oxidative phosphorylation. The channels through which protons are pumped outward are linked with spatial units, the electron-transport complexes, that are built into the inner mitochondrial membrane in the form of a mosaic, together with the F_1-ATPase through which the proton flux is reversed. These elements occur in well-defined molar ratios, and they appear to be densely packed, bound together by a small amount of phospholipid as a seal. The number of such channels that can be fitted onto the unit area of membrane is clearly limited. Because of the tight link between electron transport, proton flux, phosphorylation, and oxidation, we can therefore postulate that the capacity of mitochondria for oxidative phosphorylation must be proportional to the number of such units and hence to the surface area of the inner mitochondrial membrane.

Mitochondria and the Cell's Aerobic Potential

We have seen that all enzymes which catalyze oxidative phosphorylation are built into the mitochondria: the Krebs cycle enzyme into the matrix, electron transport carriers and F_1-ATPase into the inner membrane. Mitochondria contain little else, except the enzymes of β-oxidation of fatty acids which are again linked to aerobic metabolism. In gross terms we can therefore predict that the capacity of a cell for aerobic metabolism must be proportional to the amount of mitochondria it contains.

What is now the best morphometric parameter to relate to a cell's aerobic capacity? Since O_2 consumption and ATP formation are definitely linked with molecular complexes of the inner mitochondrial membrane, the most relevant morphometric descriptor is the surface area of the inner mitochondrial membrane, including the cristae (Fig. 5.4) which we shall call S(imi). As we have said in chapter 3, such morphometric parameters must be expressed relative to a meaningful reference parameter; since the sites of ATP consumption are distributed throughout the cell, the basic reference parameter is simply the cell volume, V(c). The capacity of a cell for oxidative phosphorylation should therefore be related to the surface density of inner mitochondrial membrane in the cell:

$$S_V(imi,c) = S(imi)/V(c) \tag{5.1}$$

which can be estimated by the simple point-counting method described in equation 3.32.

A second descriptor is the volume density of mitochondria in the cell

$$V_V(mi,c) = V(mi)/V(c). \tag{5.2}$$

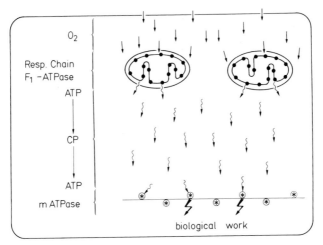

Fig. 5.4 The "flow of energy" to the sites in the cell where biological work is being done involves a flow of O_2, oxidative phosphorylation, and a flow of high-energy phosphate bonds through the ATP-creatine phosphate (CP) shuttle system.

This parameter is, in fact, essentially determined by two components: the number of cristae (that is, the surface of the inner membrane) and the volume of matrix which essentially reflects the amount of Krebs cycle enzymes present. Now it is evident that there should be a close relation between the number of elements that generate NADH (the Krebs cycle enzymes) and those that regenerate NAD^+ (the respiratory chain). It is therefore not surprising that the surface density of inner membrane with respect to the mitochondrial volume

$$S_V(imi,mi) = S(imi)/V(mi) \qquad (5.3)$$

assumes a characteristic value which is constant for a certain cell type. Thus in muscle mitochondria of different skeletal muscles from different species we find $S_V(imi,mi) = 42\ \mu m^2/\mu m^3 = 42\ m^2/cm^3$; in liver mitochondria this value is somewhat lower, namely about 25 $\mu m^2/\mu m^3$, because liver mitochondria contain more matrix, as shown in Figure 5.1. The reasons for this cell-specific difference are not yet well established.

Because the surface density of the inner membrane is characteristic for the cell type, we can use the mitochondrial volume density in the cell as a basic morphometric descriptor of the cell's aerobic capacity. This has a number of advantages: for one it can be estimated at lower powers, and it may be less affected by methodological errors because some obliquely sectioned cristae are often not easy to recognize, as seen in Figure 5.1.

One will sometimes find the mitochondrial number used as a descriptor. This is a bad parameter because it has neither a functional nor a morphometric basis. We have seen above that mitochondria may be, and often are, very long, complicated structures whose size and shape are difficult to estimate. The number and size of the profiles seen on section are therefore very difficult to interpret with respect to their spatial and functional meaning.

If we now compare a number of different cells we find that their mitochondrial content is, indeed, somehow proportional to their energetic needs. This is evident, for example, in the liver where we find two different cell types next to each other. The large hepatocytes which perform most of the liver's biochemical functions, such as protein synthesis, contain mitochondria amounting to over 20% of the cell volume. In contrast, the endothelial lining cells of the blood vessels which perform few metabolic functions have no more than 5% mitochondria. Heart muscle cells require a lot of ATP because they must contract at a high rate; in man, whose heart beats about 80 times per minute, they contain 20% mitochondria, whereas in the rat heart, which beats about 300 times per minute, the mitochondrial volume amounts to 35%.

We shall, in the following section, essentially concentrate on muscle cells and the role mitochondria play in their metabolism, for two reasons:

(1) Skeletal muscles constitute by far the largest mass of active cells of the body, nearly half the body mass in humans (Table 5.2). In the adult man we can roughly estimate that about 1.6 kg of mitochondria are contained in muscles, offering a surface of 35,000 m² or 10 acres of inner membrane to house electron-transport units!

(2) The highest levels of O_2 consumption are achieved only by strenuous muscular exercise, and under these conditions over 90% of the O_2 flow is directed to skeletal muscles.

TABLE 5.2. MITOCHONDRIAL MASS AND O_2 CONSUMPTION
IN HUMANS.

Location	Weight (g)	V_V(mi)	V(mi) (ml)	S(imi) (m²)	$\dot{V}_{O_2}$ (ml/min) Basal	Heavy work
Whole body	63,000	—	—	—	250	4,660
Skeletal muscle	31,000	0.054	1,675	35,150	50	4,500
Heart muscle	300	0.25	75	2,790	29	60
Liver	2,600	0.19	495	10,375	51	50

From Weibel (1979).

Mitochondria in Muscle Cells

Let us now look in more detail at muscle cells. They shall be at the center of our attention when we want to establish a relation between the limits of O_2 consumption and the design of the cell's respiratory units in order to test the hypothesis of symmorphosis. The reason is that we shall impose maximal O_2 consumption conditions by letting animals or humans run as fast as they can, thus stressing the aerobic capacity of their locomotory muscles to the limit.

Muscle cells consume ATP primarily in their contractile matter, the actin-myosin complex, which is built into the striated muscle cells in the form of myofibrils. These extend over the entire length of the muscle fiber and are composed of a series of symmetrical units, the sarcomeres (Fig. 5.5a). The substructure seen in these sarcomeres

Fig. 5.5 Electron micrographs of skeletal muscle cells. A longitudinal section (a) shows the organization of the contractile myofibrils (mf) into sarcomeres (S), symmetrical repeating units connected by Z-lines: the thick myosin (my) filaments extend through M- and A-band, the thinner actin filaments extend through I- and A-band; a cross-section of the A-band (b) shows that here actin and myosin interact in a very regular pattern. Mitochondria (mi), as well as the sarcotubular network (L), lie between the myofibrils; note the periodic occurrence of triads (t) where L-tubules connect to T-tubules which are invaginations of the sarcolemma. The sarcotubular system regulates Ca^{++} concentration in the myofibrils under the control of electrical signals that arise in the sarcolemma and spread into the cell along the T-tubules. Scale markers: (a) 0.5 μm; (b) 0.2 μm.

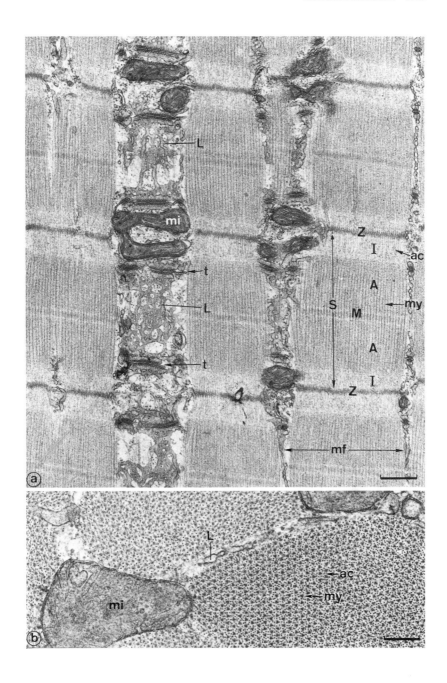

is due to the partial overlapping of actin and myosin filaments which are combined in a very regular lattice, as seen in cross-section in Figure 5.5b. One can demonstrate that the thicker myosin filaments carry a set of short processes, as shown in Figure 5.6, which can bind to the actin filaments, thus forming what is called cross-bridges. Muscle contraction is related to cyclical binding and loosening of the cross-bridge, combined with some bending movement of the myosin processes, which causes the actin and myosin filament to slide along each other. If you have ever seen a caterpillar crawl up a reed, shifting his many legs forward one after the other, you have a picture of how myosin "crawls" along actin.

ATP is required for cross-bridge cycling; the high-energy phosphate bond is cleaved when the cross-bridge detaches from the actin filament. Now this process is controlled by Ca^{++} ions whose concentration in the sarcoplasm is regulated from a highly organized system of membrane tubules that enwrap the myofibrils, the sarcoplasmic reticulum (Fig. 5.5). Calcium must be pumped into these tubules, and this also requires some ATP. In Figure 5.6 a number of additional proteins that are associated with actin to serve ancillary functions, such as Ca^{++} binding, have been omitted.

STRATEGIC DISTRIBUTION OF MITOCHONDRIA

From Figure 5.4 it is evident that the best strategic location of mitochondria should be somewhere halfway between the sites where ATP is being utilized and the entrance port for O_2 and metabolites such as glucose. However, considering that the diffusion of O_2 must be faster than that of high-energy phosphates, an optimal

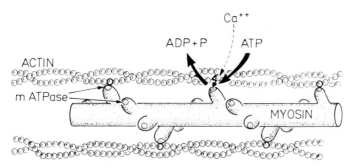

Fig. 5.6 In striated muscle ATP is used when the myosin-actin bridges cycle between being attached and loose, under the control of Ca^{++} concentration.

location would be closer to the ATP utilization site. This is indeed what one finds in many cells: in the hepatocyte of the liver, mitochondria are predominantly located amid the rough endoplasmic reticulum where most synthetic functions are performed; and in some kidney cells that actively pump ions through their membranes, mitochondria are found immediately apposed to the membrane.

In the muscle cells the optimal location is close to the myofibrils, and most mitochondria are indeed arranged as interfibrillar networks in the region of the I-band (Fig. 5.5), where they often form networks in a transverse plane. It is interesting that these interfibrillar mitochondria (which are also called central or core mitochondria) are not always evenly distributed throughout the fiber but often show a gradient of density that decreases toward the center (Fig. 5.7a). It is not known how this uneven distribution of mitochondria

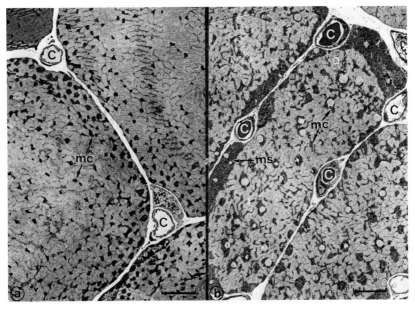

Fig. 5.7 Electron micrographs of cross-sectioned skeletal muscles show the mitochondria to be inhomogeneously distributed. In a leg muscle of a small gazelle (a) we note the density of core mitochondria (mc) to decrease from the cell periphery inward, whereas in the diaphragm of a rat (b) some fibers show thick packets of subsarcolemmal mitochondria (ms) which are missing where capillaries (C) are apposed to the cell. Scale markers: (a) 5 μm; (b) 5 μm. (From Hoppeler et al., 1981.)

might affect the supply of ATP to the myofibrils. Could it be that peripheral myofibrils perform more work than central ones? However, remember that in chapter 2 (Fig. 2.2) we have seen that ATP formed in mitochondria does not go directly to the myosin ATPase but is absorbed into a high-energy phosphate pool in which creatine phosphate serves as the main energy reservoir; it is creatine phosphate that moves about the cell and replenishes the ATP store next to the myofibril. On the other hand, we must also remember that muscle mitochondria draw their O_2 from the O_2 stores found in myoglobin, and myoglobin also facilitates O_2 diffusion. The situation is hence rather complex.

The uneven distribution of mitochondria is particularly marked in muscle cells that are notably rich in mitochondria. Here we find some 4–10% of the mitochondria concentrated beneath the cell membrane, the sarcolemma, where they form a rim of variable depth (Fig. 5.7b). The functional role of these subsarcolemmal mitochondria, which are close to the O_2 source, is not known. It is interesting to note, however, that the region of the muscle cell immediately adjacent to the capillary is free of such mitochondrial packets (Fig. 5.7b). One could therefore imagine that O_2 entering the muscle fiber directly from the capillary may diffuse into the depth of the fiber reaching core mitochondria in view of "local" production of ATP; O_2 diffusing into the interstitial space would reach the subsarcolemmal mitochondria where a large amount of ATP is generated for diffusion (via the creatine phosphate shuttle) into the fiber. Indeed, O_2 entering the cell near the subsarcolemmal packets of mitochondria barely has a chance to get into the depth of the fiber. It is conceivable — but only as a conjecture — that this distribution of mitochondria constitutes a mechanism for improving the efficiency of ATP supply to the myofibrils: high-energy phosphates and O_2 could thus diffuse independently from each other, both driven by comparatively high concentration gradients from the cell surface inward.

MUSCLE FIBER TYPES

Skeletal muscles are composites of various types of muscle fibers that differ with respect to their physiological and metabolic properties. The first distinguishing trait is the time course of their response to stimulation — either a fast or a slow twitch. Then the fibers differ with respect to the mechanism by which they generate ATP: some fibers do this mainly by oxidative phosphorylation, whereas others depend predominantly on glycolytic, that is, anaerobic, ATP production. The combination of these traits leads to the distinction of three major muscle fiber types (Table 5.3):

SO: slow-twitch–oxidative;

FOG: fast-twitch–oxidative—glycolytic;

FG: fast-twitch–glycolytic.

There have been several other classification schemes, but this one will do for our purpose.

We can distinguish these fiber types if we perform some histochemical reactions on serial sections, as shown in Figure 5.8. The fiber types first differ with respect to their staining intensity for ATPase reacted at acid pH (Fig. 5.8a); the reason for this is poorly understood, although the different fiber types contain slightly different myosin molecules. The relative capacity for oxidative phosphorylation is reflected in the staining for marker enzymes of mitochondria such as succinyl dehydrogenase (see Table 5.1), which we find to be denser in the fibers that use oxidative phosphorylation (Fig. 5.8b).

TABLE 5.3. CHARACTERISTICS OF MUSCLE FIBER TYPES.

Characteristic	SO	FOG	FG
Contraction	Slow twitch	Fast twitch	Fast twitch
Myosin ATPase (pH 4.1)	High	Low	Intermediate
ATP generation	Oxidative	Oxidative and glycolytic	Glycolytic
Succinyl dehydrogenase	High	High	Low
Glycogen content	Low	Intermediate	High
V_V(mitochondria)	$\geq 10\%$	$2-5\%$	$\leq 1\%$
Subsarcolemmal mitochondria	(+)	++	—
Fiber size	Small	Intermediate	Large
Myoglobin content	High	High	Low
Color	Red	Red	White

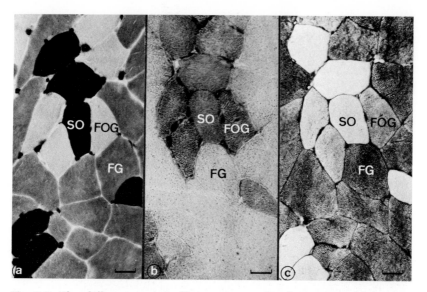

Fig. 5.8 The different muscle fiber types can be demonstrated by histochemical reaction, as shown here on three serial sections from M. semitendinosus of a cat. Besides differences in the intensity of acid ATPase reaction (a), oxidative fibers stain more intensely in the reaction for succinyl dehydrogenase, a Krebs cycle enzyme (b), whereas the PAS stain reveals the high glycogen content of glycolytic fibers (c). Scale markers: 20 μm.

It is therefore not surprising that such oxidative fibers have a higher concentration of mitochondria than the FG fibers (Table 5.3 and Fig. 5.9), although there is a very large variation. We may note on Figure 5.8b that the SDH stain shows up in the form of granules which actually correspond to mitochondria, and their histochemical stain reveals the concentration gradient of mitochondria from the periphery into the core, the packets of subsarcolemmal mitochondria appearing as black patches. It is particularly interesting that such subsarcolemmal patches occur in FOG fibers, so that we may reach the tentative conclusion that muscle cells with subsarcolemmal mitochondria might be FOG fibers. Finally, we can also stain for glycogen and will find the staining intensity to be proportional to the relative importance of glycolysis in cell metabolism (Fig. 5.8c). But there are two additional characteristics that need to be mentioned. The fibers that depend on O_2 are smaller than the glycolytic fibers. They also contain a higher amount of myoglobin, the red heme pigment that serves as O_2 store and facilitates O_2 diffusion through

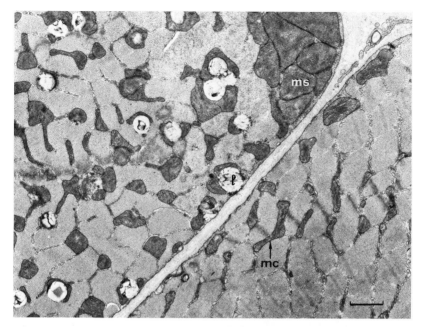

Fig. 5.9 Comparison of two fiber types from diaphragm of a dwarf mongoose (*Helogale pervula*). The core mitochondria (mc) are larger and more numerous in an FOG fiber than in the predominantly glycolytic FG fiber. Subsarcolemmal mitochondria (ms) and lipid droplets (*l*) occur only in the oxidative fiber. Scale marker: 1 μm. (From Mathieu et al., 1981.)

the cell; because of this pigment, oxidative fibers are red, whereas glycolytic fibers are white, the oldest classification of muscle fiber types.

The differentiation of various fiber types in one and the same muscle and its malleability under different conditions is, in fact, a rather interesting topic on which I could expand much more, but it would detract from the main focus of this text. All we really need to know is this: each muscle has a characteristic composition in terms of fiber types, which are even arranged in a characteristic pattern, and this depends on the type of work done by the muscle. Muscles that need to generate large forces for short periods will mostly contain "white" fibers, whereas muscles that must perform work over long periods will be made predominantly of oxidative "red" fibers. This is because glycolysis can provide ATP instantaneously, but not over a prolonged period (see chapter 2), since lactate accumulation leads to a dangerous drop of pH (acidosis) in the *milieu intérieur*. In contrast, the process of oxidative phosphorylation can go on as long as substrates and O_2 are available in adequate quantity because its breakdown products, CO_2 and H_2O, are harmless and easily eliminated. Jumps and sprints are therefore best performed by glycolytic fibers, whereas endurance runs over several kilometers need to be supported by oxidative fibers. In that respect it is interesting that the diaphragm is made only of oxidative SO and FOG fibers because it must contract incessantly to ventilate the lungs.

The distinction of fiber types is therefore important for understanding the functional differentiation of different muscles. For our purpose, however, we meet with one major difficulty, namely that the mitochondrial content is only loosely related to fiber types; it shows very large variations. But since we know that oxidative phosphorylation is limited to the mitochondria, we can still estimate the oxidative capacity of a given muscle by measuring its total content in mitochondria, averaging over all fiber types. We will have to keep in mind, however, that this does not necessarily reflect the total ATP requirement or the total work performed because white fibers call upon the fast process of glycolytic ATP production.

ARE MUSCLE MITOCHONDRIA ADAPTED TO ENERGETIC NEEDS?

Let me now finally address the question whether muscles are able to adapt their structure to the functional needs. If the hypothesis of symmorphosis is correct, then the muscles of an athlete should be different from those of a lazy-bug who never moves himself an inch further than necessary. This is indeed the case. However, the muscles of a weightlifter will also be different from those of a marathon runner. The reason for this difference is immediately evident when we consider the properties of the different fiber types.

A weightlifter must train himself to generate enormous forces. For that he needs to increase his myofibrillar mass, or rather the number and size of myofibrils that act in parallel. Accordingly his muscles become enlarged; indeed this is what happens in body-building which is induced by force training. But the weightlifter has to sustain this work for only a short period, so he can rely almost entirely on glycolysis to generate the large quantities of ATP he needs quickly. The consequence is evident: he will almost exclusively increase his FG fibers. One may have noticed that these athletes breathe heavily *after* the deed, when they need to pay off the O_2 debt incurred by oxidizing the lactate that was produced during exertion.

The situation is quite different for a marathon runner, who has to develop muscles that can endure a long, strenuous run; for that he will have to improve his capacity for oxidative phosphorylation. Long-distance runners are usually lean fellows whose muscles do not appear particularly impressive because they need not generate large forces. If we examine their muscles, however, we will find that they contain a large proportion of oxidative SO and FOG fibers.

Let us now approach the question whether the mitochondrial mass contained in muscle cells is proportional to O_2 consumption during running. Remember that we wanted to approach this question by a double strategy, comparing first individuals of similar size but different O_2 needs and then the effect of body-mass-dependent variations in O_2 consumption. Remember also that we need to base the comparison on estimates of maximal O_2 consumption, that is, on the level at which any additional energy need is covered by glycolysis.

With respect to the first approach, a number of studies have compared O_2 needs and mitochondria in long-distance runners and sedentary people. The approach is to measure maximal O_2 consumption by one of the methods described in chapter 3 while the individual runs on a treadmill at increasing speed; alternatively, one can let him pedal on a bicycle ergometer against increasing loads. In order to estimate the mitochondrial content of muscle cells, one takes a needle biopsy from a known location in one of the large leg muscles that contributes significantly to the work performed; in man one usually samples from the M. vastus lateralis, an easily accessible and major portion of the quadriceps muscle of the thigh which stretches the knee joint and is hence a major contributor to the forward thrust in running. Such biopsies are then processed for electron microscopy. The findings are rather striking. In Figure 5.10 we compare "typical" cells from a young sedentary individual, a medical student, with cells from a highly trained long-distance runner, in fact a member of the Swiss National Team of Orienteers at the peak of performance. First of all, note that the size of the myofibrils is about equal in both cases, in line with what we noted above. However, the trained runner has more and larger mitochondria; and furthermore, there are more fat droplets associated with them, a sign that he might use more fatty acids as substrate for oxidation. Such pictures are, however, not very conclusive because of the great variability in

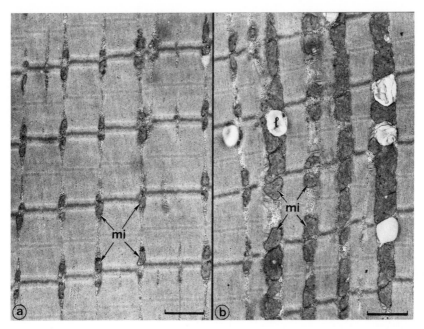

Fig. 5.10 Muscle biopsies from leg muscles show greater content in mitochondria (mi) and lipid droplets (*l*) in highly trained (b) than in untrained (a) men. Scale markers: 1 μm.

mitochondrial density that one normally finds between fibers in one and the same muscle. So we need to base our analysis on morphometric data obtained from sufficiently large samples. The result of this is shown in Figure 5.11: in highly trained athletes the volume density of mitochondria is considerably larger than in the sedentary individuals. Evidently, there is a close proportionality between mitochondrial volume density and $\dot{V}_{O_2}$max per unit body mass: in male runners both the mitochondrial content and $\dot{V}_{O_2}$max are about 1.5 times larger than in the population of male students that represent the sedentary population. A detailed study of the mitochondria revealed that the surface density of inner membrane in the mitochondria was unchanged, so that the augmentation of mitochondrial volume reflects the changes in the machinery for oxidative phosphorylation rather well. This kind of result has been obtained in several studies, and it was also shown that endurance training induces an increase of Krebs cycle enzymes and cytochromes in proportion to $\dot{V}_{O_2}$max. We can therefore conclude that the hypothesis of symmor-

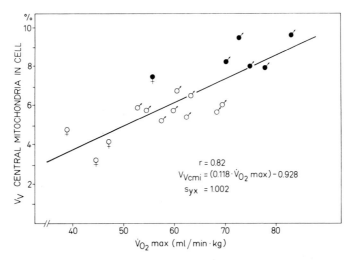

Fig. 5.11 The volume density of mitochondria in leg muscle cells is proportional to $\dot{V}_{O_2}$max in a population of untrained (open circles) and trained (full circles) humans. (From Hoppeler et al., 1973.)

phosis is supported in this case: the limit of O_2 consumption is proportional to the amount of mitochondria and associated enzymes in the muscle cells.

There is one last point we need to raise, however: does this proportion reflect a real adaptation of cell structures to energetic demands? Adaptation to an imposed stress means that the muscle cells must have augmented the units of oxidative metabolism *in response* to the stimulus and above their genetically determined complement. The comparison of athletes with sedentary students does not demonstrate adaptation, for it could well be that individuals who have more mitochondria congenitally are more likely to become competitive runners. To clarify this, H. Howald has looked at pairs of identical twins, one of whom was subjected to vigorous endurance training. Both $\dot{V}_{O_2}$max and V_V(mi,c) increased by about 15% in the trained sibling, compared with the untrained sibling. The system is, therefore, adaptable to increased energetic needs, both at the structural and the functional level. This can be confirmed if one takes repeated biopsies from individuals who undergo systematic training: as their aerobic capacity ($\dot{V}_{O_2}$max) increases, their muscles develop a proportionally larger complement of mitochondria.

Turning now to the second approach, we can ask whether the

mitochondrial mass of muscles scales in proportion to O_2 consumption when animal size varies. We have seen in chapter 2 that $\dot{V}_{O_2}$max changes with body mass to the 0.8 power (Fig. 2.9); in other terms, O_2 consumption per unit body mass changes as

$$\dot{V}_{O_2}max/M_b = a \cdot M_b^{-0.2}. \tag{5.4}$$

If mitochondrial volume density is proportional to O_2 consumption per unit body mass, then we would expect $V_V(mi,c)$ to scale also with $M_b^{-0.2}$. When we performed such a study on a series of wild African mammals that covered a weight range from 0.5 to 250 kg we found this to be the case for some of the muscles studied but not for others, as shown in Figure 5.12. Does this mean that the hypothesis of symmorphosis is not supported when we look at animals of different size? Not necessarily; maybe our basis for comparison is not correct.

One possibility is that we should have looked at the surface area of inner membranes rather than at mitochondrial volume. This did not change the result because it turned out that the inner membrane surface density within the mitochondria was constant, irrespective of animal size. But when we looked at the situation more carefully we came to suspect that mitochondrial volume *density* was not necessarily the best parameter to look at. The reason for this is that

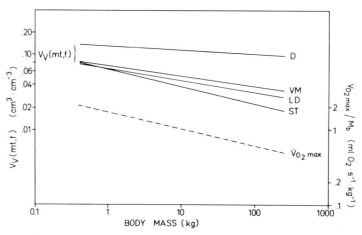

Fig. 5.12 The volume density of mitochondria in various muscles is not, in general, proportional to mass-specific maximal O_2 consumption. D = diaphragm, LD = longissimus dorsi, ST = semitendinosus, VM = vastus medialis. (From Mathieu et al., 1981.)

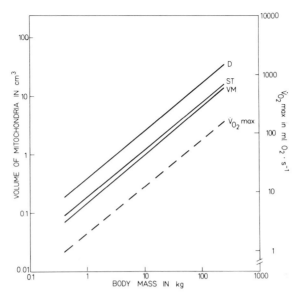

Fig. 5.13 When the total mass of the muscles is considered, the total volume of mitochondria in the muscles becomes proportional to total $\dot{V}_{O_2}$max. (From Mathieu et al., 1981.)

the total mass of a given muscle is not in all instances a fixed fraction of body mass: some muscles are relatively larger in smaller animals than others. So we reasoned that *total* maximal O_2 consumption of a running animal should be proportional to the *total* mitochondrial mass (or volume) in the muscles that contribute equivalently to running. The total mitochondrial volume in a muscle is easily obtained as the product of muscle volume and mitochondrial volume density. When we did this calculation for the muscles included in the study of African mammals, we found that total mitochondrial volume scaled in close proportion to total $\dot{V}_{O_2}$max, as shown in Figure 5.13. It thus appears that also by the second approach the limit to O_2 consumption is proportional to the mass of mitochondria in active muscles. The hypothesis of symmorphosis is hence supported by this additional evidence.

What Have We Learned?

From varied evidence we have first concluded that the enzymes involved in the process of oxidative ATP production, from the Krebs cycle to electron transfer and coupled phosphorylation, are housed in the mitochondria. We have also learned that structural organization within the mitochondria plays an eminent role in this process by assembling the elements of the electron transfer chain in a membrane across which a proton gradient can be built up as the main force for phosphorylation. From all this we have deduced that mitochondrial structure must have an important bearing on the relation between O_2 consumption and ATP flux to the energy-consuming sites.

The relation between energetic needs and O_2 consumption is perhaps not as simple as one could, at first, imagine. In the muscles we find that some fibers prefer to make their ATP from glycolysis, without taking recourse to oxidative phosphorylation. But this rapid pathway does not permit sustained work because lactate accumulation leads to dangerous acidosis. Therefore, any work that must be endured for longer periods depends on oxidative phosphorylation in mitochondria because the end products, CO_2 and H_2O, are harmless and easily eliminated. Oxidative metabolism is a "clean" source of energy, whereas glycolysis "pollutes" the internal environment with undesirable waste products.

Do mitochondria determine the size of the O_2 sink? Do they, in other words, set the limit for O_2 consumption? In order to check those questions out we have studied, along the double strategy proposed above, the relations between the mass of mitochondria in locomotory muscles and the level of $\dot{V}_{O_2}$max that the organism can achieve. We found, on the one hand, that strenuous endurance training leads to a parallel increase of both the aerobic capacity of a runner and the relative amount of mitochondria in the muscles used during running. And in comparing animals of varying size we found total $\dot{V}_{O_2}$max to be again closely related to total mitochondrial mass of locomotory muscles. This is strong, perhaps even convincing, evidence in support of the hypothesis that structural elements of cell metabolism are limiting factors for the functional capacity of the cells to generate the high-energy phosphates required to cover their energetic needs. The system is also adaptable: as the cell needs more energy, it can increase its mitochondrial complement and can thus improve its capacity for aerobic metabolism. Isn't this good evidence that the cell's metabolic machinery is built economically and that symmorphosis is a valid or at least reasonable assumption at this level of organization?

Summary

Mitochondria are small subcellular organelles, often much elongated or of complex shape, even forming networks. They are bounded by two membranes: the outer membrane establishes the interface to the cytoplasm, the inner membrane forms numerous infoldings called cristae. The inner membrane separates the matrix from the narrow intermembrane space. Mitochondria have their own DNA and ribosomes which are similar to those found in bacteria; they are able to synthesize some proteins autonomously, but also require additional proteins made in the cytoplasm. Mitochondria enlarge and multiply by growth and division.

The mitochondrial matrix houses all enzymes of the Krebs cycle, as well as some additional enzymes which catalyze β-oxidation of fatty acids or oxidation of pyruvate. The inner membrane carries the respiratory chain assemblies and the ATPase that makes ATP. The close spatial relation between matrix and the cristae of the inner membrane ensures that the NADH formed in the Krebs cycle is efficiently reoxidized to NAD^+, a necessary cofactor for the Krebs cycle enzymes. Mitochondrial structure puts order into the complex enzyme system of oxidative phosphorylation.

Oxidation-phosphorylation coupling depends on mitochondrial structure. According to the chemiosmotic theory, the respiratory chain builds up a proton gradient across the inner membrane as electrons are transferred along the chain to molecular O_2, in that three protons are pumped from the matrix to the intermembrane space for every electron transferred from NADH to O_2. The result is a high-energy intermediate state because the inner membrane is a good proton barrier. The F_1-ATPase, which is also built into the inner membrane, uses this energy to make ATP by binding a third phosphate group to ADP. Six mol ATP are made for 1 mol O_2 consumed in the respiratory chain.

The cell's potential for oxidative phosphorylation is proportional to the inner membrane surface of its mitochondria, and to the volume density of its mitochondria, because mitochondria of a given cell type contain a characteristic amount of inner membrane, for example 42 $\mu m^2/\mu m^3$ in muscle. The mitochondrial content of different cells is proportional to their energetic needs. In skeletal muscle one finds different fiber types. Fast-twitch glycolytic fibers contain few mitochondria because they cover their fast ATP needs by anaerobic glycolysis. Fast-twitch and slow-twitch oxidative fibers are rich in mitochon-dria because they depend mostly on oxidative phosphorylation; these two fiber types are responsible for endurance work.

The mitochondrial population of muscles is adapted to overall energetic needs, but the type of work required is also taken into account. Weight lifters need rapid energy and thus depend on glycol-ysis for ATP production, whereas endurance athletes produce their ATP aerobically. The mitochondrial content of muscles is propor-tional to the endurance work capacity and, specifically, to aerobic capacity, that is, to maximal O_2 consumption achieved during pro-longed work, such as running. This holds as well when animals of similar size (or humans) with different work capacity are compared, as when we look across the size range of mammals: total mitochon-drial volume of muscles is proportional to $M_b^{0.8}$, just as is maximal O_2 consumption. We conclude that the mitochondrial content of cells (and muscles in particular) is a rate-limiting factor for oxidative metabolism.

Further Reading

MITOCHONDRIA

Ernster, L., and G. Schatz. 1981. Mitochondria: a historical review. *Journal of Cell Biology* 91:227s–255s.
Grivell, L. A. 1983. Mitochondrial DNA. *Scientific American* 248:60–73.
Hinkle, P. C., and R. E. McCarty. 1978. How cells make ATP. *Scientific American* 238:104–123.
Mitchell, P. 1979. Keilin's respiratory chain concept and its chemiosmotic consequences. *Science* 206:1148–1159. (Nobel Lecture.)
Nicholls, D. G. 1982. *Bioenergetics: An Introduction to Chemiosmotic Theory.* New York: Academic.
Racker, E. 1975. Inner mitochondrial membranes: basic and applied aspects. In *Cell Membranes: Biochemistry, Cell Biology and Pathology,* ed. G. Weissmann and R. Claiborne. New York: HP Publishing, pp. 135–141.
Tzagaloff, A. 1982. *Mitochondria.* New York: Plenum.
See also "Further Reading" in chapter 4.

MUSCLE

Close, R. I. 1972. Dynamic properties of mammalian skeletal muscles. *Physi-ological Review* 52:129–97.

Franzini-Armstrong, C., and L. D. Peachey. 1981. Striated muscle: contractile and control mechanisms. *Journal of Cell Biology* 91:166s–186s. (Review.)

Gollnick, P. D., and B. Saltin. 1982. Significance of skeletal muscle oxidative enzyme enhancement with endurance training. *Clinical Physiology* 2:1–12.

Holloszy, J. O., and F. W. Booth. 1976. Biochemical adaptations to endurance exercise in muscle. *Annual Review of Physiology* 38:273–290.

Howald, H. 1982. Training-induced morphological and functional changes in skeletal muscle. *International Journal of Sports Medicine* 3:1–12.

Murray, J. M., and A. Weber. 1974. The cooperative action of muscle proteins. *Scientific American* 230:58–71.

References

MITOCHONDRIA

* Altmann, R. 1890. *Die Elementarorganismen und ihre Beziehungen zu den Zellen.* Leipzig: Veit.

* Benda, C. 1898. Weitere Mitteilung über die Mitochondrien. *Verhandlungen Physiologische Gesellschaft Berlin,* pp. 376–383.

Fernandez-Moran, H., T. Oda, P. B. Blair, and D. E. Green. 1964. A macromolecular repeating unit of mitochondrial structure and function. *Journal of Cell Biology* 22:63–100.

Hackenbrock, C. R. 1966. Ultrastructural bases for metabolically linked mechanical activity of mitochondria. I. Reversible ultrastructural changes with change in metabolic steady state in isolated liver mitochondria. *Journal of Cell Biology* 30:269–297.

Kagawa, Y., and E. Racker. 1966. Partial resolution of the enzymes catalyzing oxidative phosphorylation. IX. Reconstitution of oligomycin-sensitive adenosine triphosphatase. *Journal of Biological Chemistry* 241:2461–2466.

* Mitchell, P. 1961. Coupling of phosphorylation to electron and hydrogen transfer by a chemical osmotic type of mechanism. *Nature* (London) 191:144–148.

* Palade, G. E. 1953. An electron microscope study of the mitochondrial structures. *Journal of Histochemistry and Cytochemistry* 1:188–211.

* Sjöstrand, F. S. 1953. Electron microscopy of mitochondria and cytoplasmic double membranes. *Nature* (London) 171:30–32.

Weibel, E. R. 1979. Oxygen demand and the size of respiratory structures in mammals. In *Evolution of Respiratory Processes,* ed. S. C. Wood and C. Lenfant. New York: Dekker, pp. 289–346.

MUSCLE

Barany, M. 1967. ATP-ase activity of myosin correlated with speed of muscle shortening. *Journal of General Physiology* 50:197–218.

Billeter, R., H. Weber, H. Lutz, H. Howald, H. M. Eppenberger, and E. Jenny. 1980. Myosin types in human skeletal muscle fibers. *Journal of Histochemistry and Cytochemistry* 65:249–259.

Burke, R. E., D. N. Levine, P. Tsairis, and F. E. Zajac. 1973. Physiological types and histochemical profiles in motor units of the cat gastrocnemius. *Journal of Physiology* (London) 234:723–748.

Bylund, A. C., T. Bjurö, G. Cederblad, J. Holm, K. Lundholm, M. Sjöström, K. A. Aengquist, and T. Schersten. 1977. Physical training in man: skeletal muscle metabolism in relation to muscle morphology and running ability. *European Journal of Applied Physiology* 36:151–169.

Eisenberg, B. R., A. M. Kuda, and J. B. Peter. 1974. Stereological analysis of mammalian skeletal muscle. I. Soleus muscle of the adult guinea pig. *Journal of Cell Biology* 60:732–754.

Gauthier, G. F. 1979. Ultrastructural identification of muscle fiber types by immunocytochemistry. *Journal of Cell Biology* 82:391–400.

Gauthier, G. F., and H. A. Padykula. 1966. Cytological studies of fiber types in skeletal muscle: a comparative study of the mammalian diaphragm. *Journal of Cell Biology* 28:333–354.

Gollnick, P. D., and D. W. King. 1969. Effect of exercise and training on mitochondria of rat skeletal muscle. *American Journal of Physiology* 216:1502–1509.

Hoppeler, H., P. Lüthi, H. Claassen, E. R. Weibel, and H. Howald. 1973. The ultrastructure of the normal human skeletal muscle: a morphometric analysis on untrained men, women and well-trained orienteers. *Pflügers Archiv* 344:217–232.

Hoppeler, H., O. Mathieu, R. Krauer, H. Claassen, R. B. Armstrong, and E. R. Weibel. 1981. Design of the mammalian respiratory system. VI. Distribution of mitochondria and capillaries in various muscles. *Respiration Physiology* 44:87–111.

Howald, H. 1976. Ultrastructure and biochemical function of skeletal muscle in twins. *Annals of Human Biology* 3:455–462.

Howald, H., and J. R. Poortmans, eds. 1975. *Metabolic Adaptation to Prolonged Physical Exercise.* Basel: Birkhäuser.

Mathieu, O., R. Krauer, H. Hoppeler, P. Gehr, S. L. Lindstedt, R. M. Alexander, C. R. Taylor, and E. R. Weibel. 1981. Design of the mammalian respiratory system. VII. Scaling mitochondrial volume in skeletal muscle to body mass. *Respiration Physiology* 44:113–128.

Pernow, B., and B. Saltin, eds. 1971. *Muscle Metabolism during Exercise.* New York: Plenum.

Pette, D., ed. 1980. *The Plasticity of Muscle.* Hawthorne, N.Y.: de Gruyter.

Pette, D., W. Müller, E. Leisner, and G. Vrbova. 1976. Time dependent effects on contractile properties, fibre population, myosin light chains and enzymes of energy metabolism in intermittently and continuously stimulated fast twitch muscles of the rabbit. *Pflügers Archiv* 364:103–112.

Tomanek, R. J. 1976. Ultrastructural differentiation of skeletal muscle fibers and their diversity. *Journal of Ultrastructure Research* 55:212–227.

6

THE VEHICLE FOR
OXYGEN TRANSPORT:
BLOOD AND CIRCULATION

THE FOLLOWING TWO CHAPTERS deal with the question how O_2 is delivered to the cells in adequate quantity to cover the demands of oxidative metabolism in the mitochondria. In the present chapter I discuss the transport of O_2 from the lung into the tissues, and first ask the question why we need blood with a specialized O_2 carrier, the red blood cell.

In chapter 3 we have learned that the flow rate of O_2 mediated by blood flow is the product of blood flow rate and O_2 content of the blood which can be related to P_{O_2} through the solubility or capacitance coefficient β_{O_2}. We have also seen that the *net* O_2 flow rate — that amount of O_2 which is delivered to the tissues — is obtained by the difference in O_2 content of arterial and venous blood, multiplied by blood flow. The two important formulae that describe O_2 flow through compartment B of our model for the respiratory system (Fig. 3.1) are therefore equations 3.9 and 3.10:

$$\dot{V}_{O_2}(B) = \dot{Q}_B \cdot [C_{O_2}(a) - C_{O_2}(v)] \tag{6.1}$$
$$= \dot{Q}_B \cdot \beta_{O_2}(B) \cdot [P_{O_2}(a) - P_{O_2}(v)] \tag{6.2}$$

whereby one often writes Ca_{O_2} and Cv_{O_2} for arterial and venous O_2 content.

The major problem now is that O_2 is poorly soluble in water. If our arteries were filled with a simple aqueous solution, one liter of this "blood" would contain only some 3 ml of O_2. Even if all this O_2 could be discharged into the tissue, the heart would have to pump over 1000 liters of "blood" per minute to deliver the 3 liters of O_2 that the muscles of an athlete may need to cover the energetic demands of a strenuous run. That is clearly impossible. The strategy used to improve the situation is to add an O_2 carrier to the blood that appreciably increases its O_2 capacitance, thus reducing the blood flow required.

The O_2 carriers used to that effect are fairly large proteins that contain a metal. In some molluscs and arthropods this pigment is *hemocyanin*, a very large copper-containing molecule with molecular weight ranging from 300,000 to 9,000,000; it forms little crystals that are freely carried in solution in the blood plasma. The most extensively used O_2 carrier, which occurs in all vertebrates and many other animals, is, however, *hemoglobin*, a much smaller protein that contains iron-porphyrin rings. The hemoglobin molecule of vertebrates has a molecular weight of 66,000 daltons.

The structure of a human hemoglobin molecule, which is characteristic for all hemoglobins in vertebrates, is shown in Figure 6.1. The protein or *globin* part is made of two pairs of identical polypeptide chains: two α and two β chains each containing 141 and 146 amino acid residues, respectively. These polypeptides are folded up in a characteristic manner and assembled as a tetramer about an axis of rotational symmetry. Each of the four polypeptide chains contains one *heme*, which we had already seen to occur as a prosthetic group

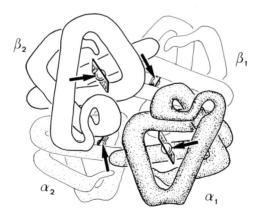

Fig. 6.1 As shown in this molecular model, the human hemoglobin molecule is made of four polypeptides—two α and two β chains, each having one heme to which O_2 can bind (arrows). (After Dickerson and Geis, 1971.)

of the cytochromes in the mitochondrial electron transport chain (Fig. 4.9). In hemoglobin the heme is used as reversible O_2 carrier because the iron can undergo cyclic changes between the reduced form, Fe(II), and the oxidized form, Fe(III); O_2 binds to the reduced form.

The presence of highly soluble hemoglobin in red cells at high concentration clearly increases blood O_2 capacity, because each mol of hemoglobin can bind 4 mol O_2. In one liter of normal human blood we find about 150 g of hemoglobin (15 g/100 ml) which can bind 8.7 mmol of O_2, thus increasing the O_2 capacity by a factor of about 30 above simple solution in water. Note that the O_2 capacity of blood is now similar to that of air, which is about 9 mmol/L.

The O_2 and CO_2 Carrier: Blood

THE STRUCTURE OF BLOOD

About 45 percent of the blood is made up of cells of different type, the remainder being plasma, an aqueous solution containing a variety of proteins, carbohydrates, lipids, hormones, and many solutes, including O_2 and CO_2. Among the cellular constituents, the red blood cells or erythrocytes are by far the most frequent, whereas the leukocytes, or white blood cells, and the blood platelets make up only a small fraction of the blood cell volume.

Erythrocytes, the cells of major concern in our context, are very unusual cells in many respects. They owe their intense red color to their high hemoglobin content of 33 g per 100 ml of erythrocytes; this means that the O_2-carrying pigment occupies about a quarter of the cell's internal space, an extraordinarily high concentration. This is only possible because in mammals the erythrocyte has eliminated all intracellular structures, organelles, ribosomes, and membranes, as well as the nucleus, and has retained only the plasma membrane with a little bit of structural protein attached to it (Fig. 6.2). In other vertebrates the nucleus is retained together with a small complement of mitochondria and other organelles. This reduction of intracellular structures in mammals is a gradual process. During erythropoiesis — the process of erythrocyte formation that occurs in bone marrow — the stem cells first multiply and then begin to synthesize hemoglobin in the course of differentiation. For this they evidently require ribosomes and messenger RNA derived from the nucleus in

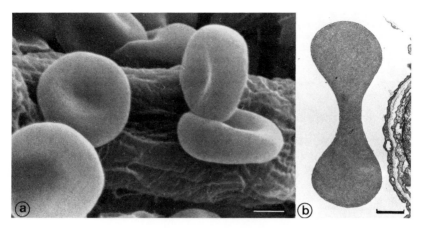

Fig. 6.2 Mammalian erythrocytes are biconcave discs, as shown for human red cells by scanning electron microscopy (a). On section (b) they are seen to be bounded by a cell membrane, but to be devoid of nucleus or organelles. Scale markers: (a) 2 μm; (b) 1 μm.

order to make the polypeptide chains; they also need mitochondria to generate the necessary ATP, and perhaps even to make the hemes. Once this is completed, the nucleus is removed, and then the cytoplasmic organelles are gradually eliminated before the newly formed red cell is released into the blood stream. However, some immature red cells may be found in the blood, mainly when, for some reason, the production of new red cells must be accelerated. Such immature cells, called reticulocytes, still contain some residual ribosomes and mitochondria among the hemoglobin mass.

A mature mammalian red cell has, in fact, lost its capacity to synthesize proteins and so on, and consequently its ability to repair whatever damage or loss of substance it may incur. It has become a vulnerable cell of limited life span which, in man, lasts about 140 days on the average. This means that about 0.7% of all erythrocytes, or $175 \cdot 10^9$ cells, must be replaced by new ones every day.

The shape of mammalian erythrocytes is also very unusual: they are circular biconcave discs bounded by a smooth cell membrane (Fig. 6.2). The erythrocyte size is tightly controlled; in man its diameter is 7.4 $\pm$ 0.2 μm and its volume 87 μm³; its thickness measures 2 μm in the thickest part but less than 1 μm in the center (Fig. 6.2). This erythrocyte shape has a number of functional consequences. On the one hand it makes for a very large surface-to-volume ratio: the

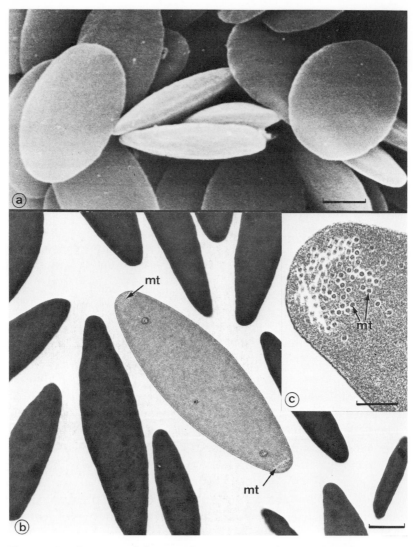

Fig. 6.3 Erythrocytes of the camel are exceptional: their shape is that of a biconvex disc, as seen in the scanning electron micrograph (a) and on section (b); their edge is reinforced by a hoop of microtubules (mt), shown at higher power in (c). Scale markers: (a) 2 μm; (b) 1 μm; (c) 0.2 μm.

erythrocyte surface of 163 μm^2 is some 70% larger than the surface of a spherical cell of equal volume. This definitely favors the exchange of O$_2$ with the surrounding plasma and it furthermore reduces the mean distance between the surface and the hemoglobin molecules.

The disc shape also offers hemodynamic advantages because the red cells can be easily deformed as they pass through the narrow capillaries in the tissue and in the lung, without being mechanically damaged; by this the effective viscosity of the blood can be reduced.

There are some interesting exceptions with respect to the shape of erythrocytes. In most mammals the osmotic pressure of blood plasma is regulated within narrow limits so that their red cells are not subjected to severe osmotic stresses. This is different in the camel, for example, which has become adapted to tolerate considerable water loss when it goes without drinking for 6 to 8 days, and part of this water is taken from the blood plasma. Now the shape and fine structure of camel erythrocytes is different from that of other mammals (Fig. 6.3): they are biconvex discs and their large circumference is reinforced by a hoop made of a bundle of microtubules; therefore camel erythrocytes can apparently shrink without major deformation when plasma osmotic pressure rises.

Since all the hemoglobin is packed into the red cells, the O_2 capacity of the blood is clearly determined by the amount of erythrocytes contained. Table 6.1 lists a number of the parameters of human blood. The number of erythrocytes contained in 1 μl (mm^3) of blood is about 5 million, slightly more in males than in females. Considering that the mean cell volume is 87 μm^3, it is easy to calculate that erythrocytes occupy some 45% of the blood volume; this important parameter is called the hematocrit. Since the size of human erythrocytes appears to vary very little, the hemoglobin content of blood is directly proportional to red cell number, or to hematocrit, and

TABLE 6.1. SOME CHARACTERISTICS OF HUMAN BLOOD.

Characteristic	Human blood	
	Male	Female
Hematocrit (%)	47	42
Number of erythrocytes (μl^{-1})	$5.4 \cdot 10^6$	$4.8 \cdot 10^6$
Hemoglobin in blood (g/100 ml)	16.3	14.5
Mean corpuscular volume (μm^3)	87	
Mean diameter (μm)	7.4 ± 0.2	
Mean thickness (μm)	2.2	
Hemoglobin in red cells (g/100 ml)	34	
(g/cell)	$3 \cdot 10^{-11}$	

amounts, on the average, to 15 g/100 ml of blood. This evidently determines the O_2 carrying capacity of blood. In *anemia* the number of red cells per unit volume of blood is reduced; there is less hemoglobin available and, accordingly, a smaller amount of O_2 can be carried.

In Table 6.2 a number of characteristics of blood in various species has been listed. We note that the size of erythrocytes in mammals varies only between 4 and 9.4 μm in diameter, resulting in a range of mean corpuscular volumes of 20–120 μm³; compared to a range in body mass from 2 g for the shrew to 4 tons for the elephant, this is evidently a small variation. Red cell size is, furthermore, not related to body mass; the red cells of the horse are smaller than those of man, but the same size as those of the mouse, whereas the goat has the smallest erythrocytes of all mammals. It also turns out that hematocrit and hemoglobin concentration are similar for all mammals, so that the O_2 capacity of mammalian blood varies by no more than ±20%. Note that the red cell dimensions are larger and more variable in other vertebrates, but even here the hemoglobin content of blood is not much lower than in mammals.

O_2 CARRIER FUNCTION OF BLOOD

We can now examine how blood can serve as an O_2 carrier to which O_2 can bind fairly easily and at high concentration, but not so tightly as to make discharge into the tissue difficult.

Oxygen occurs in the blood in two forms: (1) dissolved in the plasma and (2) bound to hemoglobin. Therefore the total O_2 content of the blood is simply the sum of the two:

$$C_{O_2}(\text{total}) = C_{O_2}(\text{sol}) + C_{O_2}(O_2Hb). \tag{6.3}$$

Dissolved and bound oxygen must be in equilibrium, and this is possible because both depend on the P_{O_2}, though in a different manner. The amount of O_2 in solution is linearly proportional to P_{O_2} (Fig. 6.4):

$$C_{O_2}(\text{sol}) = 0.003 \cdot P_{O_2} \tag{6.4}$$

where C_{O_2} is in ml O_2/100 ml blood and P_{O_2} is in torr, which means that 0.003 ml $O_2 \cdot$ torr^{-1} are added for each P_{O_2} increment of 1 torr,

TABLE 6.2. SOME CHARACTERISTICS OF BLOOD IN VARIOUS SPECIES. (MAMMALS IN DECREASING ORDER OF BODY MASS.)

Species	Erythrocytes				[Hb] (g/100 ml blood)	Hematocrit (%)
	Number ($\times 10^6$ mm^{-3})	Diameter (μm)	Thickness (μm)	Mean corpuscular volume (μm^3)		
Elephant	3.8	9.4	2.9	117	14.9	44.6[a]
Horse	9.3	5.5		50	11.1	33.4
Cow	8.1	5.9		50	11.5	40
Man (female)	4.8	7.4	2.2	87	14.5	42
Man (male)	5.4			87	16.3	47
Dog	6.3	7.0		66	14.8	45.5
Goat	16.0	4.0		19.3	10.5	33
Rabbit	5.7	7.5		61	11.9	41.5
Rat	8.9	7.5		61	14.8	46
Mouse	9.3	6.0		49	14.8	41.5
Etruscan shrew	18.2	5.5	1.15	27	17	50[b]
Frog	0.44	24.8	15.3	670	7.8	29.3
Fish (trout)	1.01	12	8	314	8.5	27.2
Bird (chicken)	2.8	11.2	6.8	127	10.3	35.6

Data from Altman and Dittmer (1971), tables 66 and 67, and

a. K. D. Bremer (unpublished results).

b. H. Bartels et al., *C.R. Acad. Sc. Paris* 286:1195–98 (1978).

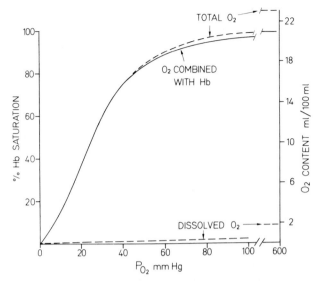

Fig. 6.4 The O_2 content of blood has two components: O_2 binding to hemoglobin follows an S-shaped curve up to full saturation; the amount of O_2 in simple solution increases linearly with P_{O_2} without limit. (From West, 1974.)

irrespective of the level of P_{O_2}. The amount of O_2 bound to hemoglobin also depends on P_{O_2}, but not in a simple fashion:

$$C_{O_2}(O_2Hb) = 4 \cdot C_{Hb} \cdot S_{O_2}(P_{O_2}) \cdot P_{O_2}. \qquad (6.5)$$

The two factors which affect this relation are, on the one hand, the hemoglobin concentration, C_{Hb}, which evidently determines the O_2 *capacity* of the blood since each hemoglobin molecule can bind up to four O_2 molecules, one at each heme, whence the factor of four. A hemoglobin concentration of 15 g/100 ml amounts to about 0.22 mmol hemoglobin per 100 ml, so that the O_2 capacity of blood is about 0.88 mmol O_2 per 100 ml; in terms of gas volume this is equivalent to 20.8 ml O_2 STPD.

The other factor determining O_2 concentration in the blood by equation 6.5, S_{O_2}, is called the O_2 *saturation* of hemoglobin, that is, the fraction of the available binding sites which are occupied by O_2. If we designate the deoxygenated and oxygenated forms of hemoglobin as Hb and O_2Hb, respectively, O_2 saturation is the ratio of the concentration of O_2Hb to that of total hemoglobin that can combine with O_2:

$$S_{O_2} = \frac{[O_2Hb]}{[Hb] + [O_2Hb]} \cdot 100\%. \tag{6.6}$$

(Note that Hb and O_2Hb actually symbolize the O_2 binding sites, four of which are assembled in one hemoglobin molecule, and that a square bracket symbolizes *concentration* of the compound bracketed.)

It turns out that S_{O_2} is a nonlinear function of P_{O_2} described by an S-shaped curve as that shown in Figure 6.4, where we find that the O_2 loading of hemoglobin increases steeply at low O_2 pressures up to about 50 torr, and then follows a shallow curve that approaches 100% saturation asymptotically. This curve is usually called the *oxyhemoglobin dissociation curve*, sometimes also the O_2 *equilibrium curve*; the latter is probably a better term because the curve, in fact, describes the level of O_2 binding to hemoglobin when the latter is in equilibrium with O_2 dissolved in plasma at a given P_{O_2}. The shape of the O_2 equilibrium curve is determined by the fact that the affinity of the hemoglobin molecule for O_2 — the "avidity" with which it binds it — decreases as one, two, or three of the four sites are occupied, due to an allosteric effect; it obviously becomes zero when all hemes have bound O_2, which occurs, however, only at very high P_{O_2} approaching 1 atm (Fig. 6.4). At a P_{O_2} of 100 mm Hg to which human arterial blood is equilibrated, 97% of the hemes have bound O_2; at 40 mm Hg, a characteristic value for venous P_{O_2} in a resting person, the saturation falls to some 70%.

Remember, however, that S_{O_2} does not allow any direct conclusions on the O_2 content of the blood unless we know its O_2 capacity, or its hemoglobin content. For normal human blood we saw that the O_2 capacity amounts to 0.88 mmol O_2 per 100 ml. But in an anemic person with a hemoglobin concentration of only 10 g/100 ml the O_2 capacity is only about 0.6 mmol O_2 per 100 ml of blood. An anemic person will therefore have in his arterial blood about the same amount of O_2 as a normal person has in his venous blood, which is saturated to only 70%. The distinction between O_2 content and saturation is therefore most important. We should also note that the *total O_2 content* of blood is the sum of the O_2 bound to hemoglobin and that dissolved in plasma as given in equation 6.3. As we increase P_{O_2} above full saturation, nothing is added to hemoglobin but we will still increase the amount of dissolved O_2 in linear proportion to P_{O_2}. In the physiological P_{O_2} range, that is, up to 100 mm Hg, the dissolved

O_2 is not much more than 1% of the total O_2; but if we breathe pure O_2 at 760 mm Hg, the dissolved O_2 amounts to about 2.3 ml or a good 10% of the total O_2 content of normal blood.

The O_2 dissociation curve is nevertheless a very useful characteristic of the O_2 binding properties of blood. For one, it is relatively easy to measure because it depends on the proportion of oxidized and reduced hemoglobin. We know that oxygen-rich arterial blood is bright red, whereas oxygen-poor venous blood is purplish. The relative amounts of O_2Hb and Hb can thus be estimated by measuring spectrophotometrically the absorptions of light beams of wave lengths of 542 nm (O_2Hb) and 555 nm (Hb).

Furthermore, it turns out that the O_2 binding properties of blood are affected by a number of different factors, and this is often reflected in characteristic shifts of the O_2 dissociation curve without changing its shape, and independent of Hb content. For example, an increase in temperature or in P_{CO_2} as well as a fall in pH all decrease the oxygen affinity of hemoglobin; the curve becomes *shifted to the right*, that is, a higher P_{O_2} is required to obtain a certain saturation (Fig. 6.5). In order to quantify this shift one estimates the so-called P_{50}—the P_{O_2} at which a saturation of 50% is achieved. For human blood at 37° C and pH 7.4 the P_{50} is 26.8 mm Hg.

The effect due to P_{CO_2} and pH was described by C. Bohr, K. A.

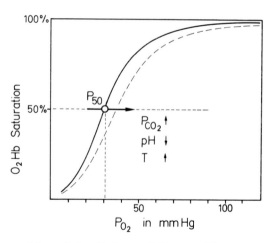

Fig. 6.5 The position of the O_2-hemoglobin equilibrium (or dissociation) curve is characterized by the P_{O_2} at which 50% saturation is achieved (P_{50}). It is shifted to the right by a fall in pH, or a rise in P_{CO_2} or temperature.

Hasselbalch, and A. Krogh in 1904 and is called the *Bohr effect*. It is probably best understood if we consider that hemoglobin can bind a number of different ligands and that this will modify its O_2 affinity. Thus hemoglobin is a powerful buffer as it can bind large amounts of H^+. It can also bind CO_2 to form a carbamino compound. Other ligands are organic phosphates, in man particularly 2,3 DPG (2,3 diphosphoglycerate), a side product of glycolysis, the mechanism by which red cells produce their ATP. The effect of these ligands on the O_2 binding properties of hemoglobin is determined by the fact that deoxyhemoglobin binds these ligands more easily than oxyhemoglobin, and that the ligand reduces O_2 affinity of hemoglobin. Furthermore, ligand binding is proportional to the ligand concentration. In a way, a number of different ligands "compete" with O_2 for binding sites on hemoglobin, although the binding sites are evidently different for the different compounds.

The effect of this on the O_2 binding properties of blood is as follows: When the pH of blood falls, hemoglobin will mop up the excess H^+ and this will reduce O_2 affinity; this is called the fixed acid Bohr effect. When the P_{CO_2} rises, two things occur: (1) part of the CO_2 will be converted to bicarbonate, as we shall see below, and this releases H^+ which become fixed to hemoglobin; (2) some of the CO_2 becomes directly bound to hemoglobin as carbamino compound. Thus the Bohr effect due to an increase in P_{CO_2} has two components, one due to CO_2 and one to fixed acid. In either case, however, the O_2 affinity of hemoglobin becomes reduced and the curve is shifted to the right, that is, a higher P_{O_2} is required to achieve a certain O_2Hb saturation (Fig. 6.6). In addition, direct CO_2 binding reduces the O_2 capacity of hemoglobin to some degree; this is called the Root effect. Lastly, the

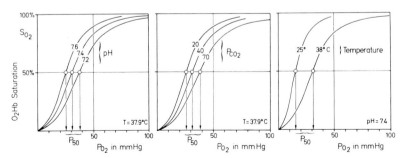

Fig. 6.6 Effects of varying pH, P_{CO_2}, and temperature on O_2Hb equilibrium curve.

effect of organic phosphate binding to hemoglobin also is a right shift of the curve because it reduces O_2 affinity. There has been some emphasis on the role of 2,3 DPG in man, because it becomes increased during exercise and during an ascent to high altitude, but these are quantitatively small effects.

It turns out that these shifts in the O_2 equilibrium curve offer advantages for O_2 exchange in the lung and in the tissue. Let us first look at O_2 delivery in the tissue. The arterial blood which enters the tissue capillaries has a P_{CO_2} of about 40 mm Hg and a pH of 7.4; its P_{50} is about 27 mm Hg and at the arterial P_{O_2} of 100 mm Hg hemoglobin is about 97% saturated. As the blood moves along the capillary it picks up CO_2 from the cells and its P_{CO_2} rises to 46 mm Hg, entailing a pH drop to 7.2; due to the Bohr effect the equilibrium curve gradually shifts to the right, which means that O_2 becomes less tightly bound to hemoglobin. Indeed, referring to Figure 6.7 we can see that this allows a greater quantity of O_2 to be liberated: at a P_{O_2} of 50 mm Hg, for example, arterial blood is saturated to 84%, whereas venous blood saturation falls to about 70%. Thus, simply by shifting the O_2 binding properties, 100 ml of blood can deliver about 0.12 mmol of O_2, or about one quarter of all the O_2 discharged into the cells, without changing the P_{O_2}. This is important because it allows the P_{O_2} in capillary blood plasma to remain relatively high, and this helps to

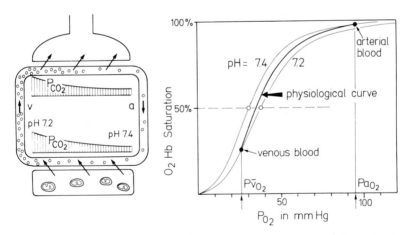

Fig. 6.7 The uptake of CO_2 in the tissue capillaries and its discharge in the lung cause arterial and venous blood to have different O_2Hb equilibrium curves. The "physiological" O_2Hb equilibrium curve in the capillaries is steeper and assists gas exchange.

drive the O_2 into the cells by diffusion. When the blood passes through the lung capillaries the reverse occurs: as CO_2 is discharged into the air, the pH rises again and the Bohr shift is now to the left (Fig. 6.7). The O_2 affinity increases gradually, allowing a greater amount of O_2 to be bound while keeping plasma P_{O_2} low, thus favoring O_2 uptake from the air.

The temperature effect shows the same tendencies. In a hard working muscle generating heat, for example, blood temperature increases by several degrees, favoring O_2 unloading from hemoglobin, whereas in the lung blood temperature returns to normal, restoring O_2 affinity.

On the whole, one therefore finds that the "physiological" dissociation curves are steeper than the physicochemical ones (Fig. 6.7), which simply means that the saturation change is relatively larger than the P_{O_2} change.

CO_2 TRANSPORT IN THE BLOOD

Although I shall discuss the respiratory system mostly in terms of O_2 transport and utilization, CO_2, the gaseous waste product of the Krebs cycle, must always be considered alongside. With respect to the carrier function of the blood it is important in two respects: (1) in assessing how the large quantity of CO_2 that is being produced during aerobic metabolism is carried to the lung for discharge into the air, and (2) in appreciating the effect of CO_2 on the O_2 transport properties of the blood, as discussed above.

CO_2 is carried in the blood in three forms: dissolved in the plasma and in the red cells, as bicarbonate ion, and bound to some proteins. The quantity of *dissolved* CO_2 is linearly proportional to P_{CO_2}, just as with O_2, but CO_2 is about 20 times more soluble than O_2, so that there is much more CO_2 than O_2 in simple solution. The CO_2 that diffuses into the red cell is rapidly converted to carbonic acid (H_2CO_3) by the action of the enzyme *carbonic anhydrase* contained in these cells. The H_2CO_3 molecule dissociates spontaneously into a *bicarbonate ion*, HCO_3^-, and H^+; bicarbonate diffuses into the plasma while H^+ is buffered, primarily by hemoglobin. The fact that deoxygenated Hb binds more H^+ than O_2Hb is important because it explains why an increase in $[H^+]$, or a fall in pH, reduces O_2 affinity of Hb, resulting in the Bohr shift.

On the other hand, the degree of O_2 saturation of hemoglobin affects the CO_2 concentration in blood at a given P_{CO_2}, a phenomenon generally called the *Haldane effect* (Fig. 6.8). It has two causes: (1) We have seen above that CO_2 binds to hemoglobin in the form of a carbamino compound, and that deoxygenated Hb binds much more CO_2 than O_2Hb; (2) deoxygenated Hb can bind more H^+ than O_2Hb, so that a greater amount of CO_2 can be converted into bicarbonate in deoxygenated blood since the additional H^+ formed can be buffered by Hb.

The physiological importance of the Haldane effect derives from the fact that the relative amount of deoxygenated Hb increases in the tissue capillaries as CO_2 is taken up from the cells; thus the CO_2 capacity of blood increases owing to the Haldane effect, and for both reasons given above. In the lung, O_2 is being loaded onto Hb. This causes CO_2 to be released from the carbamino compounds; it also reduces the buffering capacity of the blood, which can now hold less CO_2 in the form of bicarbonate. Carbonic anhydrase now converts bicarbonate to CO_2 and H_2O. Both effects favor the discharge of CO_2 from the blood into alveolar air, because they maintain a high P_{CO_2} in the pulmonary capillary blood. We should note that of the CO_2 released in the lung, about 60% comes from bicarbonate, 30% from carbamino compounds, and 10% from dissolved CO_2.

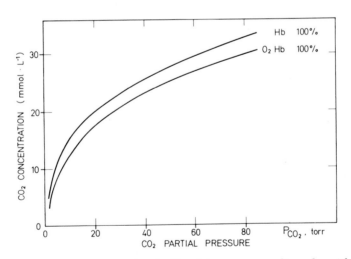

Fig. 6.8 The CO_2 concentration in blood increases nonlinearly with P_{CO_2} and depends on O_2Hb saturation (Haldane effect), the range of possible values being delimited by the curves for total oxygenation and total deoxygenation of blood. (From Dejours, 1981.)

Because of these various and complex reactions, the CO_2 content of blood is evidently not a linear function of P_{CO_2} but it is rather also described by a *CO₂ equilibrium curve*. In contrast to the O_2 dissociation curve it is, however, not a saturating function which reaches a plateau but rather increases steadily (Fig. 6.8). It also shows a shift due to the Haldane effect.

ACID – BASE BALANCE

The exchange of CO_2 has a profound effect on the acid – base status in the blood and in all the tissues of the body. Most of the CO_2 retained in arterial blood is in form of bicarbonate and is hence an important component in determining the acid–base balance of the blood in mammals.

The regulation of acid – base balance in blood and other body fluids occurs by means of a variety of buffers which are acid–base conjugates. An example is the bicarbonate buffer, where carbonic acid can reversibly dissociate into bicarbonate and H^+:

$$H_2CO_3 \rightleftharpoons HCO_3^- + H^+. \tag{6.7}$$

This reaction depends on the dissociation or equilibrium constant

$$K_1 = \frac{[H^+] \cdot [HCO_3^-]}{[H_2CO_3]}. \tag{6.8}$$

Similar relations must be considered for protein buffer systems (remember the buffering capacity of hemoglobin), for phosphate buffers, and so on, each with its own equilibrium constant. Acid–base balance, estimated by pH of the blood, depends on all these buffers acting simultaneously.

The bicarbonate buffer system is most important for respiration physiology because its effect is directly related to CO_2 exchange in the lung. The point is that, in the blood, the concentration of H_2CO_3 is proportional to the concentration of dissolved CO_2 which can be exchanged with air in the lung. Thus we can replace, in equation 6.8, $[H_2CO_3]$ by $[CO_2]_{dis}$, that of dissolved CO_2, but we evidently need to change the equilibrium constant accordingly to K_1'. Taking logarithms and remembering that pH is $-\log [H^+]$, we obtain from equation 6.8

$$pH = pK_1' + \log \frac{[HCO_3^-]}{[CO_2]_{dis}} \qquad (6.9)$$

and finally, since pK_1' is known and the concentration of CO_2 in solution is proportional to P_{CO_2}, we find

$$pH = 6.1 + \log \frac{[HCO_3^-]}{0.03 \cdot P_{CO_2}}. \qquad (6.10)$$

This is called the Henderson-Hasselbalch equation. It is of great importance in respiratory physiology because it shows two things: (1) to maintain blood pH constant, the ratio between P_{CO_2} and bicarbonate concentration must be kept constant; (2) a fall in P_{CO_2}, with bicarbonate concentration constant, will cause the blood pH to rise.

The bicarbonate concentration is regulated essentially by the kidney and the P_{CO_2} by the lung. If alveolar P_{CO_2} is reduced, for example by hyperventilation, this ratio increases and pH increases, the result being what is called *respiratory alkalosis*. Evidently, if P_{CO_2} increases, pH falls and *respiratory acidosis* ensues. If these changes are due to chronic disturbances of pulmonary ventilation, for example because of uneven ventilation and perfusion of the lung, the kidney can correct the acid–base status by excreting more or less bicarbonate.

Alkalosis and acidosis are not necessarily the result of respiratory disturbances affecting P_{CO_2}; they can also be due to *metabolic* troubles which then affect the bicarbonate concentration, that is, the numerator in the Henderson-Hasselbalch equation. There are many possibilities for that; the accumulation of acids for any reason leads to metabolic acidosis, a good example in our context being that due to the build-up of lactate in strenuous exercise where much of the energy must be supplied by glycolysis. Metabolic acidosis is also a common occurrence in uncontrolled diabetes mellitus.

Keeping blood pH constant at the normal value of, for example, 7.4 in man at 37° C is not necessarily best under all circumstances. One can ask what the ultimate goal of acid–base regulation is. The physiological events that critically depend on pH are enzyme reactions in the cells for which optimal pH ranges are known to exist. The cells therefore tend to maintain intracellular pH close to or slightly above the neutrality of water which at 37° C is at about 6.8. This is ensured if blood plasma is maintained at relative alkalinity. Figure 6.9 shows that the optimal pH levels depend on temperature because the pH of neutrality of water, pN, increases as temperature falls: it is 7.0 only at 20° C. Thus, if body temperature falls, the intracellular pH must rise in order to be maintained close to neutrality, and this will require pH of the blood to also rise in parallel. Because of the dependence of blood pH on P_{CO_2}, the P_{CO_2} in the lung must fall.

Thus acid–base regulation can follow different criteria when body or tissue temperature changes:

(1) Blood pH can be kept constant, but this will shift the cytoplasmic pH away from the optimum, with the result that enzymes will not function at their optimal level; this principle, which has been called *pH stat regulation*, may be of advantage in

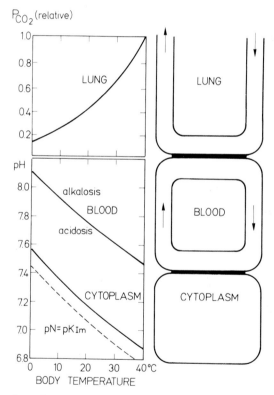

Fig. 6.9 The physiological pH of blood, regulated by changing P_{CO_2} in the lung, depends on body temperature, because the "neutral pH" in cytoplasm (pN, broken line) increases with falling temperature. (From Rahn and Reeves, 1982.)

hibernating animals since they want to preserve energy by reducing their metabolism.

(2) Cytoplasmic pH can be kept near pN to allow cell functions to maintain their normal level; this principle, called *alpha-stat regulation*, will require blood pH to rise and lung P_{CO_2} to fall as temperature falls; we find that this happens in ectotherms, that is, in animals that adjust their body temperature to that in the environment such as in amphibia or reptiles, and also when, in man, blood flows into the skin or body appendages where the temperature is lower than in the core of the body.

Moving Blood Around: Circulation

From our discussions above it has become evident that the transport of O_2 from the lung into the tissue, and for that the transport of CO_2 from the tissue to the lung as well, depends essentially on an adequate blood flow, $\dot{Q}_B$. This needs, on the one hand, a pump that drives blood around in sufficient quantity and, on the other hand, a well-designed system of pipes that directs and distributes the blood to the places where it is needed and that prevents any loss of blood while still permitting exchange of substances with the tissue. In this part I shall discuss the design and functional properties of circulation mostly in rather general terms, expanding on details only where the topic bears directly on our primary concern: the role of blood circulation in providing O_2 and substrates to the cells. I emphasize this self-imposed limitation because circulation serves many additional functions. It is, indeed, the chief integrator of body functions next to the nervous system, but to deal with all these essential aspects would clearly reach way beyond the scope of this book.

BASIC DESIGN OF THE CIRCUITRY

Blood is moved about in a circuit that can be broken into four functional components (Fig. 6.10):

pump	:	heart
distributing vessels	:	arteries
exchange vessels	:	capillaries
collecting vessels	:	veins

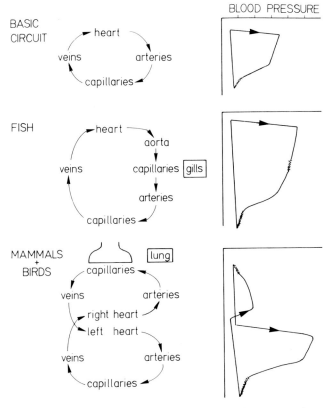

Fig. 6.10 The general design features of circulation determine the profiles of blood pressure along the circuit.

The pump is basically designed as two chambers in sequence, the atrium and the ventricle (Fig. 6.11). Blood coming from the veins is collected in the atrium and transferred to the ventricle, whose wall is a powerful muscle sleeve which contracts periodically and thus squeezes the blood out. The two openings of the ventricle are fitted with valves which give the blood stream a direction: as the ventricle contracts the valve at the arterial end opens and that toward the atrium closes; as the muscle relaxes the arterial valve closes and the blood in the atrium can flow in. The blood in the arteries is under higher pressure than that in the veins because of ventricular contraction, and this keeps the blood flowing through the circuit. This means, however, that the walls of the arteries must be strong enough to withstand this pressure. Thus, one of the basic design features of all arterial vessels is that they are enwrapped by a sleeve of smooth

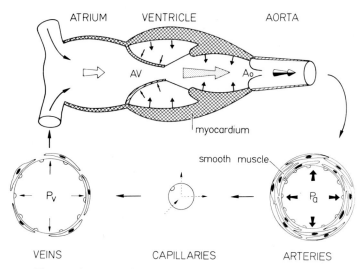

ATRIUM   VENTRICLE   AORTA

VEINS   CAPILLARIES   ARTERIES

Fig. 6.11 The unidirectional action of the heart depends on the rhythmic contraction of the myocardium of the ventricle, with alternating closing and opening of the atrioventricular (AV) and aortic (Ao) valves. The high intra-vascular pressure (P_a) in arteries needs to be counteracted by a strong wall of smooth muscle, whereas few fibers suffice in the veins due to lower pressure (P_v). Capillaries are designed for gas and solute exchange with the tissue.

muscle, combined with elastic and collagenous connective tissue fibers, whose thickness is about proportional to the internal pressure (Fig. 6.11). Exchange vessels, on the other hand, must have as thin a wall as possible so as to allow easy passage of O_2, CO_2, and many other solutes into the surrounding tissue. This means that the blood pressure must be reduced to tolerable levels before the blood reaches the capillaries. The arterial part of the circuit must therefore incorporate vessels with high resistance capable of reducing the pressure; such vessels, called arterioles, constitute, in fact, the final part of the arterial pathway, just prior to the capillaries. Veins also have some smooth muscle in their wall; but in addition they contain a sequence of little valves that help move the blood back to the heart in spite of the low pressure in these collecting vessels.

With respect to gas exchange we need two sets of vessels: those which pick up O_2 (and discharge CO_2) in the external gas exchanger and those which discharge O_2 (and collect CO_2) in the tissue. In the course of evolution several solutions have been tried. In fishes we find that the blood that leaves the heart is first pumped through the capillary network in the gill lamellae (Fig. 1.9); it then flows into the main part of the arterial tree which distributes it to the tissues for O_2 discharge, and finally it flows back to the heart. The fish heart is therefore simply made of the sequence of atrium and ventricle which pumps deoxygenated blood. But because the gill capillaries are intercalated in the arterial part of the circuit, the blood flows through them under quite high pressure (Fig. 6.10). These thin walled exchange vessels can tolerate this high pressure essentially because they are surrounded by water; perfusing the gill capillaries at high pressure is even an advantage when the fish swims in deep waters where the hydrostatic pressure of the water is very high.

In air-breathing animals the blood in lung capillaries must be under low pressure, however, and this requires a separate loop of the circulation for perfusing the lung. This has been realized in several evolutionary steps. In the frog, for example, the separation of pulmonary and body circuits is only partial (Fig. 1.12). The frog heart has two atria but only a single undivided ventricle; leaving the ventricle, however, are two main arteries: the aorta leading into the body, and the pulmonary artery reaching the lung and, in part, the skin which, as we have seen, participates in gas exchange. The oxygen-rich blood returning from the lung enters the heart through the left atrium, while the venous blood returning from the body flows into the right atrium. It is interesting that the ventricle, although it is a single chamber, pumps most of the oxygen-rich blood into the aorta, and most of the venous blood into the pulmonary artery, so that, functionally at least, the blood flows sequentially through the lung before it is pumped into the tissues.

In mammals and birds, circulation forms two completely separated loops (Figs. 6.10 and 6.12). The heart is divided into a right and left heart, each made of atrium and ventricle. The *pulmonary circulation* starts in the right ventricle and ends in the left atrium after passage through pulmonary arteries, capillaries, and veins. The *systemic circulation* begins in the left ventricle, which pumps the blood into the aorta, from where it is distributed to various organs through arteries; the systemic veins lead the oxygen-poor blood back to the right atrium, and the cycle can begin anew. The complete separation of pulmonary and systemic circulation has the big advantage that the blood can be driven through the pulmonary circulation under much lower pressure than through the systemic circulation; indeed, in mammals the right ventricle generates only about one fifth the

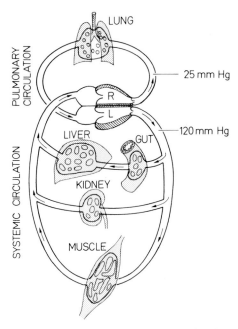

Fig. 6.12 In birds and mammals the circulating blood mass is pumped at low-pressure but in a single loop through the lung, whereas in the high-pressure systemic circulation it is directed through various pathways, such as gut-liver (splanchnic), kidney, and muscles.

pressure of the left heart, which must get the blood through all organs. This clear separation of loops also ensures that all the blood flows through the lung in each cycle, a condition that is fulfilled in the fish but only approximated in the frog.

With respect to gas exchange in mammals, the pathway for blood is simple (Fig. 6.12): O_2 uptake in the lung and O_2 delivery into the tissues are strictly in series. This is not so for the distribution of substrates, solutes, and wastes, for we find that the organs serving these functions are arranged along parallel subloops of the systemic circulation (Fig. 6.12). One such loop leads through the intestine and, from there, through the liver; it is the principal route for the uptake of substrates from food, whereby the serial passage of this blood through the liver regulates, for example, the sugar content of the blood to a constant level under the action of hormones such as insulin. This is important, for when our muscles work they will need more substrates for glycolysis and aerobic metabolism, and the blood must be able to rapidly mobilize additional glucose which is stored in the liver as glycogen. It is therefore convenient to arrange the liver in parallel to the muscles; in consequence, however, the blood takes more time to provide the muscles with more substrate than with more O_2, because it has to pass through several cycles before the newly mobilized glucose reaches the muscles. On the other hand, remember that aerobic muscle metabolism can also use fatty acids as substrates for the Krebs cycle (chapter 4), and these are, to some extent, collected by the blood in fat tissue of the skin, for example, which is also arranged on parallel subloops.

A further consequence of this system of parallel subloops is that the O_2 content of the blood collected in the veins is different for each loop because tissues extract O_2 to different degrees. The P_{O_2} in blood leaving active muscles will be much lower than that leaving quiescent organs. The blood that enters the right atrium is a mixture from all these sources. Note that the so-called *mixed venous* P_{O_2}, as it is measured in the right heart or the pulmonary artery, reflects the O_2 discharged into *all* organs and gives only limited information on that used in individual groups of muscles engaged in running, for example.

The distribution of blood flow through these different loops is regulated to need, however. Thus in man at rest, where the total cardiac output is about 5.5 liters, only about 1 liter flows through the muscles. On heavy exercise the cardiac output may rise to 20–25 liters and of this 15–20 liters flow through the muscles. After a heavy meal, on the other hand, the perfusion of the gastrointestinal tract is favored, the reason why we do not feel fit to do heavy work just after we have eaten. Conversely, we do not feel like eating when we are doing heavy exercise.

THE MAMMALIAN HEART AS A PUMP

To function as a fluid pump the heart needs a chamber that can forcefully reduce its volume, and that is bracketed by two valves which give the blood flow its direction (Fig. 6.11). The mammalian heart needs two such pumps which must act in a coordinated fashion because they are, in effect, serially inserted in a closed circuit, so that both must pump at the same flow rate. This is achieved by housing the two ventricles in the same body and allowing them to partially share the muscles that form their wall, but particularly to share the specialized tissue that regulates heart function. The two atria are likewise incorporated into the heart and are also enwrapped by the same muscle. The two tracts, right and left hearts respectively, are, however, completely separated by a ventricular and an atrial septum, both again made of muscle.

Cardiac muscle is made of chains of striated muscle cells, called myocardial cells, which differ from skeletal muscle fibers in several respects. Whereas skeletal muscle is made of long, multinucleated syncytial fibers, myocardial cells are short cylinders, each having a single nucleus (Fig. 6.13). They form contractile fibers by joining with neighboring cells at both ends, where they are mechanically firmly coupled. But they are also electrically coupled through pores that traverse both cell membranes, so that they will contract in concert. These chains of myocardial cells are partially interconnected and this results in the formation of fiber networks which encircle the ventricles in the form of well-organized sheets of spirals (Fig. 6.14a). Thus, as the muscle strands contract, the lumen of the ventricle is narrowed down, squeezing out the blood just as a sponge is squeezed

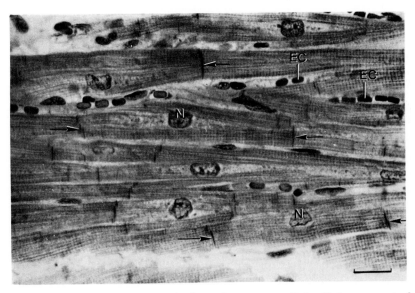

Fig. 6.13 Section of heart muscle shows how myocardial cells have a central nucleus (N) and are connected to each other in series by means of intercalated discs (arrows). Note erythrocytes in capillaries between the fibers which are partly branched. Scale marker: 20 μm.

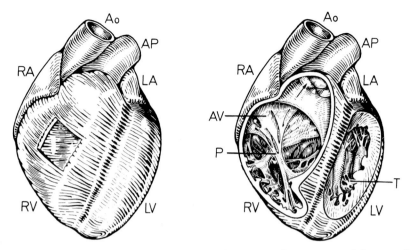

Fig. 6.14 Heart muscle fibers enwrap the ventricles in several layers of alternating direction, as shown by window in (a). The wall of the left ventricle (LV) is about five times thicker than that of the right ventricle (RV), but both form trabeculae (T) and papillary muscles (P) on which atrioventricular valves (AV) are anchored (b). Note right and left auricle (RA, LA), aorta (Ao) and pulmonary artery (AP) whose valve (arrow) is shown in (b).

out by contracting the fingers of the hand about it. The comparison with a sponge is, in fact, not totally beside the point, because the ventricle chamber is partly pervaded with bundles of myocardial fibers and much resembles a sponge (Fig. 6.14b).

The thickness of the muscle coat is proportional to the force it must generate on contraction. Thus we find, in man, that the wall of the left ventricle is about five times as thick as that of the right, because the left ventricle must generate a pressure of 120 mm Hg to drive the blood through systemic circulation, whereas about 25 mm Hg suffice to pump the blood through the lung (Fig. 6.12). In a smaller mammal, such as a rat, the proportion in the thickness of right and left heart is similar but the absolute thickness is smaller because the volume of blood that must be pumped is obviously smaller. On the whole, one finds that the total muscle mass of the heart of mammals is linearly proportional to body size, making up about 0.6% of body mass for all species, whether small or large. This may be intriguing because small animals must, in fact, maintain a higher blood flow to cover their higher metabolic needs, as we shall see below.

The heart pumps blood by cyclical contractions and relaxations of the muscle. As the ventricular muscle relaxes in the phase called *diastole,* the ventricle fills with blood from the atrium while the outflow valve is closed; in the *systole* that follows the muscle contracts forcefully, the in-flow valve closes, and blood flows out under pressure in the direction of the artery. The blood flow rate, or cardiac output, measured as volume of blood pumped per minute, is the product of two quantities: the *heart-beat frequency* and the *stroke volume,* that is, the volume of blood discharged by the ventricle in each beat. It is plausible that the stroke volume is essentially determined by the capacity of the ventricle, since we know that the heart beat empties out about 80% of the blood it contains; looking at different species we find that the stroke volume is proportional to heart size and hence linearly proportional to body mass. Heart-beat frequency, on the other hand, increases as animals become smaller. In man at rest, the heart beats at a frequency of about 70 per minute, in the elephant at 25, whereas in the rat the heart frequency is of the order of 300. In the smallest mammal, the Etruscan shrew, weighing 2 grams, heart rates of over 1000 per minute have been recorded, as we shall discuss later. In an allometric comparison one finds that heart-beat frequency, f_h, of mammals of different body mass, M_b (in kg), is described by

$$f_h = 241 \cdot M_b^{-0.25}. \tag{6.11}$$

The most important observation is that heart-beat frequency falls with the power -0.25 of body mass; it thus scales the same way as specific metabolic rate, that is, O_2 consumption per unit body mass (Fig. 2.6). Considering that stroke volume is linearly proportional to body mass, we conclude that cardiac output, the product of frequency and stroke volume, scales with $M_b^{0.75}$, that is, in proportion to total metabolic rate, as we saw in chapter 2.

Two further points need to be mentioned before we can examine cardiac output more closely. The first relates to how contraction of the heart muscle is regulated, and the second to the way myocardial cells generate the energy that the heart-beat requires.

I have said that all myocardial cells are electrically coupled by means of so-called communicating or nexus junctions, patch-like contacts between the plasma membranes where the cytoplasm of the two adjoining cells communicate through a set of channels or pores.

This allows the electrical membrane potential which triggers contraction to rapidly spread along the fiber strands, synchronizing their contraction. The myocardium also contains a set of specialized muscle fiber strands which spontaneously generate such potentials at a certain rate. These strands are arranged in two parts: one set lies in the wall of the atria and begins with the *sinus node*, a remnant of the very first muscle fibers that form in embryonic life; a second set begins with the *atrioventricular node* at the junction between atria and ventricles and spreads with several bundles throughout the ventricle walls. Both systems can generate electrical potentials independently at their own rhythm, but in the healthy heart the sinus node dictates the heart rate because the atrioventricular node responds to its impulses. Thus the sinus node is the pacemaker of the heart. Various factors control the frequency at which the sinus node fires, and thus the frequency at which the heart beats: nerve impulses from the parasympathetic vagus nerve slow it down, whereas sympathetic nerves speed it up. When we get excited—for whatever reason—our heart beats faster because the sympathetic nerves are more active; this occurs also when we run, for example. Some hormones have a similar effect; in particular adrenaline, a secretion of the adrenal gland, speeds up the heart because it is actually the substance discharged by the sympathetic nerve fibers when they fire.

Myocardial cells generate the ATP required to drive contraction exclusively by oxidative phosphorylation. This is actually not surprising if we consider that the heart must contract without interruption and is therefore an exquisite example of "endurance muscles." Myocardial cells are therefore particularly rich in large mitochondria which are evenly spread throughout the cell (Fig. 6.15). In all species myocardial cells have the highest content in mitochondria of all muscle cells, as a rule nearly twice as much as the cells of the diaphragm, another endurance muscle, and five times as much as a typical locomotor muscle.

THE RATE OF BLOOD FLOW

The *cardiac output*, $\dot{Q}_B$, is evidently the most important and most comprehensive descriptor of heart function in our context; it determines the quantity of O_2 that can be transported convectively by blood flow, once we know how much O_2 can be loaded onto the

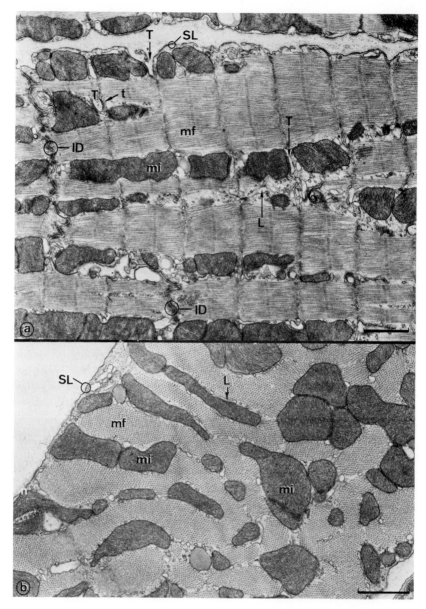

Fig. 6.15 Longitudinal (a) and transverse (b) sections of myocardial cells. The myofibrils show the same structure as in skeletal muscle (Fig. 5.5). Mitochondria are larger and more numerous. Note that the wide T-tubules (T) are located near the Z-line and that their membrane is continuous with the sarcolemma (SL); triads (t) are formed with the L-tubules. Cells in series are mechanically coupled in the intercalated disc (ID) where the myofibrils of each cell insert in the respective cell membranes which are joined by an adhesive layer. Scale markers: 1 μm.

blood. In an adult human, cardiac output at rest is of the order of 3–5 $l \cdot min^{-1}$, that is, of similar magnitude as ventilation of the lung; this is not so surprising if we consider that the O_2 capacity of blood and air are alike.

Because of the importance of cardiac output for respiratory function, we must briefly discuss how this variable can be measured. Note first that by cardiac output we mean the blood flow rate generated by either the right or the left heart; under steady-state conditions both must be the same. In fact, the flow out of the right ventricle must equal the flow through the entire lung, and the flow into the left atrium, as well as the flow out of the left ventricle and into the right atrium. If it were not so, blood would accumulate at some point in the system. Thus one can estimate cardiac output by measuring the flow rate through any one of the major parts of circulation. It is evidently convenient to look at the pathway from the right to the left heart because, as we have seen, all the blood passes through the lung in a single cycle. One method used is to inject some dye into the venous blood, as close to the right atrium as possible: after some time this dye will appear in the arterial blood, first increasing in concentration and then decreasing again; by integrating this concentration curve one can calculate cardiac output. Similarly, one can use a so-called thermodilution method where one injects a known volume of cold saline into the venous blood and follows the transient decrease in arterial blood temperature.

The most frequently used and also easiest method is to estimate cardiac output by the Fick principle, which exploits the fact that O_2 is being added to the blood in its passage through the lung, and that the same quantity of O_2 is removed (consumed) in the tissues. The Fick equation

$$\dot{V}_{O_2} = \dot{Q}_B(Ca_{O_2} - C\bar{v}_{O_2}) \tag{6.12}$$

is by now well known to us (see also chapter 3); remember that $Ca_{O_2} = \beta_B \cdot Pa_{O_2}$. Thus, clearly, if we can measure O_2 consumption, $\dot{V}_{O_2}$, and the O_2 content in arterial and mixed venous blood, we can calculate $\dot{Q}_B$, the cardiac output. Ca_{O_2} can be measured on a blood sample taken with a needle from any conveniently accessible artery. Since $C\bar{v}_{O_2}$ is the O_2 content of *mixed* venous blood, we cannot measure it in blood drawn from any vein because O_2 extraction is different in various parts. We can obtain a sample of mixed venous blood, however, if we thread a catheter through a vein until it reaches the right atrium. This procedure of cardiac catheterization is relatively harmless and widely used in clinical medicine; it was introduced by A. Cournand and D. W. Richards in 1941 in their pioneering work on pulmonary circulation. They were honored for this work with the Nobel Prize in 1956, together with W. Forssmann, a German surgeon who had done the first cardiac catheterization on himself before the Second World War.

As O_2 consumption increases in exercise, cardiac output must increase in order to allow a greater quantity of O_2 to be transported into the tissues. In a healthy young man of about 70 kg body mass, cardiac output can increase from about $5 \, l \cdot min^{-1}$ at rest to $20 \, l \cdot min^{-1}$ under strenuous exercise conditions where $\dot{V}_{O_2}max$ is reached. This is achieved by both an increase in heart rate and in stroke volume. In this young man, reasonably well trained, we would expect the heart rate to be about $60 \, min^{-1}$ at rest and to increase to $170 \, min^{-1}$ in strenuous exercise. Dividing cardiac output by heart rate, we calculate the stroke volume to be about 85 ml at rest and 120 ml in heavy exercise. The four-fold increase in cardiac output is hence achieved by increasing stroke volume by 35% and by nearly tripling heart rate.

We have seen before that the increased heart rate is primarily the result of sympathetic stimulation, an effect that is related to the "fight-or-flight" condition induced by adrenaline and the sympathetic nervous system: we become alert, the pupils of the eye open, as do the eye lids, and we prepare physically to fend off an adversary — or to flee! The increase in stroke volume is essentially a consequence of more blood returning to the heart which leads to greater filling of the ventricle during diastole. This causes the ventricle wall to be stretched more than before and in consequence it contracts more forcefully, ejecting a greater fraction of the ventricular volume; this phenomenon, which is of great functional importance, is called the *Starling law* of the heart, because it was discovered by the eminent British physiologist Ernest Starling (1866–1927). But there is an additional factor: adrenaline, the hormone whose blood level increases in the fight-or-flight condition, augments the force generated by contraction of heart muscle, and thus aids in increasing stroke volume in exercise.

The increase in cardiac output is, however, not quite proportional to the increase in O_2 flow rate required to cover the muscles' ener-

getic needs. One factor is that the distribution of blood flow is changed in exercise, in that less blood flows into the so-called splanchnic loop of circulation which perfuses the gut, thus shifting the bulk of blood flow into the muscles. The second factor is that working muscles extract more O_2 from the blood; as a consequence the P_{O_2} of mixed venous blood falls from about 40 mm Hg at rest to about 20 mm Hg in heavy exercise. Referring to Figure 6.7 one can immediately see that a much greater fraction of the blood's O_2 content is discharged to the muscle cells; this is aided, in addition, by a greater Bohr shift due to a larger quantity of CO_2 delivered to the capillary blood, as well as by the greater temperature of the blood in the working muscle due to local heat production, which also shifts the O_2 dissociation curve to the right (Figs. 6.5 and 6.6). Thus the O_2 flow rate supported by the blood is augmented in exercise by increasing the cardiac output *and* the P_{O_2} difference between arterial and venous blood, according to equation 6.3. In addition, the O_2 transport capacity of the blood can be increased to some extent by increasing the hematocrit, a process that happens particularly in some mammals that maintain an erythrocyte store in their spleen, which can be rapidly discharged into the circulating blood; in man this capacity is limited, however.

We must finally ask whether cardiac output is a limiting factor for O_2 supply to the tissues, that is, whether it is related to maximal $\dot{V}_{O_2}$. It is well known that endurance training considerably increases maximal cardiac output. High performance endurance athletes, such as professional cyclists, develop an enlarged heart which is due as well to an increase in myocardial mass as to an enlargement of the ventricle volumes, so that these athletes have a considerably enlarged stroke volume. A well-trained athlete will maintain a high blood flow at relatively low heart-beat frequencies. As shown in Figure 6.16, the maximal cardiac output of such athletes is indeed proportional to their $\dot{V}_{O_2}$max.

The second line of evidence derives from comparative studies on mammals of different body size, where one finds cardiac output to be proportional to $M_b^{0.75}$, or, in other words, proportional to O_2 consumption. As mentioned above, this is essentially the result of a higher heart rate in smaller animals, whereas the stroke volume is linearly proportional to body mass. This evidence is not quite as strong, however, because it refers to resting animals; unfortunately, data on maximal cardiac output are not available yet.

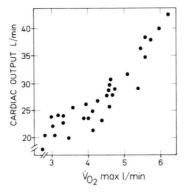

Fig. 6.16 Maximal cardiac output in man increases in proportion to maximal O_2 consumption. (From Åstrand and Rodahl, 1977.)

O_2 Transport by the Blood

Let us now summarize the various factors that determine the quantity of O_2 that can be transported by the blood from the site of uptake in the lung to the site of delivery in the tissues. If we look back at equations 6.1 and 6.2 we note that O_2 transport depends essentially on two separate forces: the *motive force* generated by the heart and resulting in a certain blood flow rate, $\dot{Q}_B$, and a *carrying force*. The latter, it turns out, is not a simple affair. It depends, on the one hand, on the partial pressures in arterial and venous blood that are the result of gas exchange in the lung and in the tissue respectively; but it also depends on the O_2 capacitance of the blood, expressed by the coefficient β_{O_2}. This coefficient is, however, not a constant; since most of the O_2 carried in the blood is bound to hemoglobin, it depends on the prevailing P_{O_2}, according to the O_2-hemoglobin equilibrium curve, and is affected by a number of other factors, such as the Bohr effect due to CO_2 loading and the temperature effect which both modify the O_2 affinity of hemoglobin. These effects play a major role in O_2 uptake and discharge in the capillaries, as we shall see. However, when the blood flows in arteries or in veins, the factors affecting O_2 affinity do not change; the O_2 content of arterial and venous blood can therefore be calculated from the P_{O_2} by considering a separate value of β_{O_2} for arterial and venous blood taken from the O_2-hemoglobin equilibrium curve, considering its position as a function of P_{CO_2}, pH, and temperature.

In measuring O_2 contents and O_2 consumption one can then calculate cardiac output by the Fick equation. This allows us to assess the

relative importance of blood flow (the motive force) and of O_2 extraction from the blood (the carrying force) in securing an adequate net O_2 transport from the lung into the tissues.

Summary

Oxygen transport through the circulation of blood depends on the O_2 carrying capacity of blood and on the blood flow rate. The O_2 carrying capacity of blood depends essentially on its content in hemoglobin, a protein of 66,000 dalton molecular weight, made of four polypeptides and containing four hemes. Each hemoglobin molecule can reversibly bind up to four O_2 molecules on its hemes. One liter of human blood contains 150 g hemoglobin and can bind 8.7 mmol O_2, the same amount as contained in air.

Hemoglobin is found in erythrocytes at a concentration of 33 g per 100 ml of cells. Mammalian erythrocytes are biconcave discoid cells, devoid of a nucleus and cell organelles, which range in mean volume from $20 - 100$ μm^3 with no apparent dependence on body size.

Oxygen binding to blood depends on P_{O_2} in a nonlinear fashion, the kinetics being described by the S-shaped O_2-hemoglobin equilibrium (or O_2Hb dissociation) curve. Dissolved O_2 is linearly proportional to P_{O_2}, but of limited importance except at very high P_{O_2} values. In arterial blood hemoglobin is 97%, in venous blood 70%, O_2 saturated. The position of the O_2Hb equilibrium curve is estimated by its P_{50}, the P_{O_2} causing 50% O_2Hb saturation. It is shifted to the right (higher P_{O_2} needed to achieve a given saturation) by an increase in temperature or in P_{CO_2}, or a fall in pH, and vice versa; the effect of P_{CO_2} and pH is called the Bohr effect. These shifts offer advantages for O_2 discharge in the tissue: as CO_2 (generated by the Krebs cycle) is taken up, the O_2 affinity of blood falls (Bohr effect) and a greater quantity of O_2 is discharged without a large change in P_{O_2}. In the lung the reverse occurs: as CO_2 is discharged, more O_2 can be bound to hemoglobin. CO_2 is transported in the blood in dissolved form as carbonic acid (bicarbonate), and bound to hemoglobin as carbamino compound. Carbonic anhydrase in red cells catalyzes the conversion of CO_2 into carbonic acid. Bicarbonate content of the blood is an important regulator of acid – base balance which greatly depends on the degree of CO_2 elimination or retention in the lung. Man maintains an arterial P_{CO_2} of about 40 torr to keep the acid – base status at an optimal level.

Blood circulates in a closed vascular system which forms two loops in series: the lesser circulation through the lung for O_2 uptake, the greater circulation through the body organs for O_2 delivery. The greater circulation consists of several parallel sub-loops for the intestinal tract, the kidney, the muscles, the brain, and so on. The arteries distribute the blood to regions of need by means of their muscle wall which allows them to change their cross-section on appropriate stimuli.

The heart provides the pump; it is made of muscle whose thickness is proportional to the work required. Cardiac output and heart beat frequency are proportional to the aerobic capacity of the body: heart frequency and cardiac output per unit body mass are proportional to $M_b^{-0.25}$ in mammals of varying size. Cardiac output increases with work, but not quite in proportion to O_2 consumption; at maximal O_2 consumption cardiac output increases by a factor of 3 whereas O_2 consumption is 10 times greater.

Further Reading

BLOOD

Bartels, H., and R. Baumann. 1977. Respiratory function of hemoglobin. In *International Review of Physiology, Respiration Physiology*, II, vol. 14, ed. G. W. Widdicombe. Baltimore: University Park Press, pp. 107–134.

MacFarlane, H. T., and A. H. T. Robb-Smith. 1961. *Functions of the Blood.* New York: Academic.

Reeves, R. B. 1977. The interaction of body temperature and acid–base balance in ectothermic vertebrates. *Annual Review of Physiology* 39:559–586.

Reeves, R. B., and H. Rahn. 1979. Patterns in vertebrate acid–base regulation. In *Evolution of Respiratory Processes*, ed. S. C. Wood and C. Lenfant. New York: Dekker, pp. 225–252.

Riggs, A. 1965. Functional properties of hemoglobins. *Physiological Reviews* 45:619–673.

Roos, A., and W. F. Boron. 1981. Intracellular pH. *Physiological Reviews* 61:296–434.

Siggaard-Anderson, O. 1974. *The Acid–Base Status of the Blood.* Copenhagen: Munsgaard.

Wood, S. C., and C. Lenfant. 1979. Oxygen transport and oxygen delivery. In *Evolution of Respiratory Processes*, ed. S. C. Wood and C. Lenfant. New York: Dekker, pp. 193–223.

CIRCULATION

Anderson, R. H., A. E. Becker, and S. P. Allwork. 1980. *Cardiac Anatomy.* London: Gower Medical Publishing.

Blomqvist, C. G., and B. Saltin. 1983. Cardiovascular adaptations to physical training. *Annual Review of Physiology* 45:169–189.

Caro, C. G., T. J. Pedley, R. C. Schroter, and W. A. Seed. 1978. *The Mechanics of Circulation.* Oxford: Oxford University Press.

Clausen, J. P. 1977. Effect of physical training on cardiovascular adjustments to exercise in man. *Physiological Reviews* 57:779–815.

Folkow, B., and E. Neil. 1971. *Circulation.* New York: Oxford University Press.

Guyton, A. C., A. E. Taylor, and H. J. Granger. 1973/75. *Circulatory Physiology.* Vol 1: *Cardiac Output and Its Regulation,* 2nd ed. Vol. 2: *Dynamics and Control of Body Fluids.* Philadelphia: Saunders.

Johansen, K. 1979. Cardiovascular support of metabolic functions in vertebrates. In *Evolution of Respiratory Processes,* ed. S. C. Wood and C. Lenfant. New York: Dekker, pp. 107–192.

Taylor, M. G. 1973. Hemodynamics. *Annual Review of Physiology* 35:87–116.

References

BLOOD

Altman, P. L., and D. S. Dittmer. 1971. *Biological Handbooks: Respiration and Circulation.* Bethesda: Federation of American Societies for Experimental Biology.

Benesch, R., R. E. Benesch, and Y. Enoki. 1968. The interaction of hemoglobin and its subunits with 2,3-diphosphoglycerate. *Proceedings of the National Academy of Sciences USA* 59:526–532.

* Bohr, C., K. A. Hasselbalch, and A. Krogh. 1904. Ueber einen in biologischer Beziehung wichtigen Einfluss, den die Kohlensäurespannung des Blutes auf dessen Sauerstoffbindung übt. *Scandinavian Archives of Physiology* 16:402–412.

Dejours, P. 1981. *Principles of Comparative Respiratory Physiology.* 2nd ed. Amsterdam: Elsevier North-Holland.

Dickerson, R. E., and I. Geis. 1971. *Struktur und Funktion der Proteine.* Weinheim: Verlag Chemie.

Hlastala, M. P., and R. D. Woodson. 1975. Saturation dependency of the Bohr effect: interactions among H^+, CO_2, and DPG. *Journal of Applied Physiology* 38:1126–1131.

Holland, R. A. B. 1969. Rate of O_2 dissociation from O_2Hb and relative combination rate of CO and O_2 in mammals at 37° C. *Respiration Physiology* 7:30–42.

Holland, R. A. B., and R. E. Forster. 1966. The effect of size of red cells on the kinetics of their oxygen uptake. *Journal of General Physiology* 49:727–742.

Lenfant, C., P. Ways, C. Aucutt, and J. Cruz. 1969. Effect of chronic hypoxic hypoxia on the O_2-Hb dissociation curve and respiratory gas transport in man. *Respiration Physiology* 7:7–29.

Malan, A., T. L. Wilson, and R. B. Reeves. 1976. Intracellular pH in cold-blooded vertebrates as a function of body temperature. *Respiration Physiology* 28:29–47.

Moll, W., and H. Bartels. 1968. Oxygen binding in the blood of mammals. In *Oxygen Transport in Blood and Tissue*, ed. D. W. Lübbers, U. C. Luft, G. Thews, and E. Witzleb. Stuttgart: Thieme, pp. 39–47.

* Perutz, M. F. 1970. Stereochemistry of cooperative effects in haemoglobin. Haem-haem interaction and the problem of allostery. The Bohr effect and combination with organic phosphates. *Nature* 228:726–733.

Rahn, H., and R. B. Reeves. 1982. Hydrogen ion regulation during hypothermia: from the Amazon to the operating room. In *Applied Physiology in Clinical Respiratory Care*, ed. O. Prakash. The Hague: Martinus Nijhoff, pp. 1–15.

Reeves, R. B., J. S. Park, G. N. Lapennas, and A. J. Olszowka. 1982. Oxygen affinity and Bohr coefficients of dog blood. *Journal of Applied Physiology* 53:87–95.

Schmidt-Nielsen, K. 1979. *Animal Physiology*. 2nd ed. Cambridge: Cambridge University Press.

West, J. B. 1974. *Respiratory Physiology: The Essentials*. Baltimore: Williams & Wilkins.

CIRCULATION

Åstrand, P. O., and K. Rodahl. 1977. *Textbook of Work Physiology*. New York: McGraw-Hill.

Cournand, A. 1957. Pulmonary circulation; its control in man, with some remarks on methodology. *Science* 125:1231–1235. (Nobel Lecture.)

* Cournand, A., and H. A. Ranges. 1941. Catheterization of the right auricle in man. *Proceedings of the Society for Experimental Biology and Medicine* 46:462.

Richards, D. W. 1957. Right heart catheterization: its contributions to physiology and medicine. *Science* 125:1181–1185. (Nobel Lecture.)

* Richards, D. W., Jr., A. Cournand, R. C. Darling, W. H. Gillespie, E. de F. Baldwin. 1942. Pressure of blood in the right auricle, in animals and in man under normal conditions and in right heart failure. *American Journal of Physiology* 136:115–123.

7

DELIVERING OXYGEN TO THE CELLS

IN DISCUSSING THE ROLE of structural design in the delivery of O_2 to the cells we must consider two factors: (1) those features which allow the blood flow to be distributed to the various organs and tissues in an appropriate amount, and (2) the design properties which determine gas exchange between the blood and the cells.

The vasculature sets up a system of vessels which should permit the blood flow required to ensure the metabolic activity of the cells in the various parts of the body in proportion to the functional demands imposed on them. But there is only one organ which keeps its metabolic activity nearly constant all the time: the brain. All other organs will go through phases of rest and of accrued activity, and it never happens that all organs are at peak activity simultaneously. One of the most important functions of the vasculature is therefore the distribution of blood flow according to need.

On the other hand, it is evident that each sector of the vasculature, for example, the subloop leading through a certain muscle group (Fig. 6.12), must be made of such a size as to allow the blood flow required when that part of the body needs the maximal amount of blood flow to perform at its peak metabolic activity, even though, most of the time, this will not be exploited. Thus we must expect — if the principle of symmorphosis holds — that the vascular supply of an organ is commensurate with the needs for blood flow imposed by the metabolic activity of its cells. In that respect, however, we must remember that blood serves more functions than to carry O_2, although this function may be particularly critical.

Distributing Blood to the Tissues: Design of the Vasculature

The arteries that distribute the blood to the tissues have an elastic wall which contains smooth muscle fibers (Fig. 6.11). This is important in two respects: first, in regulating blood pressure, and second, in regulating the distribution of blood to the various organs.

The heart pumps the blood into the arteries in short forceful bursts; during systole the blood pressure in the ventricle increases rapidly to over 120 mm Hg and then falls back to nearly 0 mm Hg in diastole. This is the origin of the pulse wave. If we measure blood pressure in an artery of the arm, we find that it varies between 120 mm Hg during systole and 80 mm Hg in diastole; the amplitude is hence much smaller than that observed at the exit of the ventricle. The pulse wave is damped because the ventricle pumps its stroke volumes into a large vessel, the aorta, whose highly elastic wall becomes stretched in systole, stores some of the energy gained in the process, and gives it back to the blood during diastole. All arteries exert this effect to a certain extent, and when the blood reaches the microvessels in the tissues the pulse wave is still there but has a much reduced amplitude.

Blood vessels also have an effect on the absolute magnitude of blood pressure because they offer blood flow a certain resistance which depends on the dimensions of the tubes. The flow $\dot{q}$ of a fluid of viscosity η through a tube of length l and radius r is described by Poiseuille's law (Fig. 7.1)

$$\dot{q} = \frac{\pi}{8 \cdot \eta} \cdot \frac{r^4}{l} \cdot \Delta p. \tag{7.1}$$

Blood flow through a system of tubes of finite diameter thus inevitably results in a pressure drop along the way. Because the resistance to flow is proportional to the fourth power of the radius, a small change in the caliber of the vessel must have a profound effect on the pressure drop.

One problem in designing a system of branched arteries that distributes the blood into the various parts of the body is to avoid too large a drop in pressure before the blood reaches its destination; this can evidently be achieved by keeping the diameter of the vessels large, but not too large because this would make the blood volume

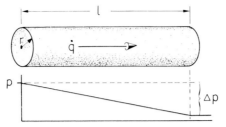

Fig. 7.1 When fluid flows along a tube the pressure falls as a function of flow resistance.

that is contained in arteries — and must be moved by the action of the heart — very large, and this would cost more energy. It turns out that the body has succeeded in optimizing the diameter of all the branches of the arterial tree so as to require the minimum energy to pump the blood into all tissues. The largest pressure drop occurs in the very last segments of the arterial tree, the arterioles, which lead directly into the microvascular units, the capillary networks we shall describe below.

The arteries that arise from the aorta form tree-like structures made of branches of different diameter and length that all end in over 100 million end twigs, the arterioles, before they feed their blood into the capillaries. Figure 7.2 shows a short sequence of such branches which will allow me to discuss some of the essential consequences of this design.

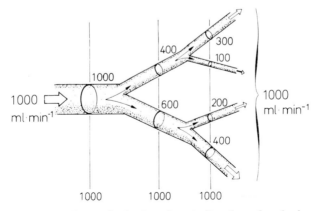

Fig. 7.2 In a system of branched tubes, flow is distributed to the branches as a function of local resistance, but total flow through the total cross section at each level remains constant.

After each branching the number of segments has doubled. If we pump blood into the main branch at a rate of, say, $1 \, 1 \cdot min^{-1}$ the same quantity must flow out at the ends. In fact, we must postulate that the same flow must also cross the total cross section of the tree at any point from left to right. Since the diameters of the branches are different we would, however, expect the flow to divide unevenly at each branch point, because a smaller vessel has a higher resistance, as we conclude from Poiseuille's law. This then shows that the distribution of blood to various parts of the body is determined by the cross section of the arterial branches leading to them. If one looks at the real arterial tree, one finds that the size of an artery is indeed proportional to the blood flow required by the tissue it supplies.

This system also offers possibilities for regulating the regional blood flow according to needs. The sleeve of circular smooth muscle in the arterial wall allows the vessel diameter to be regulated, essentially under the influence of the autonomous (sympathetic and parasympathetic) nervous system. A reduction in the diameter of some arteries allows more blood flow to other parts of the body. Thus, following a meal we find more blood to flow into the gut and less into the muscles, which explains why we should not go for a run right after eating. Regional blood flow can, in principle, be measured the same way as cardiac output, that is, by a dye dilution method, injecting the tracer into the artery supplying the region; the main problem is that the drainage of the blood into the veins is not always simple. An alternative approach is to inject into the aorta a small but known quantity of radioactive particles of such a size that they get trapped in the microvasculature. The blood flow through a particular group of muscles, for example, can then be calculated from the measurements of the radioactivity retained in that region.

The Microvascular Unit

The arterial blood enters the tissue with a P_{O_2} of 95 mm Hg and an O_2 content of 20 vol % (20 ml O_2 STPD in 100 ml of blood) which is mostly bound to hemoglobin. The blood that drains into the vein has a P_{O_2} of 40 mm Hg and an O_2 content of 14 vol %, values which can be considerably lower in a working muscle. Thus a significant amount of O_2 has been rapidly discharged, aided, as we have seen, by the simultaneous uptake of CO_2 which reduces O_2 affinity of hemoglo-

bin. All this happens while the erythrocytes traverse the capillaries in less than 1 second; it evidently depends on an adequate design of the vessels which bring the blood into close proximity of the cells that avidly take up the O_2 delivered.

The morphological basis for gas exchange in the tissue is the *microvascular unit*, as it is shown in Figure 7.3 for skeletal muscle and explained in diagram form in Figure 7.4. The unit begins with an arteriole which is, in fact, the end twig of the arterial tree and is therefore provided with a thin but compact sleeve of smooth muscle fibers allowing regulation of blood flow. Indeed, the arterioles constitute the major resistance vessels, for we find the largest drop in blood pressure to occur in arterioles (Fig. 6.10), just prior to discharge of the blood into the capillary network. The connection from the arteriole to the actual exchange vessels, the capillaries, is established by short precapillaries which have an incomplete muscle sleeve, but may have a slightly thickened ring of muscle at their end, a sphincter that is presumably capable of restricting blood flow into part of the capillary network, or even of shutting it off altogether. Characteristi-

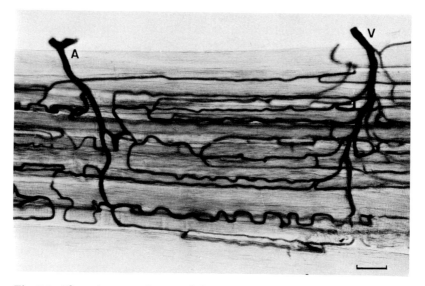

Fig. 7.3 The microvasculature of skeletal muscle, extending from arteriole (A) to venule (V), is revealed by perfusion of stained gelatin. Note that capillaries course predominantly parallel to muscle fibers, and that the capillary density increases somewhat toward the venule. Scale marker: 100 μm.

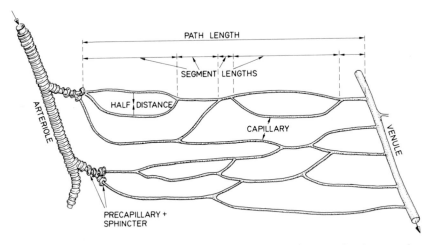

Fig. 7.4 The microvascular unit is built of a capillary network whose path length from arteriole to venule is an important characteristic. (From Weibel, 1979.)

cally, the capillaries form a network made of a varying number of segments that split up and join again. Toward the venous end capillaries merge to form postcapillaries and finally venules that drain the blood into veins.

The design of this microvascular unit obeys a number of basic rules:

(1) The capillary wall structure is continuous, in order to confine the blood to the vascular compartment even in the finest vessels, but it is minimal in order to facilitate exchange of substances with the cells.

(2) The shape of the capillary meshwork reflects the shape of the associated cells or cell groups, as a result of close apposition of the capillaries to the cells they supply.

(3) The density of the meshwork is proportional to the metabolic needs of the cells, both with respect to O_2 and to other materials delivered by the blood.

CAPILLARY WALL STRUCTURE

Figure 7.5 shows a cross section of a capillary as it is found in muscle tissue. Its wall is basically made of two layers, an endothelial cell and a basement membrane. The *endothelial cell* can be described as a thin flat cell whose nucleus is usually flattened and enwrapped by a thin layer of cytoplasm only; in the region of the nucleus the cell is 1 – 2 μm thick. The major part of the cell is made of greatly attenuated cytoplasmic extensions no more than 0.1 μm thick, and sometimes even thinner, but extending to an average radius of about 20 μm from the nucleus. These extensions are built essentially of two plasma membranes with some cytoplasmic ground substance in between; they typically contain very few organelles (an occasional small mitochondrion and here and there a few ribosomes with some endoplasmic reticulum) but are often richly endowed with membrane vesicles implicated in transendothelial transport of macromolecules, a process called micropinocytosis or, more accurately in this context, cytopempsis. The endothelial lining is complete because these extensions reach out until they meet another one; along these intercel-

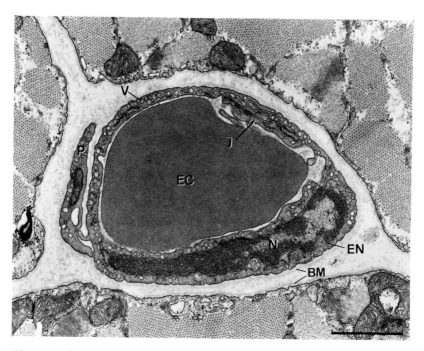

Fig. 7.5 This electron micrograph shows a muscle capillary cut in cross section and containing an erythrocyte (EC). Its wall is made of an endothelial cell (EN) which contains a nucleus (N) and numerous vesicles (V), and forms a tortuous intercellular junction (J). It is enwrapped by a basement membrane (BM) which is associated with a pericyte process (P). Scale marker: 1 μm. (From Weibel, 1979.)

lular junctions the plasma membranes of the two cells become closely apposed and joined to each other by a band-like complex of molecular bridges, called tight junction or *zonula occludens*. However, it appears that this complex forms a rather leaky seal of the intercellular cleft so that passageways are established which allow ions and even some smaller macromolecules to "leak" out from the plasma into the interstitial space.

The structure of the squamous extensions shows some particularities depending on the tissue they supply; thus in muscle — as, by the way, in the lung — the lining is continuous without gaps (Fig. 7.5), whereas in other organs such as kidney, intestine, and some glands, fenestrae of about 50 nm diameter are formed which penetrate the depth of the endothelium and are closed off only by a thin diaphragm, somehow like a thin plasma membrane. In the sinusoidal capillaries of the liver, wide canaliculi extend right through the endothelium, giving the plasma broad and possibly direct access to the surface of the liver cells. It is likely that such specializations are related to particular requirements for transendothelial exchange of macromolecules or even larger particles; they probably play an insignificant role in the exchange of O_2 and CO_2 between the blood and the cells, as these gases can freely diffuse through the cytoplasmic leaflets.

With a few exceptions (liver, some endocrine glands) the capillary *basement membrane* forms a continuous lining of the entire outer surface of the endothelium to which it adheres tightly; it is a thin sheet made of proteoglycans and a special type of collagen and allows solutes and even small macromolecules to pass freely.

Most capillaries also have an additional set of cells called *pericytes* that partially enwrap them with long processes and are closely associated with the basement membrane (Fig. 7.5). Pericytes appear to have contractile properties and are thought to be a type of smooth muscle whose long and thin extensions encircle the capillary, and may serve as a sparingly applied mechanical support for these very thin-walled vessels which must withstand the small but positive pressure under which blood flows through.

ARCHITECTURE OF THE CAPILLARY NETWORK

In the microvascular unit, capillaries form networks built of segments of different lengths (Fig. 7.4). Thus a red blood cell which enters the microvascular unit from the arteriole can take several routes until it reaches the venule. The representation of a "microvascular unit" shown in Figure 7.4 is, in fact, somewhat simplified, because such units are not sharply defined: the capillary networks from adjoining units are connected by capillary segments, as well. In consequence, the capillary networks of a given tissue usually form a large continuum into which arterioles deliver blood at several points, and from which multiple venules drain blood.

The geometry of the capillary network is dictated by the shape and arrangement of the cells it supplies. In intestinal villi it closely follows the epithelial lining; in glands it forms baskets around the acini, the groups of cells that produce the secretory product and are arranged like berries at the end of branched epithelial ducts. In skeletal muscle, the tissue with which we are mostly concerned, the capillaries are predominantly oriented parallel to the muscle fibers (Fig. 7.3) with some transverse connections here and there.

One can approach the problem of how to characterize the microvascular unit quantitatively in a number of different ways. One approach is to analyze the *architecture of the network* by noting the number of segments used to build it, as well as the length of the segments (Fig. 7.4). The network is furthermore characterized by the number of nodes, the branch points where three segments come together; in terms of blood flow through this network, however, it is important to note also whether such nodes are points of divergence or convergence, that is, whether the bloodstream separates or whether two streams join. While one can surely make this kind of distinction in first approximation by simply looking at the sequence of segments from arteriole to venule and by considering the angles at which segments meet, one may easily be deceived; a stringent analysis requires this pattern to be worked out by looking directly at blood flow under the microscope, an undertaking which is not that easy. Such studies have been done mostly on a flat leg muscle of the frog, and there one finds that up to nine segments were used to make a path from arteriole to venule, depending on the total length of the path, which ranged from 1 to 7 mm in this case. The number of divergent branch points decreased along the path, whereas that of convergent nodes increased, as one would expect. The average path length was 3.6 mm and required four segments of average length 0.9 mm. These numbers and dimensions may well be different for other muscles, although the pattern of capillary arrangement is very similar even in mammalian muscle. It seems, however, that the total path length is considerably smaller in mammalian muscle; data on the rat show it to be of the order of 0.5 to 1 mm, although a similar number of segments is used to make the network. In the capillary network of monkey muscle shown in Figure 7.3 the path length is about 0.5 mm, subdivided into roughly four segments, on the average.

CAPILLARY DENSITY IN THE TISSUE

One can take another approach to characterize the capillary network, and this is to estimate the *capillary density*, that is, the amount of capillary blood available for gas exchange with the cells. The capillary density also tells us something about the distances between capillaries, that is, in fact, how far O_2 has to diffuse into the tissue. This is the approach chosen by August Krogh (1874 to 1949) in his classical work *Anatomy and Physiology of Capillaries* (1922, 1929), who, in fact, has laid all the ground work for the present treatise. In studying capillary density of muscles the usual approach is to cut a transverse section (Fig. 7.6) and to count how many capillaries are found per mm² of cross-sectional area, the measurement resulting in a number per unit area, $N_A(cap)$. For skeletal muscles this is a reasonable approximation of capillary density because the capillaries are quite well aligned with the cylindrical muscle fibers (Fig. 7.3). Krogh has therefore proposed that the capillary density estimates the cross-sectional area of an average tissue cylinder surrounding the capillary and hence supplied with O_2 from this capillary, a very fruitful concept indeed. Let us look at this more closely.

Figure 7.7 represents an idealized piece of muscle tissue with parallel straight capillaries at equal distances. On the cross sections one can mark out the boundaries of a hexagonal lattice with one capillary in the center of each hexagon; in the tissue each capillary is hence contained in the axis of a hexagonal prism. Such a prism can be approximated by a right circular cylinder whose radius R_k is such that the area of the circular cross section is equal to the area of the hexagon. Now the average area of the hexagon, $\bar{a}$, is directly derived from the capillary density estimated on cross sections:

$$\bar{a} = 1/N_A. \tag{7.2}$$

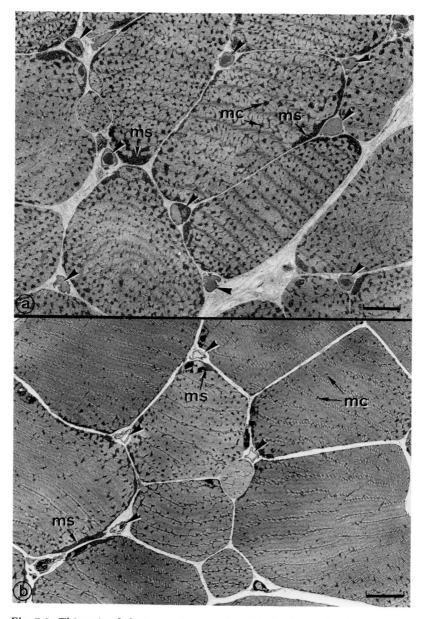

Fig. 7.6 This pair of electron micrographs of skeletal muscles from a small gazelle shows the relation between capillaries (arrow heads) and mitochondria (m): in the diaphragm (a) both capillaries and mitochondria are more numerous than in semitendinosus (b). (From Hoppeler et al., 1981b.) Scale markers: 10 μm.

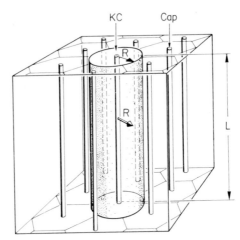

Fig. 7.7 Model of capillaries that are completely parallel and evenly spaced is highly idealized. Each capillary (Cap) is conceived to supply a prismatic or cylindrical sleeve of tissue called Krogh cylinder (KC) of radius R, the half-distance between capillaries.

With a capillary density of about 400 mm^{-2}, a typical value for human leg muscles, we find $\bar{a}$ to be about 2500 μm^2, which results in an average radius R_k of the cylindrical unit of about 28μm. If one now takes this cylinder to be about as long as the average total path length from arteriole to venule, that is, L ~ 0.5 to 1 mm, we have a reasonable approximation of the tissue unit that is supplied with O$_2$ by one capillary path. In recognition of Krogh's pioneering work such a cylindrical unit is commonly called a *Krogh cylinder*. Subsequently we shall see that this concept is a good first approximation, which has allowed a number of important conclusions to be drawn, but which definitely needs some refinement.

One point of criticism is that the capillaries are, of course, not straight tubes (see Fig. 7.3). Furthermore, their density, as observed on cross sections, varies a great deal: if one compares cross sections through muscles of different fiber-type composition (Fig. 7.6), one notes much fewer capillaries to surround glycolytic than oxidative fibers. One has therefore introduced a second descriptor of capillary density, the number of capillaries per number of muscle fiber, N_c/N_f, and has found this ratio to be about 2.5 for oxidative and 1 for glycolytic muscles, on the average. It is, however, rather difficult to make use of such information in analytical models of the type of Krogh cylinders, and it does not overcome the difficulty that capillaries are not straight tubes, a fact that cannot be adequately assessed on cross sections of muscle.

A NEW LOOK AT CAPILLARY DENSITY

Let us therefore take a fresh approach and see whether there is not a better way of characterizing capillary density. What kind of morphometric information do we really need to characterize O_2 delivery to the cells? For one we would like to know how much blood is exposed to the cells for gas exchange. This is described by the ratio of *capillary blood volume to cell volume*; referring back to chapter 3 we find this volume ratio to be a volume density (capillary blood volume per cell volume) for which we have used the symbol

$$V_V(cap,cell) = V(cap)/V(cell) = P(cap)/P(cell) \qquad (7.3)$$

and which we can, in fact, estimate simply by a point-counting method, recording points of a random test grid that fall on capillaries, $P(cap)$, and on cells, $P(cell)$, respectively (Fig. 3.10, equation 3.31). The nice thing about this method is that it is not affected by the preferentially longitudinal arrangement of capillaries. The capillary volume density per cell is indeed a very valuable descriptor of the situation because we can now also relate the capillary blood volume to the mitochondria it serves, since we had used, in chapter 5, the mitochrondrial volume density in the cells, $V_V(mi,cell)$, as the basic morphometric descriptor of the cell's aerobic capacity. Since $V_V(cap,cell)$ and $V_V(mi,cell)$ have the same reference volume, their ratio tells us how much blood is used to supply O_2 to a unit mitochondrial volume.

Another important descriptor of O_2 supply to the cells is the *capillary surface area* across which O_2 diffuses into the cells, for we have seen before that the interface area between two compartments determines the exchange rate by diffusion. If we also choose the cell volume as the reference space, we can estimate the capillary surface density

$$S_V(cap,cell) = S(cap)/V(cell) \qquad (7.4)$$

from intersections between the test grid and the capillary surface trace on a section (Fig. 3.10; equation 3.32). This method cannot be used indiscriminately on muscle tissue, however, because it is affected by the orientation of the capillaries with respect to the sections; equation 3.32 only holds for truly random sections, so that measurements done on muscle cross sections will be biased, as discussed below.

In terms of estimating O_2 diffusion into the cells, or, more accurately, to the mitochondria in the cells, we would also want to estimate some characteristic mean distance, δ, that O_2 has to travel from the capillary wall to the mitochondria where it is consumed. This distance is poorly defined as yet; it depends importantly on the distribution of mitochondria within the cell, and we saw that it is not always homogeneous (Fig. 5.7); but it also depends on the model we choose to describe O_2 diffusion. In first approximation, however, δ must be somehow related to the radius R_k of the Krogh cylinder, that is, the cylinder of tissue (or cells) that surrounds a unit length of capillaries. In fact, R_k is something like a mean half distance between capillaries (Figs. 7.4 and 7.6) and is therefore related to the total length of capillaries in the unit tissue volume, or the *capillary length density*. If we choose again the cells as reference space, the morphometric descriptor is capillary length density per cell volume

$$J_V(cap,cell) = J(cap)/V(cell). \tag{7.5}$$

(In stereology we use the symbol J to mean length of a curve in space, to distinguish it from the symbol L used for length of test lines, as in equation 3.32.) It is not difficult to see that the mean cross-sectional area of the tissue cylinder that surrounds a capillary (now not necessarily straight) is directly obtained as the reciprocal of J_V: a volume per length is an area. We can therefore calculate an approximate radius of the Krogh cylinder from

$$\hat{R} \approx [\pi \cdot J_V(cap,cell)]^{-1/2}. \tag{7.6}$$

The capillary length density $J_V(cap)$ is a rather comprehensive descriptor of capillary density in the tissue, because it is also directly connected to the capillary volume and surface densities. Capillaries are cylindrical tubes whose diameter is much smaller than their length and also varies only within narrow limits (from 5 to 10 μm) since it has its lower limit in the size of the red blood cells. If we can estimate the average capillary cross section, $\bar{a}_c$, and the average capillary circumference, $\bar{b}_c$, we can obtain the capillary volume and surface density from

$$V_V(\text{cap}) = \bar{a}_c \cdot J_V(\text{cap}) \tag{7.7}$$

$$S_V(\text{cap}) = \bar{b}_c \cdot J_V(\text{cap}). \tag{7.8}$$

In consequence, we observe that all important descriptors of capillary density in the tissue — capillary volume, capillary surface, mean radius of the Krogh cylinder — depend on one essential variable: the capillary length density, $J_V(\text{cap})$.

How can we estimate $J_V(\text{cap})$? Stereology again offers a simple method (Fig. 7.8). If we cut a plane section across the tissue, the thin curved "filaments" (or capillaries) will appear as transsections; the number Q of such transsections found per unit section area A, that is, the transsection density, Q_A, is directly proportional to the length density in the volume, J_V. If the capillaries are randomly oriented in space, we have

$$J_V = 2 \cdot Q_A. \tag{7.9}$$

But this method is very sensitive to orientation. If, for example, all capillaries are parallel (Fig. 7.8c), a *longitudinal* section, that is, one

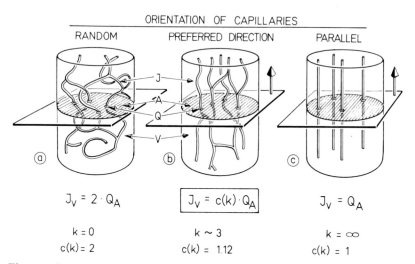

Fig. 7.8 Estimating capillary density on cross sections depends on the degree of capillary orientation.

parallel to the course of the capillaries, will not generate any transsections at all; but if we cut a *transverse* section we have

$$J_V = Q_A.$$ (7.10)

If in this case of parallel capillaries we were to cut a large number of
randomly oriented sections, we would again have $J_V = 2 \cdot Q_A$. How
can we solve this problem?

Let us suppose we suspect that the capillaries show some unknown
degree of preferred orientation and that we can determine its direction, marked by the arrows in Figure 7.8; in the case of muscle we
will suspect, on the basis of information taken from specimens such
as Figure 7.3, that capillaries orient themselves preferentially parallel to the muscle fibers. We now cut sections perpendicular to that
direction and count the transsections per unit area, Q_A. In very
general terms we can now say that the relation between J_V and Q_A
must involve a coefficient c(k) (Fig. 7.8b) which lies somewhere
between 2, if the capillaries are random, and 1, if they are completely
aligned. The value of c(k) is completely defined by the *degree* of
orientation estimated by an orientation parameter k which is something like the standard deviation of an orientation distribution. In
trying to work out this orientation distribution for muscle capillaries,
we find values of k between 3 and 8 and this yield values of c(k) of the
order of 1.12 to 1.05.

One may notice that Q_A is nothing else than the "capillary density," N_A, discussed above. The main progress made in this evaluation of methods is that we now know how to calculate the length
density of the capillary network from these data, by multiplying N_A
with a factor between 1.05 and 1.1; the difference of 5% between
these values is small and, for most purposes, unimportant. But we
have also learned that it makes more physiological sense to express
Q_A (or N_A) per unit *cell* cross-section because this allows us to relate
these data to the mitochondria that the capillaries supply with O_2.
We have also seen that the calculation of J_V opens the possibility of
estimating the capillary volume and surface available for gas exchange, as well as a realistic value of the Krogh cylinder radius. Some
typical values have been calculated in Table 7.1 in order to show the
relationship between these descriptors.

TABLE 7.1. **MORPHOMETRIC DESCRIPTORS OF MUSCLE CAPILLARIES** (expressed per unit muscle cell volume) derived from capillary counts on cross sections. Orientation factor $c(K) \sim 1.1$ and capillary radius of 3 μm were assumed.

$N_A(cap)$ (mm^{-2})	$J_V(cap)$ (cm/cm^3)	$V_V(cap)$ (%)	$S_V(cap)$ (cm^2/cm^3)	R_k (μm)
400	$44 \cdot 10^4$	1.2	83	27
800	$8.8 \cdot 10^4$	2.5	166	19
1,200	$13.2 \cdot 10^4$	3.7	249	16
1,600	$17.6 \cdot 10^4$	5.0	331	13

VARIATION OF CAPILLARY DENSITY

We have already observed, in relation to Figure 7.6, that the capillary density may vary considerably from place to place, between muscles, and even within one and the same muscle. The variability of capillary density between muscles of the same animal is evident in Figure 7.6, where we compare the diaphragm with a leg muscle (M. semitendinosus) of a small gazelle, both pictures taken at the same magnification. In the diaphragm we find 9 capillary transsections within the frame of the picture, but only 4 in that of the leg muscle. When averaged over many similar micrographs, the capillary density $N_A(cap,cell)$ is 1800 and 530 respectively for these two muscles; the length density comes out to be $19.8 \cdot 10^4$ and $5.8 \cdot 10^4$ cm, or roughly 20 and 6 m, per cm³ of muscle fiber tissue, so that the mean Krogh cylinder radius is estimated at 12.7 μm and 23.4 μm, respectively (Fig. 7.9).

What is behind this difference? In chapter 5 we saw that the diaphragm is composed exclusively of oxidative fibers, whereas the semitendinosus muscle has a mixed fiber population with many glycolytic fibers. Accordingly, the muscle fibers of the diaphragm contain 2–3 times as many mitochondria as those of the semitendinosus. In this particular gazelle the mitochondrial volume density amounted to 18% in the diaphragm and to slightly over 5% in semitendinosus (Fig. 7.9). Let us now see what this means. The difference in capillary density causes the mean cross-section of Krogh's cylinder to be about 3 times smaller in the diaphragm than in semitendinosus. If we look at a unit capillary length of, say, 0.5 mm

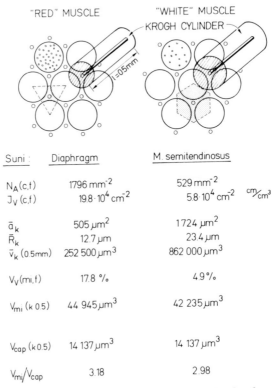

Fig. 7.9 Comparison of highly oxidative "red" muscle (diaphragm) with less oxidative "white" muscle (semitendinosus), shown in Figure 7.6, reveals that the ratio of mitochondrial to capillary volume is constant.

—the order of magnitude of the path length from arteriole to venule
—the volume of the Krogh cylinder is 252,000 μm^3 and 862,000 μm^3 respectively, thus much larger in semitendinosus. However, it turns out that in either case the total amount of mitochondria contained in this cylinder is about the same, namely 45,000 and 42,000 μm^3, a figure which we obtain by multiplying the cylinder volume with the mitochondrial volume density (Fig. 7.9). This is a remarkable finding because it suggests that the length density of the capillaries is matched to the quantity of mitochondria it must supply with O_2, so that each μm^3 of capillary blood serves about 3 μm^3 of mitochondria.

Evidently, what we have just seen relates to a particular example, so the question is whether it reflects a general principle. In Figure 7.10 we have made an attempt to see whether the relationship between mitochondrial and capillary density checks out when we compare muscles taken from a wide variety of mammals, from the shrew to the cow, and including some samples of heart muscle with its notoriously high mitochondrial content. We see that the capillary density increases systematically as the mitochondrial density increases. From these wider data we can calculate that, on the average, each μm^3 of capillary blood is related to about 2.6 μm^3 of mitochondria, very much in agreement with the conclusion we reached above.

CAPILLARY DENSITY AND O_2 NEEDS

The last question then is whether the capillary supply of muscles is proportional to their O_2 needs; we would, indeed, suspect this since we have shown in chapter 5 that the muscles' mitochondrial volume is proportional to $\dot{V}_{O_2}max$. The approach we have taken is to see whether the total capillary length of some typical muscles scales

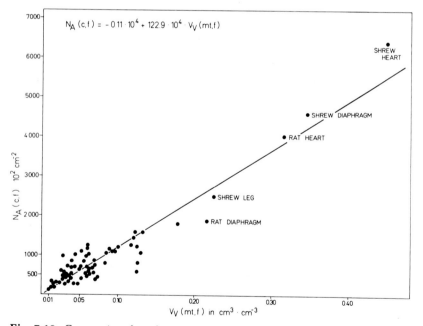

Fig. 7.10 Comparing data from a large range of animals and muscle types reveals that the capillary density, expressed as number of capillaries per cm² of muscle cross section, $N_A(c,f)$, increases in proportion to the mitochondrial volume density. (From Hoppeler et al., 1981b.)

similar to $\dot{V}_{O_2}$max when we compare animals of different body size. Figure 7.11, which is analogous to Figure 5.13, shows the result. The allometric regression lines are nearly parallel to that of $\dot{V}_{O_2}$max. The length of the capillary network, and by that the volume of blood contained in the muscles, is hence proportional to the O_2 flow required to drive muscles under conditions of limiting oxidative metabolism.

There is, however, one point in these data which is slightly disturbing: the relation between capillary length and mitochondrial volume density shows an unusually large scatter (Fig. 7.10), larger than one would expect from measurement errors. One reason for this appears to be that glycolytic fibers (see chapter 5) have a larger supply of capillaries than one would expect considering their low mitochondrial content. But these cells produce just as much ATP, only they do it mostly anaerobically through glycolysis. We have seen in chapter 4 that this process is wasteful with substrates and generates

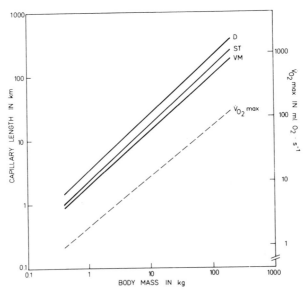

Fig. 7.11 When one calculates total capillary length (in km!) in three muscles of African mammals, one finds it to increase about in proportion to $\dot{V}_{O_2}$max, similar to what was shown for mitochondria in Figure 5.13. D = diaphragm, ST = semitendinosus, VM = vastus medialis. (From Hoppeler et al., 1981b.)

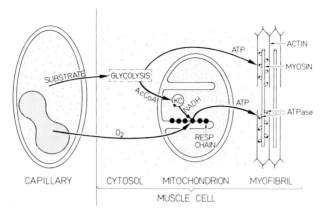

Fig. 7.12 For energy supply from capillary blood to the myosin ATPase in the muscle cells two metabolic pathways must be considered: the oxidative pathway via the mitochondria needs primarily O_2, whereas the glycolytic pathway depends on substrate supply. (From Weibel et al., 1981.)

lactate which must be removed. The blood capillaries here serve primarily to supply the cells with substrates for glycolysis and to remove lactate, rather than to furnish O_2 to the few mitochondria present. In appreciating the functional role of blood capillaries we must therefore consider their dual function as conveyors not only of respiratory gases but also of substrates and wastes (Fig. 7.12); looking at only one aspect, their respiratory role, is an oversimplification, although the supply of O_2 in sufficient quantity may still be the most critical factor determining the design of microvasculature, because the O_2 stores in the cells are much more limited than the stores of substrates, for example.

O_2 Flow from Blood to Cells

WORKING OUT THE PRINCIPLES

We should now consider the factors which determine the flow of O_2 from the capillary blood into the cells, and eventually to the mitochondria, the metabolic sinks into which O_2 disappears. To put ourselves into the picture, look at Figure 7.13: O_2 leaves the blood plasma and diffuses through the tissue spaces into the cells, where it meets mitochondria that may absorb some of it in the process of

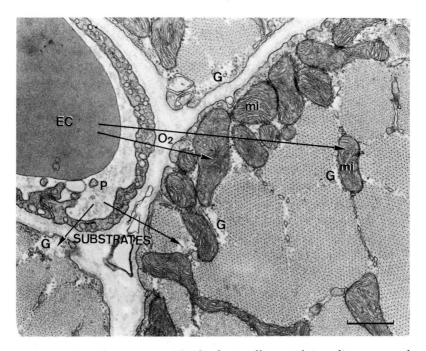

Fig. 7.13 This electron micrograph of a capillary with its adjacent muscle fibers shows the pathways for O_2 supply from the erythrocyte (EC) to the mitochondria (mi) and for substrates from the plasma (P) to intracellular glycogen deposits (G). Scale marker: 0.5 μm.

oxidative phosphorylation. A first question is: how far can O_2 penetrate into the cell?

We shall look at this question by means of the simple model shown in Figure 7.14. The primary determinant of O_2 flow rate into the tissue by diffusion is evidently the head pressure, that is, the P_{O_2} in the capillaries, which starts out at about 95 mm Hg near the arteriole and falls eventually to 40 mm Hg or less as the blood reaches the venule. Remember that the nonlinear shape of the O_2Hb dissociation curve and the Bohr shift keep the capillary P_{O_2} relatively high in spite of O_2 discharge, which means that the drop in P_{O_2} along the capillary is not a linear function of distance; but more about this later.

The second determinant of O_2 flow is the rate at which the cell, or rather its mitochondria, consumes O_2. From what we have seen in chapter 5 we suspect that this rate must be somehow proportional to the quantity of mitochondria in the cell. Let us assume for the moment that mitochondria are finely and homogeneously distributed throughout the cell; in this case we can expect the unit cell volume, say 1 μm^3, to consume O_2 at a constant and even rate which we may call $\dot{m}_{O_2}(C)$. This is definitely an oversimplification, as we shall see later.

In the simple model of Figure 7.14 we furthermore assume the cell to be exposed to a capillary on one side but to extend indefinitely in direction x, again a gross oversimplification, but it allows us to work out some of the basic principles which establish a certain P_{O_2} profile throughout the cell.

Consider first diffusion of O_2 that occurs from an initial segment of the capillary (point 1) where $P_{O_2} \sim 90$ mm Hg. In the absence of O_2 consumption — that is, when $\dot{m}_{O_2}(C) = 0$ — a linear P_{O_2} gradient (curve 11) becomes established which depends exclusively on the diffusion coefficient K (Krogh's diffusion coefficient, which is the product of solubility and diffusion constant). If O_2 is being consumed in the cell, at a constant rate $\dot{m}_{O_2}(C) > 0$ at all points, the P_{O_2} gradient falls more rapidly and follows a parabolic curve (12) which is determined by K and $\dot{m}_{O_2}(C)$; if $\dot{m}_{O_2}(C)$ is smaller the curve is less steep (13), if it is larger the curve is steeper (14). In terms of supplying O_2 to the mitochondria it is important to note that at some distance x_0 the P_{O_2} will have fallen to zero so that all the tissue beyond that region is anoxic, that is, does not receive any O_2. The location of this point,

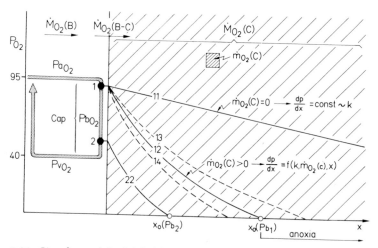

Fig. 7.14 Simple model of slab-like "cell" (cross-hatched) supplied by capillary (Cap) to show profile of P_{O_2} as function of distance into cell.

and by that the depth to which O_2 can penetrate into the cell, depends on the diffusion coefficient K, on the rate of O_2 consumption, $\dot{m}_{O_2}(C)$, and, on the O_2 head pressure in the capillary, Pb_{O_2}, such that

$$x_0 = \sqrt{2\,K \cdot \frac{Pb_{O_2}}{\dot{m}_{O_2}(C)}}. \tag{7.11}$$

Toward the end of the capillary (point 2) Pb_{O_2} is low and anoxia is reached after a shorter distance (curve 22).

This very simple model can, clearly, do no more than elucidate a few of the basic principles that govern O_2 flow into the tissue. To learn more we must now examine O_2 supply in the Krogh cylinder model, where we expect O_2 to diffuse radially into the tissue or cell sleeve that surrounds an axial capillary. Radial diffusion follows somewhat different functions than those shown in Figure 7.14 for linear diffusion, but the principle is the same: the P_{O_2} is highest near the capillary and falls off along the radial distance r, and it falls more rapidly as $\dot{m}_{O_2}(C)$ becomes larger (Fig. 7.15).

If we look at two similar radial discs located at two points along the capillary path (Fig. 7.16), it is evident that they will be exposed to a different Pb_{O_2} since O_2 is extracted from the blood along the way. Even though $\dot{m}_{O_2}(C)$ may be the same in both discs the P_{O_2} profile will be different because of the lower head pressure in the second disc along the line. And thus at equal distances r the P_{O_2} will decrease as we move along the tissue cylinder from the arteriolar to the venular

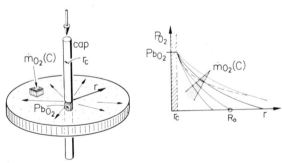

Fig. 7.15 More realistic model of "cell sleeve" around capillary considers radial diffusion of O_2. As local O_2 consumption — $\dot{m}_{O_2}(c)$ — increases the P_{O_2} profile is steeper.

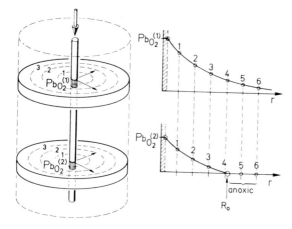

Fig. 7.16 In a given segment of the Krogh cylinder the P_{O_2} profile also depends on the distance along the capillary, since capillary Pb_{O_2} as head pressure for diffusion falls as blood flows through, owing to O_2 extraction.

end. The anoxic region will begin at a shorter distance from the capillary in the second slice.

O_2 DELIVERY INTO THE KROGH CYLINDER

Let us now see how the various factors involved affect the delivery of O_2 into the Krogh cylinder and, in particular, what kind of spatial P_{O_2} distribution results. The Krogh cylinder model shown in Figure 7.17 is thought to represent one capillary path from arteriole (a) to venule (v); note that its dimensions have been purposely distorted: relative to the diameter shown, it should in reality be about ten times as long. Consider first the distribution of P_{O_2} in the blood along the capillary path. For that purpose I have plotted, beneath the cylinder, the relation between P_{O_2} and O_2 saturation (or O_2 content) which, as we saw in chapter 6, depends on the O_2Hb equilibrium curve shown as fine lines for three different pH values (Bohr effect). I have based this plot on data measured in a goat running on a treadmill at $\dot{V}_{O_2}$max. The plot makes two assumptions: (1) the quantity of O_2 delivered in each unit length of the path is constant, so that saturation decreases linearly from about 97% in arterial to 28% in venous blood; (2) the CO_2 uptake along the path is also constant so the P_{CO_2} increases linearly, and pH decreases linearly from 7.4 to 7.2, the measured

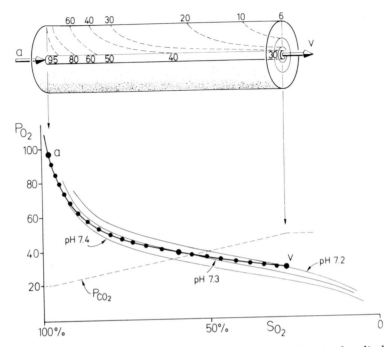

Fig. 7.17 Conventional representation of P_{O_2} profiles in the Krogh cylinder (top) as a function of the distance along the capillary shows cone- or funnel-shaped surfaces of equal P_{O_2}. Uptake of CO_2 by the blood causes blood pH to fall along the capillary, with the result that the Bohr shift causes capillary P_{O_2} to remain relatively high (bottom).

values. The "physiological O_2Hb equilibrium curve" resulting from this is shown as a heavy dotted line. It can be seen that, because of the Bohr effect, the capillary blood maintains a relatively higher P_{O_2} toward the venous end; in fact, after the first third of the path the P_{O_2} falls very little. The effect is appreciable, for in the end part of the capillary path the P_{O_2} is maintained above 30 torr, a good 40% higher than would result without Bohr shift.

The P_{O_2} profile in the Krogh cylinder is established by radial diffusion of O_2 from the capillary, and the factors governing this process are essentially those elaborated above in relation to Figure 7.14: they depend on the diffusion constant K, on the rate of O_2 consumption, $\dot{m}_{O_2}(C)$, and on the capillary P_{O_2}. These factors determine to which radial distance R_0 O_2 can diffuse, or, in other words, beyond which the tissue must be anoxic. The following relationship, due to Krogh, describes the situation:

$$P_{O_2}(cap) = \frac{\dot{m}_{O_2}(C)}{2\,K} \left[R_0{}^2 \cdot \ln \left(\frac{R_0}{r_c} \right) - \frac{R_0{}^2 - r_c{}^2}{2} \right]. \tag{7.12}$$

From the data on maximal O_2 consumption one can calculate that $\dot{m}_{O_2}(C)$ should be of the order of 0.05 to 0.1 ml $O_2 \cdot min^{-1} \cdot ml^{-1}$ in muscle tissue. Taking the capillary radius r_c to be 3 μm and assuming $K = 2 \cdot 10^{-18}$ ml $\cdot min^{-1} \cdot cm^{-1} \cdot mm\ Hg^{-1}$, we find R_0 to be of the order of 50 to 25 μm for $P_{O_2}(cap)$ values of 40 mm Hg or less, the typical values at the venous end of capillaries. Note that we had calculated above, on the basis of morphometric data, the radius of Krogh cylinders to be of the order of 25 μm or less (Table 7.1). The tissue unit for O_2 supply from one capillary is hence smaller than the critical radius calculated by Krogh's equation. We would therefore not expect anoxic regions to occur, except at very high rates of O_2 consumption and then only near the venular end.

Radial diffusion of O_2 and gradual loss of O_2 along the capillary path result in an interesting P_{O_2} profile in the tissue sleeve around the capillary (Fig. 7.17): considering points of equal P_{O_2} (isobars), we see that these do not lie on cylindrical surfaces but on a "cone" or "funnel" that tapers toward the venular end. This has led to the postulate that the tissue located near the venular end of the capillary path is less well supplied with O_2 than other parts of the muscle, and that critical levels of O_2 content may be reached in this region under certain conditions. If we consider that the capillaries follow along the muscle fibers, this may mean that certain segments of the fiber can work less well than others because they cannot produce ATP in sufficient amount. Clearly, this is not very good because, evidently, the strength of a chain is as good as that of its weakest link. However, this need not be so.

If we look at Figure 7.3 we observe that the number of capillaries coursing alongside the muscle fibers increases as we move from the arteriolar to the venular end. Consequently, the capillary density increases as the P_{O_2} falls (Fig. 7.18), and the distance R into the cells that must be furnished with O_2 from one capillary decreases. The Krogh cylinder should therefore be tapering toward the venule and perhaps be replaced by a model we could call the Krogh cone because it still obeys the same laws as his cylinder model. The evidence

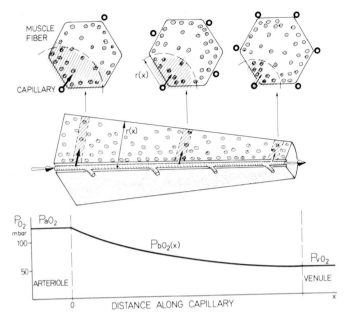

Fig. 7.18 Because the capillary density appears to increase toward the venular end of the capillary path it might be more appropriate to consider a cone-shaped Krogh model, where the fraction of the cell that must be supplied with O_2 from one capillary becomes smaller as P_{O_2} falls along the capillary.

supporting this new model is still scanty and mostly qualitative, so that we don't really know how R decreases along the capillary path. It would be nice to think the boundary of the Krogh cone should follow approximately one of the P_{O_2} isobar surfaces shown in Figure 7.17 for this would assure homogeneous oxygenation of the muscle fibers along their length. If this should turn out to be the case, we could conclude that the capillary density is adapted to the tissue's O_2 needs not only globally but also locally. But clearly this is mere speculation at present.

In spite of this refined model we are still left with the fact that the P_{O_2} near the capillary, that is, near the cell surface, is higher than it is deeper in the cell. This is perhaps not so important for oxidative phosphorylation because this process can apparently operate even at a rather low P_{O_2} of only a few torr. However, in the center of the muscle fiber there is clearly less O_2 available than at the periphery. But now we must remember that the mitochondria are not evenly spread throughout the muscle cells: in Figures 5.7 and 7.6 we have seen that the mitochondrial density decreases from the periphery to the center of the fiber; it looks almost as if the local mitochondrial density were matched to the P_{O_2} and thus to the O_2 content prevailing at different distances from the capillary. But here again the data that would establish such a match beyond speculation are still lacking.

In any event, we can draw two important conclusions from this radial distribution gradient of mitochondria: (1) The local $\dot{m}_{O_2}(C)$ is not constant throughout the cell but decreases as we move away from the capillary and this causes the P_{O_2} profile to become flatter, as shown by the broken curve in Figure 7.15, thus allowing P_{O_2}, the driving force for O_2 diffusion, to remain relatively higher in the deeper parts of the cell. (2) There is more ATP generated in the peripheral parts of the cell, so that the ATP concentration decreases toward the center; this may cause high-energy phosphates to move inward, using the creatine phosphate transfer system mentioned in chapters 2 and 5, a hypothetical feature which could again improve energy supply to the center of the cells because it would be effected by parallel (and independent) diffusion of both O_2 and energy-rich phosphates (Fig. 7.19).

But there is still another factor which helps to bring O_2 into the deeper parts of the muscle cells: the presence of *myoglobin*, a small hemoglobin molecule of molecular weight 17,000 daltons, containing one heme and thus representing about a quarter of the hemoglobin

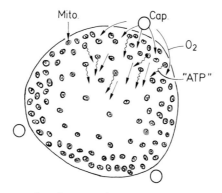

Fig. 7.19 The uneven distribution of mitochondria in the muscle cells (see Fig. 5.7) may cause local O_2 consumption to be higher near the capillaries than further away. This may also cause high-energy phosphates (ATP) to spread from the cell periphery inward.

tetramer (Fig. 6.1). Like hemoglobin, myoglobin can bind O_2 reversibly. One proposed function for myoglobin — which is present at much higher concentration in oxidative than in glycolytic fibers and causes the red color of the former — is to serve as a cellular O_2 store which could even out fluctuations in O_2 supply and on which the cell draws at the onset of oxidative phosphorylation. However, the second function, discovered by P. Scholander in 1960, is perhaps more important: it is the fact that diffusion of O_2 through a solution of hemoglobin is much greater than through water. This phenomenon is called *diffusion facilitation*; its importance lies in the fact that facilitation is greater the lower the P_{O_2}.

Scholander's classical experiment is worth a brief account. He absorbed water, plasma, or hemoglobin solutions in a highly porous membrane which he fitted between two chambers. On one side of the membrane was air, on the other a vacuum, so that the gases of the air, N_2 and O_2, diffused through the membrane. If the membrane contained water and plasma, the ratio of O_2/N_2 diffusing across was constantly 0.5, a predictable value. If the membrane contained hemoglobin, however, the amount of O_2 flowing through was doubled, whereas N_2 diffusion was unchanged: the ratio O_2/N_2 was 1. Thus hemoglobin facilitates O_2 diffusion specifically, and it could be shown that this is related to reversible binding of O_2 to the heme.

The really interesting things happened when Scholander reduced the pressure of the air in the chamber from 1 to $\frac{1}{3}$ atmosphere or less: the O_2/N_2 ratio increased dramatically when the pressure fell, resulting in an up to eightfold increase of diffusion facilitation for O_2. Thus clearly, the ability of hemoglobin, and myoglobin as well, to facilitate diffusion of O_2 increases as the P_{O_2} decreases. The physiological consequences of this effect are now evident: while myoglobin may facilitate diffusion of O_2 throughout the fiber, this effect becomes particularly marked when the P_{O_2} has fallen to very low values of, say, 10 torr or less; as a result, the P_{O_2} profile is lifted upward in the region of its tail. In Figure 7.20 I have tried to summarize these various effects on the P_{O_2} profile along a radial distance r from the capillary. The family of fine curves indicates how different levels of $\dot{m}_{O_2}(C)$ would lead to a drop of P_{O_2} (compare Fig. 7.15). Assuming $\dot{m}_{O_2}$ to be proportional to V_{vmi}, and knowing that V_{vmi} decreases along r, the actual P_{O_2} profile would follow the heavy curve as it is affected by lower and lower values of $\dot{m}_{O_2}$. Notice that this extends the P_{O_2} profile further into the cell as compared to the case where $\dot{m}_{O_2}(C)$ is evenly

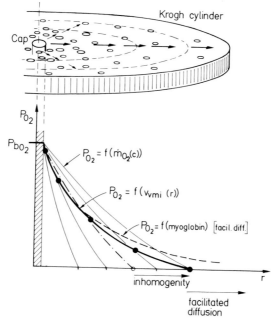

Fig. 7.20 Combined effect of inhomogeneity of local O_2 consumption and of facilitated diffusion of O_2 due to myoglobin may carry O_2 deeper into cell than expected from basic models.

distributed throughout the cell, shown by the dotted curve. When the P_{O_2} has fallen to low values, facilitated diffusion becomes a significant factor, and the P_{O_2} profile is extended even deeper into the cell as shown by the broken curve. Facilitated diffusion will have a particularly pronounced effect in the parts of the cells lying along the end part of the capillary path where P_{O_2} is low to begin with (Fig. 7.17).

Indeed, it appears that many tricks are used to overcome a seemingly difficult problem, namely that of preventing the P_{O_2} in the cell from falling to zero, and thus keeping the "fire of life" burning all through the cell, even though some of the boundary conditions would tend to extinguish it. The shape of the O_2 Hb equilibrium curve, as well as the Bohr and temperature shifts, keep the capillary P_{O_2} relatively high all along the capillary, while still allowing a large quantity of O_2 to be discharged. And as the O_2 molecules diffuse radially into the cell, the P_{O_2} is again prevented from falling too rapidly because of inhomogeneous distribution of mitochondria and because of facilitated diffusion. And then, also, the density of capillaries increases as P_{O_2} falls along the capillary, thus adjusting the size of the cell compartment to be supplied with O_2 from one capillary to the O_2 available. This part of the system appears, indeed, well designed.

Summary

The distribution of blood to the various organs depends on the distribution of resistances among the vessels of the arterial tree. The resistance in a tube is proportional to the fourth power of the vessel radius (Poiseuille's law); the circular smooth muscle sleeve of arteries allows this radius to be finely regulated, down to the smallest branches, the arterioles.

Gas exchange in the tissues occurs in capillaries, whose walls are completely lined by greatly attenuated endothelial cells; capillaries are enveloped by a basement membrane and may be provided with pericytes, branched cells whose slim processes are contractile. Capillaries form networks whose architecture depends on the shape of the cells or tissue units that are supplied. They are organized into microvascular units which begin at the arteriole and end at the venule. The total path from arteriole to venule is of the order of 0.5–1 mm in mammalian muscle, where the capillary network aligns preferentially along the muscle fibers.

Capillary density in the tissue determines the amount of blood available for gas exchange and the distance that O_2 has to diffuse into the tissue. In muscle this is often characterized by estimating the number of capillaries per mm² of muscle cross-section. A better descriptor is the capillary length density, that is the capillary length per unit tissue volume, a parameter that can be estimated by stereological methods. The results of either estimate are used to describe tissue gas exchange in terms of the Krogh cylinder model, that is, by determining the dimensions (radius and length) of the tissue cylinder that must be supplied with O_2 from one capillary. In mammalian muscle the radius of the Krogh cylinder is of the order of 12–25 μm, its length 0.5–1 mm.

In muscle capillary density shows considerable variation, from a few hundred to a few thousand per mm² of cross-section. This is directly related to the cells' O_2 needs because capillary density is linearly proportional to mitochondrial volume density in muscle cells. One finds that there is consistently 1 μm^3 of capillary blood for every 3 μm^3 of mitochondria in the muscle cells. This holds from the skeletal muscles of man to the heart of the Etruscan shrew. The relation of capillary to mitochondrial density shows considerable local variations; one reason is that capillaries serve other functions than to supply O_2, such as the provision of substrates or the removal of wastes (lactate) and heat.

The flow of O_2 into the tissues occurs by diffusion; the driving force is provided by the P_{O_2} in the capillary which falls along the capillary path from arterial to venous P_{O_2}. This fall is somewhat attenuated by the Bohr effect due to CO_2 uptake from the cells. In the cells of the Krogh cylinder the P_{O_2} falls with the radial distance from the capillary, as a function of O_2 consumption. The combination of axial and radial fall in P_{O_2} along the Krogh cylinder endangers O_2 supply to the peripheral parts of the terminal segment of the cylinder. This is avoided by a number of design features of the system: the capillary density increases toward the venous end of the microvascular unit, so that the Krogh cylinder tapers and therefore is more appropriately described by a cone model; the mitochondria are unevenly distributed within the cell, showing a higher concentration near the capillary; muscle cells contain myoglobin which facilitates O_2 diffusion when the P_{O_2} is very low. It appears that many tricks are used to prevent P_{O_2} in the cell or rather near the mitochondria from falling to zero.

Further Reading

Burton, A. C. 1972. Physiology and Biophysics of the Circulation: An Introductory Text. 2nd ed. Chicago: Year Book.

Crone, C., and N. A. Lassen, eds. 1970. The Transfer of Molecules and Ions between Capillary Blood and Tissue. Proceedings of the A. Benzon Symposium 2. Copenhagen: Benzon Foundation.

Hudlická, O. 1973. Muscle Blood Flow: Its Relation to Muscle Metabolism and Function. Amsterdam: Swets and Zeitlinger.

——— 1982. Growth of capillaries in skeletal and cardiac muscle. Circulation Research 50:451–461.

——— 1984. Growth and development of microcirculation. In Handbook of Physiology: Microcirculation. Washington: American Physiological Society (in press).

* Krogh, A. 1922. *Anatomy and Physiology of Capillaries.* New Haven: Yale University Press. (2nd ed. 1929.)

Romanul, F. C. A., and M. Pollock. 1969. The parallelism of changes in oxidative metabolism and capillary supply of skeletal muscle fibers. In *Modern Neurology,* ed. S. Locke. Boston: Little, Brown, pp. 203–213.

Weibel, E. R. 1979. Oxygen demand and the size of respiratory structures in mammals. In *Evolution of Respiratory Processes,* ed. S. C. Wood and C. Lenfant. New York: Dekker, pp. 289–346.

Wittenberg, J. B. 1970. Myoglobin-facilitated oxygen diffusion: role of myoglobin in oxygen entry into muscle. *Physiological Reviews* 50:559–636.

References

Andersen, P., and J. Hendriksson. 1977. Capillary supply of the quadriceps femoris muscle of man: adaptive response to exercise. *Journal of Physiology* (London) 270:677–690.

Brown, M. D., M. A. Cotter, O. Hudlická, and G. Vrbova. 1976. The effects of different patterns of muscle activity on capillary density, mechanical properties and structure of slow and fast rabbit muscles. *Pflügers Archiv* 361:241–250.

Bruns, R. R., and G. E. Palade. 1968. Studies on blood capillaries. I. General organization of blood capillaries in muscle. *Journal of Cell Biology* 37:244–276.

Cole, R. P. 1983. Skeletal muscle function in hypoxia: effect of alteration in intracellular myoglobin. *Respiration Physiology* 53:1–14.

Fletcher, J. E. 1980. On facilitated oxygen diffusion in muscle tissues. *Biophysical Journal* 29:437–458.

Gray, S. D., and E. M. Renkin. 1978. Microvascular supply in relation to fiber metabolic type in mixed skeletal muscles of rabbits. *Microvascular Research* 16:406–425.

Hammersen, F. 1968. The pattern of the terminal vascular bed and the ultrastructure of capillaries in skeletal muscle. In *Oxygen Transport in Blood and Tissue,* ed. D. W. Lübbers, U. C. Luft, G. Thews, and E. Witzleb. Stuttgart: Thieme, pp. 184–197.

Hermansen, L., and M. Wachtlova. 1971. Capillary density of skeletal muscle in well-trained and untrained men. *Journal of Applied Physiology* 30:860–863.

Hoppeler, H., O. Mathieu, R. Krauer, H. Claassen, R. B. Armstrong, and E. R. Weibel. 1981a. Design of the mammalian respiratory system. VI. Distribution of mitochondria and capillaries in various muscles. *Respiration Physiology* 44:87–111.

Hoppeler, H., O. Mathieu, E. R. Weibel, R. Krauer, S. L. Lindstedt, and C. R.

Taylor. 1981b. Design of the mammalian respiratory system. VIII. Capillaries in skeletal muscles. *Respiration Physiology* 44:129–150.

Ingjer, F. 1979. Effects of endurance training on muscle fibre ATP-ase activity, capillary supply and mitochondrial content in man. *Journal of Physiology* (London) 294:419–432.

* Krogh, A. 1919. The number and distribution of capillaries in muscles with calculations of the oxygen pressure head necessary for supplying the tissue. *Journal of Physiology* (London) 52:409–415.

Ljungqvist, A., and U. Gunnar. 1977. Capillary proliferative activity in myocardium and skeletal muscle of exercised rats. *Journal of Applied Physiology* 43:306–307.

Mathieu, O., L. M. Cruz-Orive, H. Hoppeler, and E. R. Weibel. 1983. Estimating length density and quantifying anisotropy in skeletal muscle capillaries. *Journal of Microscopy* 131:131–146.

Myrhage, R., and O. Hudlická, 1976. The microvascular bed and capillary surface area in rat extensor hallucis proprius muscle (EHP). *Microvascular Research* 11:315–323.

—— 1978. Capillary growth in chronically stimulated adult skeletal muscle as studied by intravital microscopy and histological methods in rabbits and rats. *Microvascular Research* 16:73–90.

Plyley, M. J., and A. C. Groom. 1975. Geometrical distribution of capillaries in mammalian striated muscle. *American Journal of Physiology* 228:1376–1383.

Plyley, M. J., G. J. Sutherland, and A. C. Groom. 1976. Geometry of the capillary network in skeleton muscle. *Microvascular Research* 11:161–173.

Romanul, F. C. A. 1965. Capillary supply and metabolism of muscle fibers. *Archives of Neurology* 12:497–509.

Schmidt-Nielsen, K., and P. Pennycuik. 1961. Capillary density in mammals in relation to body size and oxygen consumption. *American Journal of Physiology* 200:746–750.

* Scholander, P. F. 1960. Oxygen transport through hemoglobin solutions. *Science* 131:585–590.

Simionescu, N., M. Simionescu, and G. E. Palade. 1973. Permeability of muscle capillaries to exogenous myoglobin. *Journal of Cell Biology* 57:424–452.

Tyml, K., C. G. Ellis, R. G. Safranyos, S. Fraser, and A. Groom. 1981. Temporal and spatial distributions of red cell velocity in capillaries of resting skeletal muscle, including estimates of red cell transit times. *Microvascular Research* 22:14–31.

Weibel, E. R. 1979. Oxygen demand and the size of respiratory structures in mammals. In *Evolution of Respiratory Processes*, ed. S. C. Wood and C. Lenfant. New York: Dekker, pp. 289–346.

Weibel, E. R., C. R. Taylor, P. Gehr, H. Hoppeler, O. Mathieu, and G. M. O. Maloiy. 1981. Design of the mammalian respiratory system. IX. Functional and structural limits for oxygen flow. *Respiration Physiology* 44:151–164.

Whalen, W. J., D. Buerk, and C. A. Thuning. 1973. Blood-flow-limited oxygen consumption in resting cat skeletal muscle. *American Journal of Physiology* 224:763–768.

Wittenberg, B. A., J. B. Wittenberg, and P. R. B. Caldwell. 1975. Role of myoglobin in the oxygen supply to red skeletal muscle. *Journal of Biological Chemistry* 250:9038–9043.

Wolff, J. R., C. Goerz, T. Bär, and F. H. Güldner. 1975. Common morphogenetic aspects of various organotypic microvascular patterns. *Microvascular Research* 10:373–395.

8

DESIGN AND DEVELOPMENT
OF THE MAMMALIAN LUNG

FOR THE NEXT FEW CHAPTERS we shall be concerned with the question how to get O_2 from the environmental air into the blood at an adequate rate. This transfer occurs by diffusion, so in principle all we need to do is to establish a gas exchanger in which air and blood come into very intimate contact over a sufficiently large area, for we had seen before that the rate of O_2 diffusion is increased if the barrier that separates air and blood is made thinner and of larger expanse. The problem is that the requirements for a large surface and a thin barrier are apparently rather excessive. To ensure an O_2 flow rate of up to 3 liters per minute, required by the muscles of a runner, the air–blood contact surface must be about the size of a tennis court, and the barrier separating air and blood should be 50 times thinner than a sheet of air-mail paper! Furthermore the gas at the barrier surface must be rapidly replenished with O_2 from the environmental store, and blood must be allowed to flow past the barrier at a high rate. Clearly, all this poses a number of quite formidable engineering problems which we should now examine.

The first problem is how to build an extremely thin barrier which can completely and tightly separate air and blood, and can remain intact for a life time in spite of its being exposed to blood under pressure on one side and to environmental air on the other. The barrier must be able to control its permeability to fluids, for example, and to rapidly repair any damages that may result from a variety of possible insults. This calls for a lining by live cells in the form of two epithelial—that is, confluent and sealed—cell layers, one on the air side and the other toward the blood. Such cell layers can control the transit of water and solutes and can repair damages because of their capacity to synthesize proteins and lipids as well as to replace injured cells by cell division.

Since these cell layers must be very thin, they must be supported by a scaffold of connective tissue fibers which give the lung mechanical strength. But these fibers should not hinder gas exchange; they must therefore be reduced to a minimum but still be strong enough to withstand the various forces that act on them, and this requires a rather clever design tending to find an optimal compromise between two conflicting conditions.

The last problem is how to rapidly exchange the two media on either side of the thin barrier, air and blood, and mainly how to ensure that this occurs as evenly as possible over the entire large surface.

It turns out that the solution to these problems is to subdivide the gas exchange barrier into a large number of small units which are suspended on a strong three-dimensional fiber system. Even ventilation of these units is made possible by wrapping the barrier around the sac-like terminations of a heavily branched airway tree. The pulmonary arteries and veins form similar trees whose end-twigs converge in capillary networks that are wrapped around the terminal airway units.

Thus the basic structure of the lung looks like three well-matched interdigitating trees, one each for air, venous, and arterial blood, which converge in the small gas exchange units at their end branches. This is the result of a well-ordered process of morphogenesis during early development. The tree-like structure introduces a natural hierarchy of elements as we go from the central airways and blood vessels to the terminal branches. In gross terms we must distinguish two *functional zones* which result from differentiation during the later stages of development: the central parts of the trees are made of a set of branched conduits — bronchi, arteries, veins — whose function is to guide and distribute air and blood to the peripheral units where they are brought into very close contact so as to allow gas exchange. We call the entire complex of gas exchange units the *respiratory zone* of the lung, and the set of conduits with their associated structures the *conducting zone*.

The systematic development of a complex of branched trees combined with the differentiation of functional zones along the pathway make for a high degree of structural order. This is perhaps not conspicuous at first glance because this entire complex must develop into a confined space, the chest cavity, which it will, eventually, fill completely. But we shall see later on that this does not prevent the lung from adhering to some very strong engineering rules in building a functionally well-proportioned system — just as a good architect can design beautiful and functionally satisfying buildings in spite of the many constraints imposed by landscape, city planning, and preexisting structures.

Development of the Lung

Before describing some of the essential steps that lead to the development of the mammalian lung, let me recall a few basic facts about the structure of the lung and its location in the body, facts which are the ultimate result of the developmental steps I shall describe subsequently.

First, the airways of the lung communicate with the upper part of the digestive tract through the larynx. This indicates that airways and intestine have a common origin; indeed, we shall show that the airways derive directly from the gut anlage.

The second important point is that the lung fills the chest cavity; it is, however, not directly connected with the chest wall, but is rather separated from it by the narrow pleural space which is filled with a little bit of fluid and bounded toward both the lung and the chest wall by an epithelial lining, the pleural mesothelium, features which allow the lung to move within the chest. The pleural space is part of the embryonic body cavity or coelom, the space that separates the gut wall from the body wall; considering the gut origin of the airways, it is therefore likely that the lung incorporates parts of the splanchnopleura, the bounded mesenchymal layer that enwraps the gut toward the coelom.

Third, the pulmonary circulation runs from the right ventricle to the left atrium; the pulmonary arteries and veins must therefore connect with the heart through connective tissue bridges, one leading from the ventricular outflow tract into the lung, the other connecting the lung to the left atrial wall, connections which must be established during development. A result of this close relation between heart and lung is the fact that both are housed within the chest cavity, separated only by a thin fiber bag, the pericardium. But both the heart and the lung are anchored on the body wall through the posterior mediastinum, the complex of structures that extends from the neck to the diaphragm, and lies between the lungs, the spine, and the heart. This is, then, the general anatomic situation that must be achieved by lung development.

When the lung begins to develop, the embryo must have reached the stage where an intestinal tube has formed from the entoderm, the foregut being that part of the tube which lies cranially to the intestinal loop (Fig. 8.1). The head has formed, and the buccal cavity is connected to the foregut through the perforated buccopharyngeal membrane. The heart loop has been displaced ventrally, and its atrial and ventricular parts are in the process of separation into the four chambers, left and right atrium, and left and right ventricles, respectively. The two sinus horns, the entrances into the right atrium, straddle the gut just anterior to the intestinal loop, since they collect

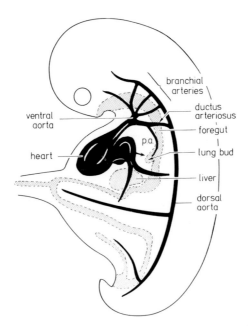

Fig. 8.1 The first stages of lung morphogenesis occur during the fourth week of human fetal development; they involve the formation of a lung bud from the foregut and the outgrowth of a pulmonary artery from the sixth branchial artery on each side. The arrow indicates the origin of the pulmonary veins.

the blood from the body wall (cardinal veins) and from the intestine (vitelline vein); this arrangement of the main body veins and the development of the liver around the vitelline veins gives rise to the separation of the chest and abdominal cavities through the formation of the diaphragm. At this stage the ventral aorta which arises from the still common ventricle splits into two main branches that follow the foremost part of the foregut and give rise to six pairs of branchial arteries which cross the side of the foregut to reach the dorsal aorta; note that this is the vascular pathway in fishes where the branchial or gill arteries perfuse the gills (Fig. 1.9), one of the best examples for the theory that our phylogenetic ancestry is duplicated during ontogenetic development.

At about this stage the foregut begins to form two little ventrolateral buds, the anlage for the two lungs, and a longitudinal groove, the anlage of the trachea (Fig. 8.2a). If we first look at the development of the trachea, we will see that it becomes separated from the esophagus by a septum that begins to form at the root of the lung buds by fusion of epithelial ridges and then extends cranially; this is of importance because it explains the mechanism by which esophagotracheal fistulae, a relatively common malformation of the newborn, can be formed, namely by incomplete fusion of the epithelial ridges from which the septum is progressively made. When the septum is complete, the larynx forms as a gate between "food ways" and "air ways."

Meanwhile the lung buds grow laterally, pushing outward the splanchnopleural mesenchyme that enwraps the gut. They then begin to branch, forming, in the human fetus, first two branches on the left and three branches on the right side; it is important to note that these first branchings involve not only the epithelial tube but also the splanchnopleural wrapping, so that we end up, at this early stage, with the formation of the five lobes that are typical of a human lung: two on the left and three on the right (Fig. 8.2b). In animals this pattern may be different in that most mammals form a fourth lobe on the right, whereas in small rodents (mice and rats) the left lung forms a single lobe.

Once branching is initiated it goes on and on, but now only the epithelial tubes divide within the mesenchymal bed of the splanchnopleura. Very soon the final shape of the lung emerges (Fig. 8.2c) because the lung develops into the space which is available, essentially to the side of the spine, the foregut, and the heart.

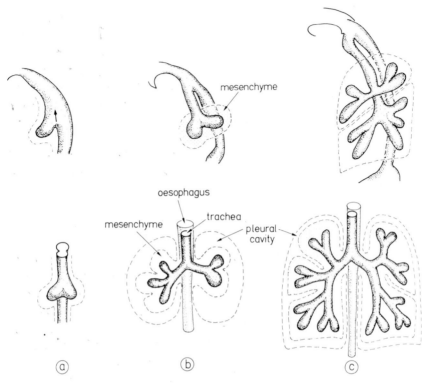

Fig. 8.2 Lateral and frontal view of a developing human lung during the fourth (a), fifth (b), and sixth (c) fetal week.

This process is paralleled by the development of the main pulmonary vessels, starting from the "fish type" vasculature that we found to develop first (Fig. 8.1). When the original ventral aorta separates into the ascending aorta and the pulmonary artery, the latter ends at the sixth branchial arches. An arterial bud originates from the right and left sixth arch on each side and grows along the trachea toward the lung anlage, where it connects with the vascular plexus of the splanchnopleura that enwraps gut and lung beds, as we shall see below. Simultaneously, a venous bud arises from the wall of the left atrium, grows toward the lung anlage, and also connects with the vascular plexus. The pulmonary loop of the circulation (Fig. 6.12) has now been established; however, it is still not completely separated from the systemic circulation. The fact is that one of the sixth branchial arteries (the left one) maintains its connection to the dorsal aorta and becomes, as the ductus arteriosus Botalli, an important pathway for shunting blood from the — yet inactive — lung to the tissues of the body that need a lot of O_2. The ductus arteriosus Botalli is closed only after birth, that is, after the lung begins to supply the blood with O_2. A second shunting pathway is preserved in the form of a hole in the atrial septum, the foramen ovale, so that part of the right atrial blood is shunted into the left atrium.

The development of the lung is determined by a number of fundamental principles which we now need to consider in some detail.

The *pattern of lung development* is determined by the branching pattern of the epithelial airway tube, which is the "pacemaker" of the process. The tubes grow in length owing to rapid proliferation of the epithelial cells; mitoses occur everywhere along the tube, but they are particularly frequent at the tubes' endings, the so-called bronchial buds, which are slightly widened. The tubes then divide at these buds into two daughter branches, a process which is called *dichotomy* ("splitting into two"). Note that by dichotomy the number of airway branches is doubled with each generation, a feature which we shall exploit in chapter 11 when we try to set up a model for the airway tree.

Although *airway development* appears to be the decisive morphogenetic factor in shaping the lung, it has been shown that the epithelial airway buds will only divide if they are in intimate contact with the mesenchyme. If a terminal bud is freed of its mesenchymal coat, it grows in length but does not divide until it becomes enwrapped by mesenchyme again. Conversely, mesenchyme removed from a bud and implanted on the epithelium of the trachea leads to the formation of a new bud which continues to divide like a terminal bronchial bud. This indicates that the process of airway division is induced by some mesenchymal factors which are, however, unidentified as yet. It is therefore safe to conclude that the development of a well-designed lung depends on the interaction between epithelium and mesenchyme, a principle which also holds for many other developmental processes throughout the body.

The *pulmonary vasculature* is a derivative of the mesenchyme. In an early embryo the foregut — as the entire intestinal tube — is enwrapped by a vascular plexus which is fed from the aorta and drained into the major veins. The lung buds which develop from the foregut epithelium carry this plexus along; it forms the basis for the development of the pulmonary vasculature because the ingrowing

pulmonary arteries and veins connect with it. The original connection to the aorta is, however, retained and eventually develops into
the bronchial arteries, the vessels that nourish the major conducting
airways in a mature lung. In the course of development of an airway
tree this plexus wraps around all branches, and some paths become
enlarged to arteries or veins. Note, however, that this process allows
a closed circuit to be maintained at all times with blood flowing from
the pulmonary artery through the plexus into the veins. The blood
flow is, however, relatively small because a good part of the blood is
shunted into the systemic circulation through the ductus Botalli and
the foramen ovale.

The mesenchyme that enwraps the airway tubes and contains the
vasculature develops into a complex *supporting structure* for the
lung and its elements (Fig. 8.3). In a general way, we can distinguish
the following features. We find that those airways which do not
further branch become enwrapped by a dense sheath of mesenchyme from which smooth muscle fibers, strong connective tissue
fiber sheaths, and, in part, cartilage will develop, thus forming all
elements of the bronchial wall. The larger vessels — arteries and
veins — also become enwrapped with condensed mesenchyme
which will form smooth muscle fibers in varying amount. The remaining loose mesenchyme forms sheaths that enwrap and separate
the airway units that result from branching. These sheaths are all
connected directly or indirectly to the splanchnopleura and are thus
the anlage for a complex system of connective tissue septa which, as
we shall see, transmit the ventilatory pull of the pleura into the
depths of the lung. Note that this is the developmental basis of the
fiber continuum that pervades the entire lung and is a major factor
determining the lung's mechanical properties (see chapter 10).

The branching of airways, as the main determinants of lung structure, results in an organ whose elements are *space-filling* with no
gaps between the units. Indeed, we shall see later that even the
mesenchymal sheets which separate the units in the early fetal lung
(Fig. 8.3) become reduced to minimal connective tissue strands hard
to see in a histological section. It is hard to visualize a dichotomous
branching process in three dimensions that results in this kind of
space-filling structure. One is, however, immediately reminded of
the beautiful and fascinating fractal trees that Benoit Mandelbrot has
constructed; the one shown in Figure 8.4 looks remarkably like a
two-dimensional lung. In fractal trees the dimensions of the branches

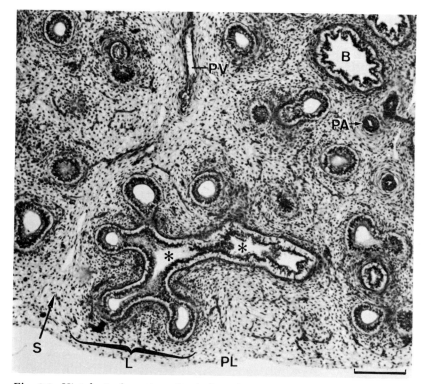

Fig. 8.3 Histological section of subpleural part of human fetal lung (about twelfth week) shows the beginning differentiation of the epithelial tube into bronchi (B) and peripheral branches (*). A lobule (L) is bounded by the septum (S) and the visceral pleura (PL). Note the location of a pulmonary artery (PA) and vein (PV). Scale marker: 200 μm.

become smaller with each generation according to a logarithmic rule, a morphogenetic principle akin to the natural growth rule that causes the nautilus to make its beautiful spiral shell. One can, in fact, recognize the so-called logarithmic spiral of the nautilus in the fractal tree of Figure 8.4, as well. The principle of the fractal tree allows the branches to undergo an infinite number of divisions, expanding gradually into the interstices; but only at the limit will the tree fill the entire area completely and homogeneously, without any gaps.

The fractal tree hence appears as an excellent model to describe the formation of an orderly, space-filling lung, particularly since we shall see in chapter 12 that the progression of airway dimensions

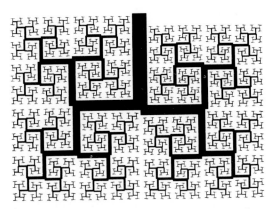

Fig. 8.4 Fractal tree model of Benoit Mandelbrot simulates space-filling branching of airway tree. (From Mandelbrot, 1983; copyright © 1983 by W. H. Freeman and Company.)

does, indeed, follow a logarithmic rule. However, the fractal model cannot elucidate the actual principles that govern growth and division in the real lung. Fractal structures are abstractions, precise mathematical constructions, that admit no compromise, no interference from external factors or constraints. But this is precisely what the developing airway tree has to meet: it develops into a given space whose odd shape is determined by the design of the chest wall, the liver, the heart, and so on, and simply has to reach into every available corner. The result is an *irregular dichotomous tree* with paths of different length, but the dimensions of the branches — length and diameter — are still regulated according to strict physical rules.

Lung Histogenesis: Differentiation toward Gas Exchange

The organ that results from the early developmental processes described in the previous section does not look like a lung at all. Its "airways" are branched tubes with a narrow lumen lined by a rather thick columnar epithelium (Fig. 8.3), a picture easily mistaken by a student of histology as a section through a gland. This stage in the development of the lung is therefore commonly called the *pseudoglandular stage;* it is reached by about 17 weeks of gestation in man, and, for comparison, by about 17 days in rats.

This initial development of a spatial system of tubes is then followed by a sequence of histological changes that gradually transform
the lung into a gas exchanger. But note that this still occurs in utero,
while the fetus receives its O_2 supply from the placenta.

In this period of differentiation the conducting airways develop
their characteristic high columnar epithelium; the mesenchymal
sheath begins to form strands of smooth muscle and a strong external
fiber sheath which incorporates, in the larger bronchi, some plates of
cartilage. Gradually we also observe small submucosal glands to
appear in the wall of larger bronchi. By about 25 weeks the conducting airways have developed their full complement of accessory
structures: they can secrete mucus and have developed the potential
for moving a mucus blanket outward by the action of ciliated cells.
Simultaneously, the conducting blood vessels develop their accessory wall, the sheath of smooth muscle being particularly conspicuous in the pulmonary arteries (Fig. 8.3.). It is also of interest that
lymphatic vessels form in this period in the mesenchymal bed associated with pulmonary arteries and veins, thus forming the potential
for draining interstitial fluid, or lymph, out of the lung.

We should be mostly concerned, however, with the differentiation
steps that establish the potential for gas exchange between air and
blood. This essentially requires three processes to occur simultaneously: (1) the epithelial lining of the peripheral airways must be
attenuated; (2) the capillaries must come into close contact with the
epithelium; and (3) the connective tissue or mesenchymal elements
must be reduced to a minimum. This is achieved in three steps, two
of which occur before birth, whereas the final transformation into a
mature lung happens during early postnatal life.

Between the 18th and 25th gestational week in the human fetus, or
from day 18–20 in the rat, the pseudoglandular terminal airways
begin to widen and the lung reaches its canalicular stage. At this
stage begins the differentiation of the epithelial cells into two types
with different function (Fig. 8.5): one cell type gradually becomes a
thin squamous cell whereas the other begins to develop into a
cuboidal secretory cell capable of synthesizing phospholipids which
the lung will need at birth in order to reduce surface tension as the air
spaces fill with air. At the end of this development the peripheral air
spaces have become wide, mostly due to the reduction of the mesenchyme to a slim layer (Fig. 8.6); they have reached what is called the
saccular stage, a structural pattern that will remain essentially unchanged until birth.

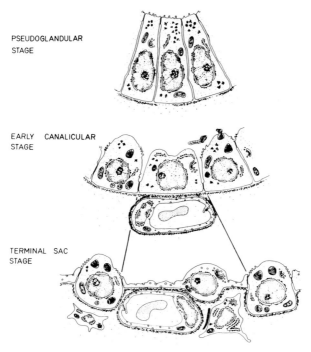

PSEUDOGLANDULAR
STAGE

EARLY CANALICULAR
STAGE

TERMINAL SAC
STAGE

Fig. 8.5 Epithelial transformation in a developing lung from a high columnar epithelium of uniform cell population in the glandular phase to a
cuboidal epithelium with two distinct cell types in the canalicular phase. In
the saccular phase the prospective lining cells (type I) become flattened and
broadened so that a thin barrier to the capillary is formed. Note that secretory type II cells with lamellar bodies occur as of the canalicular phase.
(From Burri and Weibel, 1977.)

Meanwhile the capillaries have also undergone changes. The
rather loose network found scattered in the mesenchyme during the
pseudoglandular stage has gradually become denser and has moved
closer to the airway canaliculi. But only in the saccular stage do we
find the capillaries very closely apposed to the thin squamous lining
cells, separated from the epithelium only by a thin basement membrane (Figs. 8.5 and 8.6). Evidently, a thin air–blood barrier has now
been achieved; the lung could potentially serve as a gas exchange
organ from this stage on. It is important to note that in this saccular
stage each saccule is surrounded by its own closely apposed capillary
network. The septum that separates two adjacent saccules therefore

contains two capillary networks, as well as some mesenchyme (Figs. 8.6 and 8.7).

Throughout this development the "airways" of the lung are filled with fluid, partly formed by exudation from the blood and partly by secretion from the secretory cells in the conducting airways and in the saccules. This lung fluid communicates with the amniotic fluid in which the fetus is bathed, and indeed appears to flow out at a steady rate, perhaps pumped out by "breathing" movements of the chest wall. Thus, some of the fetal lung secretions appear in the amniotic fluid and can therefore be studied by taking a small sample of this fluid through amniocentesis, the widely used clinical procedure of tapping the amnion cavity with a needle. This has become an impor-

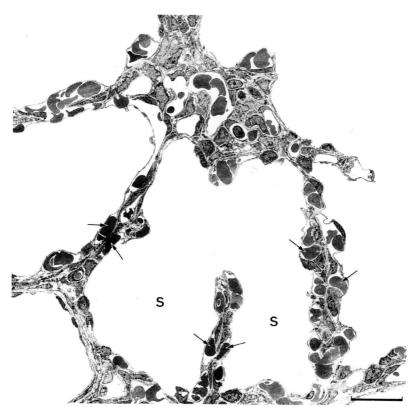

Fig. 8.6 Rat lung at birth is made of wide saccules (S) separated by septa containing two capillary networks (paired arrows). Scale marker: 20 μm. (From Burri, 1974.)

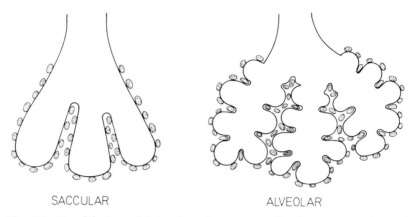

SACCULAR   ALVEOLAR

Fig. 8.7 Simplified model to show how a saccular lung is transformed postnatally into an alveolar lung.

tant diagnostic intervention in recent years because it allows the obstetrician to assess whether the fetal lung is mature for air breathing, which is only the case if the secretory cells of the saccules produce enough surfactant phospholipids to allow the air spaces to remain open when they fill with air, as we shall see in chapters 9 and 11.

The Lung at Birth and Its Postnatal Maturation

When the baby is born the lung is still in its saccular stage; however, it has reached a first mature state allowing it to function as a gas exchanger. If the secretory cells have produced sufficient surfactant, the first breath will expand the saccules with air and they will remain patent. When the umbilical cord has been tied, cutting off the O_2 supply from the placenta, the ductus Botalli and the foramen ovale are closed so that pulmonary circulation becomes fully established. We will in this stage see that the saccular surface is densely covered by blood-filled capillaries with a very thin tissue barrier separating air and blood (Fig. 8.6); O_2 can now freely diffuse into the blood, and the purplish color of the newborn baby turns pink. All is well.

In the weeks that follow, the lung will have to undergo a sequence of structural changes which result in a considerable enlargement of the gas exchange surface and a further substantial thinning of the air–blood barrier. The process can be described as the transformation of the simple saccules into alveolar ducts of rather complex surface, resulting in a so-called *alveolar lung* (Fig. 8.7).

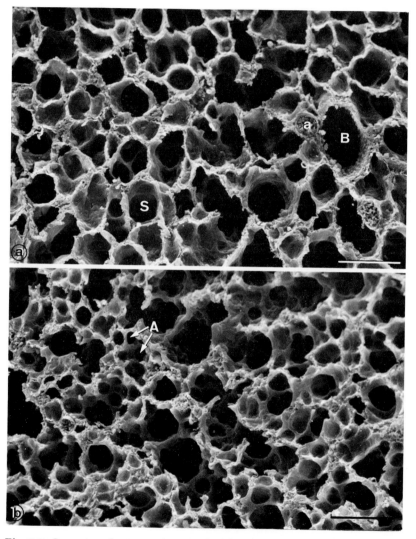

Fig. 8.8 Scanning electron micrographs of rat lungs during postnatal maturation. The wide air spaces on day 4 (a) are saccules (S), whereas on day 8 (b) the smaller units are alveoli (A). Note bronchiole (B) with associated pulmonary artery (a). Scale markers: (a) 100 μm; (b) 100 μm. (Courtesy Dr. P. Burri.)

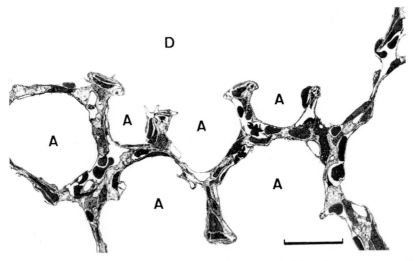

Fig. 8.9 Thin section of rat lung on day 13 of postnatal development. Alveoli (A) have been formed around the duct (D) and the septa contain only one capillary. Scale marker: 20 μm. (Courtesy Dr. P. Burri.)

Alveoli are little pockets that form in large number in the wall of the peripheral airway channels; they are densely packed, similar to the cells in a honeycomb, and are separated by a thin septum that contains capillaries. The formation of these alveoli occurs rather rapidly; in the rat it takes only about five days (from the 5th to the 10th day after birth) to complete the transformation, but in man it seems to take comparatively longer. By this process the peripheral airway surface becomes scalloped (Fig. 8.8), and this evidently increases the gas exchange surface area. This transformation is accompanied by substantial changes in the structure of the septa between air spaces. Whereas in the saccular lung each of these septa contains two capillary networks, one for each adjacent saccule (Fig. 8.6), the septa between alveoli contain only one single capillary network which is now exposed to two alveoli (Fig. 8.9).

The formation of alveoli leads to a drastic and precipitous increase of the lung's internal surface area: from day 4 to 13 in the rat the lung volume doubles as body weight doubles with growth, but the gas exchange surface enlarges disproportionately by a factor of five (Fig. 8.10). After that period the gas exchange surface continues to enlarge at a more steady pace as the lung and the body grow.

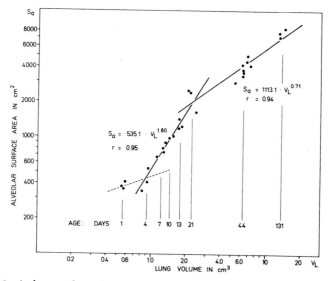

Fig. 8.10 As lung volume increases during early postnatal growth the alveolar surface is enlarged in three steps with a particularly prominent increase between days 4 and 21 in the rat.

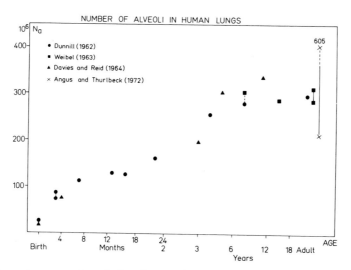

Fig. 8.11 Increase of total alveolar number with age in man. It appears that by age 6 years all alveoli of an adult lung have been formed.

The growth pattern of the human lung appears to be similar, only it takes much longer, as one would expect. The newborn lung is also essentially saccular with very few shallow alveoli. The transformation into an alveolar lung occurs during the first few months; subsequently the lung grows by both expansion and by addition of new units until the final number of about 300 million alveoli is reached at about the age of 5–6 years (Fig. 8.11).

Summary

The design of the lung as a gas exchanger between air and blood requires a large number of microvascular gas exchange units to be arranged in such a way that they can be efficiently ventilated with air and perfused with blood. Gas exchange requires a large surface of air–blood contact and a very thin barrier which must be made of cells to control its permeability to fluids. The solution is to arrange the gas exchange units around the terminal branches of a highly branched airway tree. The microvascular units extend between the terminal branches of the arterial and the venous tree, which are patterned according to the airway tree.

During lung development, a left and right bronchial bud are formed at the distal end of the trachea, which has developed from a ventral groove in the foregut. The two buds branch laterally into the mesenchymal bed of the lung anlage, expanding it into the chest cavity. Branching is by dichotomy. The pulmonary arteries grow into the lung anlage from the sixth branchial artery and form a capillary network around the proliferating bronchial tubes; the pulmonary vein grows in from the left wall of the atrium of the heart and connects to the capillary network. Thus, the pattern of lung development is determined by the branching pattern of the airway tubes, but this depends on a close interaction with the mesenchyme. The pulmonary vasculature derives from the mesenchyme, as do all the supporting structures that the lung needs.

During lung histogenesis the different functional parts differentiate. Up to 17 weeks of gestation in man the lung is in its pseudoglandular stage, where all airways are made of a columnar epithelium. After 18 weeks the most distal branches of the airway tree widen (canalicular stage) and the epithelium begins to differentiate toward the epithelial mosaic of the gas exchange region, made of attenuated *lining cells and cuboidal secretory cells which prepare for the secretion of surfactant. The more central airway tubes differentiate toward bronchi and bronchioles. After 25 weeks the terminal branches are wide (saccular stage), the epithelium thin, and the capillaries closely approximated to the epithelium of each saccule. The walls between saccules are thin but contain two capillary networks.*

At birth the lung is still in its saccular stage, but it is adequately designed to take up gas exchange. The saccules can be expanded with air upon the first breath if the secretory cells have produced enough surfactant. The barrier is thin and O_2 can diffuse into the blood. In the weeks that follow, the saccules transform into alveolar ducts by forming a very large number of alveoli, small pouches in the wall of the saccule. This causes the gas exchange surface to increase drastically; now the septa between alveoli have only a single capillary network which is in contact with alveolar air on both sides.

Further Reading

Burri, P. H. 1984. Lung development and histogenesis. In *Handbook of Physiology: Respiration*, vol. 4, ed. A. P. Fishman and A. B. Fisher. Washington: American Physiological Society (in press).

Burri, P. H., and E. R. Weibel. 1977. The ultrastructure and morphometry of the developing lung. In *Development of the Lung*, ed. W. A. Hodson. New York: Dekker, pp. 215–268.

Hamilton, W. J., and H. W. Mossman. 1972. *Human Embryology: Prenatal Development of Form and Function.* 4th ed. Cambridge: Heffer & Sons. Baltimore: Williams & Wilkins.

Hodson, W. A. ed. 1977. *Development of the Lung.* New York: Dekker.

Rudolph, A. M., and M. A. Heymann. 1974. Fetal and neonatal circulation and respiration. *Annual Review of Physiology* 36:187–207.

Weibel, E. R. 1980. Design and structure of the human lung. In *Pulmonary Diseases and Disorders*, ed. A. P. Fishman. New York: McGraw-Hill, pp. 224–271.

References

*Alescio, T., and A. Cassini. 1962. Induction in vitro of tracheal buds by pulmonary mesenchyme grafted on tracheal epithelium. *Journal of Experimental Zoology* 150:83–94.

Bartlett, D., Jr. 1970. Postnatal growth of the lung; influence of exercise and thyroid activity. *Respiration Physiology* 9:50–57.

Boyden, E. A., and D. H. Tompsett. 1961. The postnatal growth of the lung in the dog. *Acta Anatomica* 47:185–215.

Burri, P. H. 1974. The postnatal growth of the rat lung. III. Morphology. *Anatomical Record* 180:77–98.

Burri, P. H., and E. R. Weibel. 1977. The ultrastructure and morphometry of the developing lung. In *Development of the Lung*, ed. W. A. Hodson. New York: Dekker, pp. 215–268.

Burri, P. H., J. Dbaly, and E. R. Weibel. 1974. The postnatal growth of the rat lung. I. Morphometry. *Anatomical Record* 178:711–739.

Kauffman, S. L., P. H. Burri, and E. R. Weibel. 1974. The postnatal growth of the rat lung. II. Autoradiography. *Anatomical Record* 180:63–76.

Mandelbrot, B. B. 1983. *The Fractal Geometry of Nature.* 2nd ed. of *Fractals: Form, Chance and Dimension* (1977). San Francisco: Freeman.

Reuck, A. V. S. de, and R. Porter, eds. 1967. *Development of the Lung.* London: Churchill.

Spooner, B. S., and N. K. Wessels. 1970. Mammalian lung development: interactions in primordium formation and bronchial morphogenesis. *Journal of Experimental Zoology* 175:445–454.

Weibel, E. R. 1963. *Morphometry of the Human Lung.* Berlin: Springer.

9

LUNG CELL BIOLOGY

As a gas exchanger, the lung's main role is to establish a large surface of contact between air and blood. Gas exchange occurs by diffusion and is hence a passive process, governed by the P_{O_2} gradient from air to blood; the lung takes no active part in transferring O_2 to the blood. Why, then, does the lung need cells?

In the preceding chapter we have seen that the lung is formed by growth, proliferation, and transformation of a complex population of cells derived from the epithelial anlage of the foregut and from the mesenchymal bed into which it develops. What has been achieved in development must be maintained, repaired, adjusted all through life, and this needs to be done by live cells, capable of reacting to all sorts of stimuli. Although the lung's cardinal function, gas exchange, is essentially a passive phenomenon, it can only be maintained if a whole number of ancillary functions are performed by cells. Part of the cost of pulmonary gas exchange is hence borne by the varied activities of lung cells.

For one, adequate permeability barriers must be maintained between the blood space, the air space, and the interstitial fluid that bathes the connective tissue elements, because the thin air–blood barrier must be kept dry at all times. We find that both the blood vessels and the air spaces are lined by confluent cell layers, sealed by intercellular junctions: a continuous endothelium made of flat cells coats the interior of the blood vessels from the right ventricle through the pulmonary arteries, the capillaries, and the veins to the left atrium; the epithelium which lines the air spaces from the trachea out to the alveoli is made of a mosaic of different cell types serving a number of different functions. These layers regulate the transit of water and solutes because their cell membranes have quite specific permeability properties and are also endowed with the capability to actively pump certain ions to maintain a favorable ion equilibrium.

To maintain a mechanically stable and clean lung also necessitates a number of metabolic functions. The connective tissue fibers of the interstitium must be continuously renewed by fibroblasts secreting the fiber material. The air spaces, exposed to our environment, must be kept clean; cells of the airway epithelium intervene in this process by secreting a sticky mucus to the airway surface and by propelling it outward in a continuous stream driven by kinocilia, thus removing fine dust particles that enter the lung with inhaled air. Even the alveolar surface is lined by a thin layer of fluid secreted by cells; we shall see that it serves a double function: to shield the delicate epithelial cells and to reduce surface tension. Not all intruders are, however, intercepted by this cleansing mechanism, and thus the lung needs to maintain an internal defense system of cells capable of fending off potentially noxious elements of many kinds. Among them are macrophages that take up foreign matter and digest it as far as possible; a variety of other cells of the general defense system of the body are found in the interstitium, such as lymphocytes, leukocytes, and plasma cells which secrete specific antibodies.

And finally, for gas exchange to function properly, ventilation and perfusion of the many millions of respiratory units should be matched as well as possible, and this calls for a potential for active regulation of airway and blood vessel caliber imparted by smooth muscle sleeves around the various conducting channels.

To serve all these functions the lung maintains a rich population of cells of different specializations. Their varied metabolic functions are often called "nonrespiratory," but, in fact, they are essential though ancillary functions for respiration; they serve no other purpose than to make gas exchange efficient. In the following sections I shall not discuss all of the 40 different cell types that can be identified in the lung but shall rather discuss the organization of the cell population in quite general terms, and then have a closer look at the cells of the respiratory zone, in order to finally examine how they react to severe injury.

Organization of the Lung's Cell Population

The lung's cell population is organized according to three basic principles: (1) it is divided into *layers* which form the barrier between air and blood, namely, epithelium, interstitium, and endothelium; (2) it is differentiated according to location in the *hierarchy* of lung structures, basically with respect to conducting or respiratory structures; and (3) it forms *mosaics* of cells with different functions that must be performed in concert. My choice of the subdivision into layers as the primary principle for structuring this discussion is to some extent arbitrary, but it has some logical basis in lung development since the epithelium derives, as we have seen, from the intestinal entoderm, whereas the vascular wall and the interstitial tissue derive from the mesenchymal bed.

AIRWAY EPITHELIUM

All airways—from the trachea to the alveoli—are lined by an uninterrupted confluent epithelial cell sheet. By calling this cell sheet confluent I mean that each cell is completely in contact with the cells that surround it so that there are no gaps in the lining. Confluency is a basic histological property of all epithelia, and the epithelia of the lung make no exception. Figure 9.1 summarizes the main design features of a simple epithelium as it prevails, in principle but with variations, in the pulmonary airways. The cells are arranged in a tightly packed layer on top of a basal lamina that constitutes the boundary toward the subjacent interstitial or connective tissue space. By this arrangement one can distinguish three different faces of their plasma membrane: the *basal face* is attached to the basal lamina so that the epithelium is anchored on the connective tissue; the *apical face* is in contact with the space bounded by the epithelium and carries a number of specializations, such as kinocilia, by which the cell interacts with this space; the *lateral faces* are in close contact with the adjacent cells and are provided with cell junctions by which the cells interact with each other.

The cell junctions we need to be concerned with are of three kinds. In surface epithelia the predominant junction is the *terminal bar* or *tight junction* which is also called the *zonula occludens*. It is functionally most important because it constitutes the seal of the intercellular cleft and thus imparts the epithelium with its essential

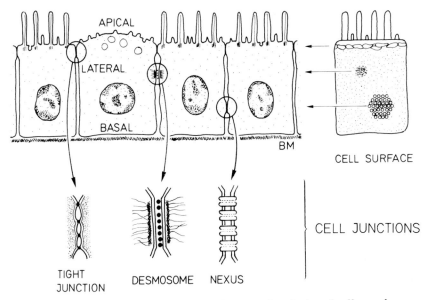

Fig. 9.1 Organization of epithelial cell layer with polarity of cell membrane and cell junctions.

barrier property between two functional compartments: the interstitial space and the outer world, the air space in our case. The terminal bars are always found at the boundary between apical and lateral cell face. They are tight junctions for two reasons: (1) they encircle the cells completely; (2) the membranes of the two adjoining cells become partly fused in the form of a ribbon of fine ridges (Fig. 9.1) so that the passage of molecules, or even of ions, is severely, though not always completely, restricted. By virtue of these tight junctions the cells proper now become the main pathway for the transit of matter across the epithelial barrier, and thus they can control this transit through the selective permeability of their membranes.

A cell junction which is often confounded with the zonula occludens because of its similar appearance is the *nexus* or *gap junction* which is found in the lower part of the lateral cell faces. Here the two cell membranes become closely apposed—but not fused—in the form of a small patch in which one finds a regular array of protein particles that span the two membranes and contain a narrow channel that connects the two cytoplasmic spaces. A nexus is thus a set of pores through which the cells can selectively exchange ions and small molecules so that they become electrically and metabolically coupled.

Finally, the cells must be coupled mechanically and this is served by small patch-like adhesions called *desmosomes* or *macula adhaerens*. Here the membranes are "glued" together by an interposed thin disc, and one finds that the filaments of the cytoskeleton insert symmetrically on the cytoplasmic face of the membranes, forming a condensed patch of filamentous material.

The nature of these junctions is the same in all epithelia, but there are large variations with respect to their quantitative development depending on functional requirements. In the airway epithelia of the lung all three types of junctions exist; however, nexus and desmosomes are usually rather small. In contrast the terminal bars are provided with junctions that are quite tight so that small macromolecules cannot traverse the intercellular pathway. This is true even for the rather thin epithelium that one finds in alveoli.

Though derived from one and the same anlage, the airway epithelium modifies its differentiation characteristics as we proceed from large bronchi over bronchioles to the alveolar region (Fig. 9.2). A simple epithelium, as represented schematically in Figure 9.1, exists as a lining of smaller bronchioles (Fig. 9.2): as we move upward toward larger bronchi, the epithelium becomes higher and some basal cells appear, making the epithelium pseudostratified; at the point of transition into the gas exchange region, that is, at the entrance into the complex of alveoli, the epithelium abruptly becomes extremely thin.

Figure 9.2 also shows that the epithelium is not made of a uniform cell population but that it is, at each level, rather a mosaic of at least two cell types, in that secretory cells are interspersed into the complex of lining cells. There are also some additional rarer cells, such as neuroendocrine cells that are capable of secreting some mediators into the blood, or so-called brush cells whose precise function is not yet understood.

If we now first have a closer look at the epithelium of conducting airways, we see that the lining cells are provided with a tuft of kinocilia at their apical cell face, whereas the secretory cells are goblet cells that produce and discharge to the surface a sticky mucus (Fig. 9.3). This mucus spreads out as a thin blanket on top of the cilia and is capable of trapping dust particles that are still contained in the air entering the lung. Kinocilia are organelles of movement that are

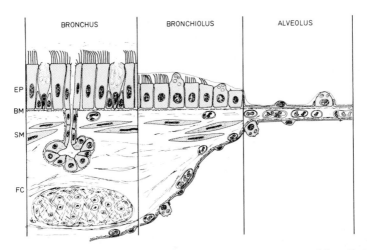

Fig. 9.2 Change of airway wall structure at the three principal levels. The epithelial layer (EP) gradually becomes reduced from pseudo-stratified to cuboidal and then to squamous, but retains its organization as a mosaic of lining and secretory cells. The smooth-muscle layer (SM) disappears in the alveoli. The fibrous coat (FC) contains cartilage only in bronchi and gradually becomes thinner as the alveolus is approached. BM = basement membrane. (From Burri and Weibel, 1973.)

known to beat rhythmically in a given direction and at a frequency of about 20 Hz; some protozoa, such as paramecia, use such cilia to move through water. In the airway epithelium the cilia are oriented in such a fashion that their beat is directed outward. It is now interesting that the cilia of airway epithelia develop at their tip fine claws with which they can grasp the mucus blanket in the phase of their forward beat, whereas on their return to the upright position they glide past the mucus blanket. The result of this is that the mucus blanket, together with the trapped foreign material, moves outward or "up the airways" in a steady stream, a feature appropriately called the "ciliary escalator." Since the lining by ciliated cells is uninterrupted from the bronchioles, up the bronchi to the trachea this "mucociliary escalator" ends at the larynx, so that the normal fate of bronchial mucus is to be steadily discharged into the pharynx whence it is swallowed, usually unnoticed. Only when an excessive amount of mucus accumulates in the trachea—for example, from irritation in a very dusty environment or from bronchitis—do we have to assist the system by coughing.

The secretory cell population of the conducting airways shows a number of specialized features which I shall only mention briefly. In major bronchi some of the secretory cells form actual small glands which are located in the connective tissue wall of the bronchus (Fig. 9.2). In the smaller bronchioles one finds a peculiar secretory cell called the Clara cell whose function is unknown.

The epithelial lining of alveoli is altogether different from that of conducting airways. The lining cells are very thin squamous cells, evidently without cilia. The secretory cells are cuboidal and produce phospholipids that can reduce the surface tension of the extremely thin fluid layer of low viscosity that covers the alveolar epithelium. We shall have a closer look at these important cells later on.

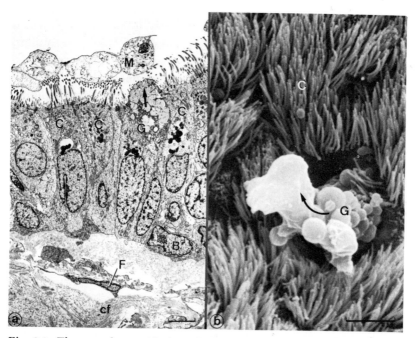

Fig. 9.3 The pseudo-stratified epithelium of a small bronchus is made of three cell types: ciliated (C), goblet (G), and basal (B) cells, as seen in (a) on an electron micrograph of a thin section. The epithelial surface, viewed with the scanning electron microscope in (b), is provided with tufts of kinocilia (C); a mucus droplet is seen to be released from the top of a goblet cell (G). Note in (a) a group of macrophages (M) situated on top of the cilia as markers of the mucus blanket; the connective tissue space beneath the epithelium contains fibroblasts (F) and fibers (cf). Scale markers: (a) 5 μm; (b) 5 μm.

VASCULAR ENDOTHELIUM

All blood spaces are lined by a continuous sheet of endothelial cells, from the heart cavities to the capillaries in the gas exchange region of the lung and all other organs. Histologically the endothelium is a simple squamous epithelium in that the cells are attached to a basal lamina and are joined to each other by intercellular junctions, just like the epithelia discussed above. There are some notable differences, however. For one, the tight junctions are leakier than in epithelia: in the capillaries and in small venules they seem to allow a rather free and uninhibited exchange of water and solutes between the blood plasma and the interstitial space; whether this is similar in larger vessels is yet unknown. Second, in each type of blood vessel the endothelium is made of a uniform type of cells, all alike in structure and in function. However, there are distinct differences in the structure and function of the endothelia in the capillaries and in the conducting vessels—arteries and veins. Whereas the capillary endothelial cell (which we shall consider in detail later) appears like a simple lining cell with a small potential for metabolic activity, that of arteries and veins is endowed with a much richer complement of cellular organelles that can perform various synthetic and metabolic functions. For example, it is known that the vascular endothelium of the lung is capable of metabolizing appreciable quantities of blood-borne fat. It also contains an enzyme that converts angiotensin I, which is produced in the plasma by the action of renin, to angiotensin II, an important regulator of blood pressure. Although this interesting function of lung vessels has received a lot of attention, I shall not discuss it further; it does not seem directly related to our broader purpose, the discussion of the lung's role as a gas exchanger.

INTERSTITIAL CELLS

In the mature lung the interstitial or connective tissue space—which derives from the mesenchyme and is hence connected to the pleura—is rather small, but it serves two principal functions: (1) to mechanically join and support the various structural elements by means of an elaborate fiber system, and (2) to establish a fluid space between the airway epithelium and the vascular endothelium that is related to lymph.

The interstitial cell population serves these two functions: fibroblasts and smooth muscle cells contribute to the mechanical support function, whereas a number of cells of the defense system are contained in the fluid space, often close to the pathways for draining lymph out of the lung.

Like all structures of our body, the collagen and elastic fibers of the lung are subject to continuous turnover, breakdown, and renewal, albeit at a slow rate. This is performed by fibroblasts which are closely apposed to the fibers, following them with long, partly branched extensions (Fig. 9.4). They are also equipped with the organelles that synthesize the fiber material: ribosomes and endoplasmic reticulum for making the proteinaceous precursors of the fibers (tropocollagen, for example) and Golgi complexes for producing the proteoglycans that are an important part of the fibers.

Smooth muscle cells occur in many places in the lung; they serve an important support function because they can modulate their tension. They are elongated and sometimes branched cells whose cytoplasm is nearly filled with filaments which can contract (Fig. 9.5). It is now known that, in all cells, the potential for contraction is due to the presence of actin and myosin which occur in different arrangement. In striated muscle (heart and skeletal muscles) they

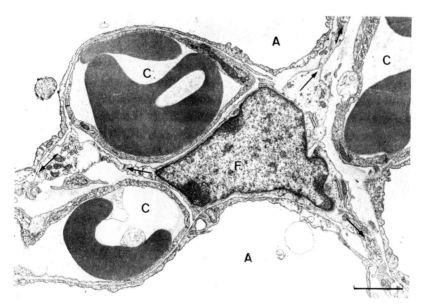

Fig. 9.4 A fibroblast (F) in the alveolar septum of the human lung shows several cytoplasmic branches (arrows) that extend over long distances through the interstitial space. Scale marker: 2 μm.

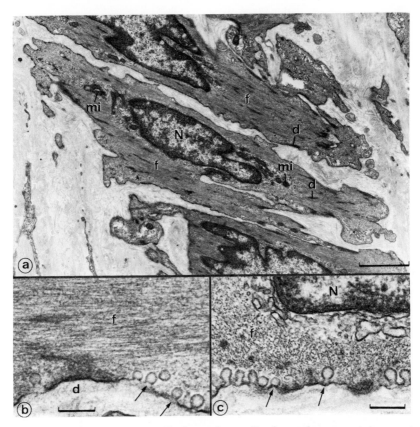

Fig. 9.5 Smooth muscle cells from the wall of a pulmonary artery cut longitudinally (a) through the nucleus (N). The cytoplasm contains mitochondria (mi) and dense bundles of filaments (f) shown in longitudinal and transverse section in (b) and (c) respectively. Note pinocytosis vesicles (arrows) and dense bodies (d) at the plasma membrane and in the interior. Scale markers: (a) 2 μm; (b, c) 0.2 μm.

occur as two separate sets of filaments, highly ordered into sarcomeres (Fig. 5.5); for each myosin filament there are three actin filaments. In smooth muscle cells actin is much more abundant than myosin and their mutual arrangement is different. The process of contraction of smooth muscle cells is much slower; whereas striated muscle contracts, upon stimulation, in a twitch — a brief contraction followed immediately by relaxation — smooth muscle responds to stimulation by a slow sustained contraction, gradually increasing the tension, followed by a slow relaxation; this can often occur rhythmically. In addition, smooth muscle possesses the mechanical property of tonus, a condition of persistent contraction independent of external stimuli by which they can modulate their elastic properties: the higher the tonus the greater the force required to stretch the fiber. In the lung, it is this latter property which is most important, particularly in the wall of smaller pulmonary arteries where the smooth muscle forms circular sleeves: the arterial cross-section depends on the balance of the distending force due to blood pressure and the narrowing force due to smooth muscle tonus; by increasing the tonus of a given vessel wall its cross section becomes smaller and the flow resistance increases. It is noteworthy that low local O_2 tensions cause a higher smooth muscle tone, and thus the blood flow into lung

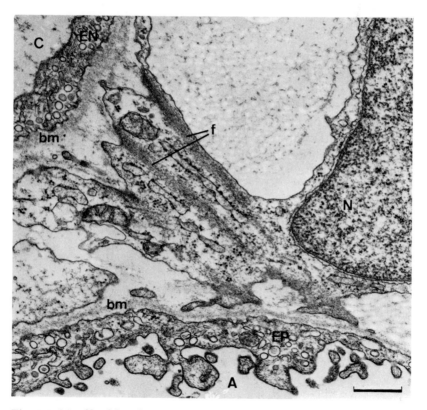

Fig. 9.6 Myofibroblast from alveolar septum contains filament bundles (f) that extend between the basement membranes (bm) of the epithelium (EP) and the capillary endothelium (EN). Scale marker: 0.5 μm.

regions which receive less O_2 due to poor ventilation becomes reduced, as we shall see.

Smooth muscle cells occur in the lung not only in vessel walls but also as more or less circular sleeves in all conducting airways, from bronchi to bronchioles, where they regulate the local resistance to air flow by changing the cross section of the tube. In asthma, resistance to air flow is impeded partly because of an excessive contraction of these cells. But smooth muscle fibers also penetrate into the gas exchange region as small bundles in the free edge of alveolar walls toward the alveolar duct, as discussed in chapter 11.

Recent studies have shown that virtually all cells contain actin and myosin and are thus invested with contractile properties. This is particularly true of some fibroblasts whose long extensions may be so rich in fine filaments that they have been called myofibroblasts. This has been demonstrated for lung fibroblasts in alveolar walls, in particular, where short filament bundles are seen to be contained in cytoplasmic branches that bridge the interstitial space from the epithelial to the endothelial basal lamina (Fig. 9.6). We shall discuss the possible functional importance of this arrangement later on. It suffices to say at this point that the mechanical properties of the lung depend not only on the inert fiber system but also on a rich complement of cells with contractile properties that range from fibroblasts to myofibroblasts and smooth muscle cells.

DEFENSE CELLS

Because of its large internal surface open to outside air, the lung is exposed to multiple potential hazards and must therefore maintain an elaborate defense system. This begins with the mechanical cleansing devices in the nasal cavity, followed by the mucociliary escalator discussed above; but not everything noxious is intercepted on the way in, so that a whole set of defense cells must be maintained deep in the lung tissue. Most of these cells occur as free cells in the interstitial space, but one cell type, the alveolar macrophage, performs its function on the outer surface of the alveolar epithelium, that is, in the alveolar lining layer.

The organism knows two ways for fending off hazardous material: (1) direct or nonimmune defense performed essentially by macrophages; and (2) immune defense where specialized cells become programmed to produce antibodies to foreign material, which then leads to their destruction or elimination.

Let us first discuss the nonimmune defense mechanism which consists in having macrophages ingest and, if possible, digest the undesired material. The process of ingestion or phagocytosis involves movements of the cell periphery, mediated by the cell's contractile material, actin and myosin. In cells preparing for phagocytosis one finds that thin flap-like extensions of the peripheral cytoplasm are formed that begin to enwrap the foreign body; in Figure 9.7 we see such flaps or lips formed around part of an erythrocyte which is — erroneously — contained in alveolar fluid. As the lips close a membrane-bounded pocket has formed which contains the foreign body but is now an internal compartment of the cell. The next process is to discharge the content of lysosomes into this pocket, which is called a phagosome. Lysosomes are small membrane-

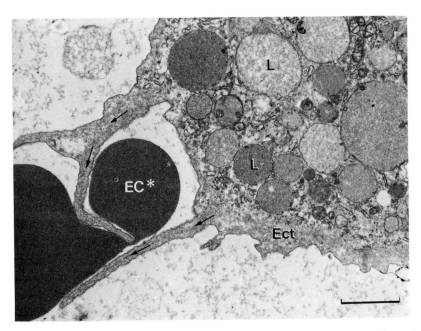

Fig. 9.7 Alveolar macrophage in the process of phagocytosis. Leaflets of ectoplasm (Ect) reach out (arrows) and engulf part of an erythrocyte (EC*). The cytoplasm contains numerous lysosomal vesicles (L) of varying size and content. Scale marker: 2 μm.

bounded granules that occur in most cells; they contain a set of powerful hydrolytic enzymes, proteins which are synthesized in the rough endoplasmic reticulum and packaged in the Golgi complex. There are about 20 or more such enzymes which are capable of breaking down (catabolizing) most organic materials, so that the foreign body, at least if it is organic in nature, is quickly disassembled.

It is evident that such a destructive process must take place in a strictly controlled environment within the cell, lest the enzymes would also attack precious cells or other components of the organism. The break-down products are either discharged, if they can be reutilized by the organism, or stored within the cell in membrane-bounded granules called residual bodies. Prolonged and sometimes permanent intracellular storage of foreign materials that cannot be digested is an important process in the lung because much of the dust we inhale in our civilized environment is nondigestible. This is particularly true of carbon dust as it is found in smoke or soot; over a lifetime, city dwellers and smokers therefore accumulate in their lungs considerable amounts of carbon dust which becomes permanently deposited in phagocytic cells of the interstitium, forming black patches beneath the pleura and along the bronchi. Mineral dusts have essentially the same fate but they are not as harmless as carbon; thus quarry workers or stone masons can be affected by a disease called silicosis, a progressive destruction of lung structure followed by scarring which is due to the constant irritation caused by stored silica particles. A much feared disease of the same nature is asbestosis, which can even cause lung cancer; it is observed in people working with asbestos, a fibrous mineral used extensively in insulating materials. Both silicosis and asbestosis are predominantly occupational diseases because intense exposure to the dust is necessary; they could largely be avoided if appropriate precautionary measures were followed, which often are not.

In the lung, direct defense by phagocytosis plays a major role. It is primarily performed by a specialized group of cells found in a strategically favorable location: alveolar macrophages which sit directly on the alveolar surface (Fig. 9.8), so that they can intercept particles that become deposited on that surface. These cells are free cells that are capable of actively moving over the surface by ameboid movement. They do so by means of the same contractile machinery that allows them to ingest particles: they extend a cytoplasmic flap, called

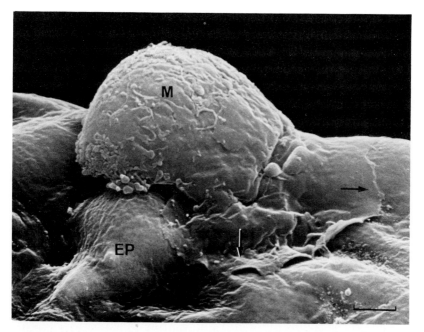

Fig. 9.8 Alveolar macrophage (M) seen in the process of crawling over the epithelial surface (EP) by extending its advancing lamella (arrows). Scale marker: 3 μm.

an advancing lamella, in the direction of their movement, dragging behind the main part of the cell body with the nucleus and the cytoplasmic organelles, lysosomes and all. Thus they police the entire alveolar surface, searching out contaminants that need to be removed; it is interesting that they do not depend exclusively on random searching strategies but are attracted chemotactically to certain compounds.

Macrophages are not of pulmonary origin. They rather derive from the bone marrow, circulate in the blood as monocytes, and settle in the lung secondarily. It is noteworthy that the turnover of alveolar macrophages is rather rapid, so that a continuous influx of new cells from the blood is required. The fate of macrophages is varied: some of them leave the peripheral air spaces via the bronchi, where they are transported out of the lung by the mucociliary escalator; others may return to the interstitium and either settle there, or leave via lymphatics.

I shall not discuss the immune defense mechanism in any detail, for there is nothing specifically pulmonary about it. As in all organs, the pulmonary interstitium contains a set of free cells that derive from the lymphatic system, in particular lymphocytes and plasma cells. In the lung these cells are concentrated mostly in the connective tissue envelopes of bronchi and blood vessels, where one also finds lymphatic vessels. The actual immune defense is performed partly by the lymphocytes and partly by the plasma cells which produce specific antibodies. This defense depends on a process of learning, however; it can only respond to intruders which are known to the body and for which it has had a chance to program specific defense cells. The process is highly sophisticated and can be studied in any modern immunology textbook.

Defense cells do not originate in the pulmonary interstitium; rather, they are brought in by the blood, macrophages from the bone marrow and immune defense cells from lymphatic tissue in various locations — lymph nodes, lymphoepithelial organs, or spleen. These cells must leave the pulmonary interstitium again, and preferably through escape routes different from their entrance pathway so as not to contaminate the blood. One escape route has already been mentioned: many of the defense cells that reach the airway surface are wasted and transported out of the lung through the mucociliary escalator. This is true as well for alveolar macrophages as for macrophages, leukocytes, or immune defense cells that have traversed the epithelium of conducting airways to perform their defense function there.

The escape route for defense cells in the pulmonary interstitium is established through the system of lymphatic vessels that drains interstitial fluid (lymph) toward central veins where it is discharged into the blood. Lymphatics are vessels that are bounded by an endothelium which is, however, somewhat different from that of blood vessels. They start with blind ending lymph capillaries, fairly wide vessels provided with a "leaky" endothelium through which interstitial fluid and free cells can easily penetrate. In the lung, such lymph capillaries are found near the acini, but they do not penetrate into the delicate alveolar septa. They are located in "fluid sumps" in the loose connective tissue sheaths around conducting blood vessels or bronchi and in septa connected to the pleura. These are also the regions where one finds interstitial defense cells which, normally, are also not found in alveolar septa.

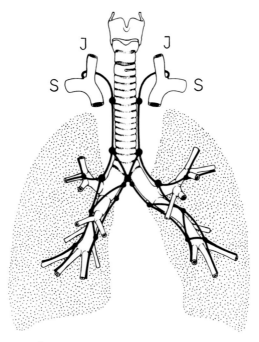

Fig. 9.9 Schematic diagram of the distribution of lymph nodes and main lymphatic channels along the bronchial tree, ending on either side in the corner between the subclavian (S) and jugular (J) veins. (From Weibel, 1980.)

Lymphatic vessels form loose meshworks that follow in their centripetal path the trees of airways and blood vessels, and this directs them toward the pulmonary hilum. There they merge into larger trunks which follow the trachea to eventually connect with the left and right subclavian veins, at the point where these are joined by the jugular veins (Fig. 9.9).

Two points are important: (1) the lymph always flows in a centripetal direction thanks to numerous valves that are found in the larger lymphatic vessels which, by the way, also have a loose smooth muscle coat; (2) the lymph flow is directed through a sequence of *lymph nodes* (Fig. 9.9) which function as biological filters in that they can intercept foreign materials, damaged cells, and, most importantly, macrophages that have ingested foreign indigestible material. The lymph that is eventually delivered back to the blood — note that lymph derives from interstitial fluid which is a blood filtrate — is clean. On the other hand, one will find, in all lymph nodes along the path, variable deposits of macrophages which store indigestible foreign materials, such as carbon and mineral dusts. The passage of macrophages and immune defense cells through the lymph nodes plays another important role, however: it conveys antigens to the pools of immunocompetent cells in the lymph nodes, which can program new immune defense cells for future tasks.

A Closer Look at the Cells of the Gas Exchange Region

BASIC DESIGN OF A GAS EXCHANGE BARRIER

Efficient gas exchange in the lung depends, as we have said repeatedly, on designing a very thin barrier of very large surface between air and blood. Nevertheless, this barrier must be built of the three minimal tissue layers: an endothelium lining the capillaries, an epithelium lining the air spaces, and an interstitial layer to house the connective tissue fibers. The guiding principle in designing these cells must evidently be to *minimize thickness* and *maximize extent*. However, there is definitely a limit to this, set by the need to make the barrier and its constituent cells strong enough to resist the various forces that act on it — capillary blood pressure, tissue tension, and surface tension, in particular. Furthermore, the barrier must remain intact for a lifetime, and this requires continuous repair and turnover of the cells and their components.

The barrier that separates air and blood is so thin than one can just see it in a light micrograph but cannot resolve its different layers. In fact, there was a long dispute as to whether the alveoli are lined with an epithelial layer or not until, in 1953, Frank Low presented the first electron micrographs of lung tissue on which he could unambiguously demonstrate that both the capillaries and the alveoli were lined by continuous cell sheets.

In spite of this delicacy of tissue structure we find that $\frac{3}{4}$ of all the lung cells by volume or weight are contained in the gas exchange region, usually called lung parenchyma (Table 9.1). We also note that epithelium and endothelium make up about $\frac{1}{4}$ each of the tissue barrier in the alveolar walls, whereas interstitial cells amount to 35%; the interstitial space with the connective tissue fibers comprises no more than 15% of the barrier, an astonishingly low value which calls for very clever design features, as we shall see in chapters 10 and

TABLE 9.1. ESTIMATED CELL VOLUMES IN THE HUMAN LUNG.

Cell or tissue	Volume (ml)	Percent septal tissue
Tissue (excl. blood)	284	—
Nonparenchyma	99	—
Alveolar septa	185	—
Cells	213	—
Nonparenchyma	50	—
Alveolar septa	163	—
Parenchymal cells	163	—
Alveolar epithelium type I	23	12.6
Alveolar epithelium type II	18	9.7
Capillary endothelium	49	26.4
Interstitial cells	66	35.8
Alveolar macrophages	7	3.9

11. The important population of alveolar macrophages, discussed above, contributes some 4% of the barrier tissue or 1% of lung weight.

THE CELLS LINING THE BARRIER

If we now first look at the cell layers bounding the barrier, we note that by far the major part of the barrier surface is lined, both on the air and on the blood side, by simple layers of squamous cells. This histological description is sufficient for the endothelium whose cell population is uniform. The epithelium, however, is a mosaic of different cell types, and one therefore finds a small fraction of the total surface — only a few percent (Table 9.2) — to be occupied by secretory cells; one usually calls the squamous lining cells type I and the secretory cells type II alveolar cells or pneumocytes. A very rare third cell, the brush cell, is also found in some specific regions near the terminal bronchiole; I shall not deal with it, for its function is as yet unknown.

The squamous lining cells (the capillary endothelium and the type I epithelial cells) show very similar design features (Fig. 9.10). In terms of cell biology they are rather simple cells. Their small compact nucleus is surrounded by a slim rim of cytoplasm where one finds a modest basic set of organelles: a few small mitochondria, some

TABLE 9.2. MORPHOMETRIC CHARACTERISTICS OF CELL POPULATION IN LUNG PARENCHYMA.

Cell population	Percent of total cell number[a]			Average cell volume (μm^3)			Average apical cell surface (μm^2)		
	Human	Baboon	Rat	Human	Baboon	Rat	Human	Baboon	Rat
Alveolar epithelium									
Type I	8	12	8	1,764	1,224	915	5,098	4,004	4,518
Type II	16	8	14	889	539	366	183	285	62
Endothelium	30	36	45	632	365	336	1,353	1,040	946
Interstitial cells	36	42	30	637	227	615	—	—	—
Alveolar macrophages	10	2	3	2,492	1,059	665	—	—	—

Data from Crapo et al. (1982) and Haies et al. (1981).
a. Total cell numbers: human, $230 \cdot 10^9$; baboon, $48 \cdot 10^9$; rat, $0.9 \cdot 10^9$.

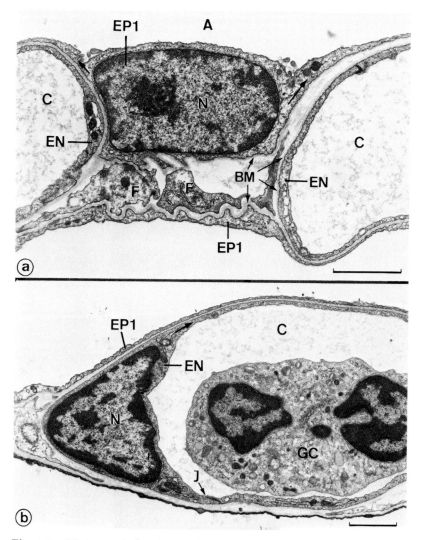

Fig. 9.10 (a) A type I alveolar epithelial cell (EP1) from human lung. The nucleus (N) is surrounded by very little cytoplasm which extends as thin leaflets (arrows) to cover the capillaries (C). Note the basement membranes (BM) of the epithelium and endothelium (EN) which become fused in a minimal barrier. Interstitial space contains fibroblast processes (F). (b) An endothelial cell (EN) of capillary (C) is similar in basic structure to a type I epithelial cell (EP1). The nucleus is enwrapped by little cytoplasm but thin leaflets extend as capillary lining (arrow). Note the intercellular junction (J) and a white blood cell (granulocyte, GC) in the capillary. Scale markers: 2 μm.

cisternae of endoplasmic reticulum with a few ribosomes indicating a limited potential for protein synthesis, and a small Golgi complex with associated vesicles. This is the picture of a quiescent cell with no great metabolic activity.

At the edge of the perinuclear region a very attenuated cytoplasmic leaflet emerges (Fig. 9.10) and spreads out broadly over the basal lamina. This leaflet is made essentially of the two plasma membranes of the apical and basal cell face (Fig. 9.1), respectively, with a very small amount of cytoplasmic ground substance interposed (Fig. 9.11). Here one rarely finds any organelles, except for numerous microvesicles that are implied in the transcellular transport of macromolecules; they may be partly responsible for keeping the barrier "dry," that is, for regulating its fluid content, as we shall discuss in chapter 10.

As one would expect, terminal bars are formed where the cytoplasmic leaflets of epithelial cells, or of endothelial cells, meet. Here

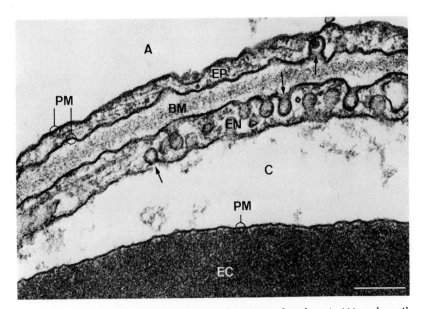

Fig. 9.11 Thin, minimal tissue barrier between alveolar air (A) and capillary blood (C) is made of cytoplasmic leaflets of epithelium (EP) and endothelium (EN), joined by fused basement membranes (BM). Note that the epithelial and endothelial leaflets are bounded by plasma membranes (PM), as is the erythrocyte (EC). Arrows point to pinocytotic vesicles. Scale marker: 0.2 μm.

there is a notable difference between these two linings in that the tight junction between epithelial cells constitutes a powerful seal of the intercellular cleft, whereas that in the endothelium is rather leaky, allowing a nearly uninhibited exchange of water, solutes, and even some smaller macromolecules between the blood plasma and the interstitial space.

There is another notable and important difference between these two basically similar lining cells: their size. Although the capillary surface is some 10–20% smaller than the alveolar surface, the capillary endothelial cells are about four times more numerous than type I cells; this means that the surface covered by one type I epithelial cell must be about four times larger, namely 4000–5000 μm^2 as compared to about 1000 μm^2 in endothelial cells (Table 9.2). In some texts one may find the type I cell called the "small alveolar cell" because of its small nucleus; clearly this is a misnomer, as the type I cell is a rather large cell indeed, both with respect to surface and to cell volume (Table 9.2).

If one looks at the surface of the alveolar epithelium either in scanning electron micrographs (Fig. 9.12) or in silver impregnated specimens where the terminal bars are revealed, one notes that the patches covered by single type I cells are much smaller than the 4000–5000 μm^2 given above, a number derived by dividing the total alveolar surface by the total number of type I cell nuclei; the one large type I cell seen in Figure 9.12 has an area of only about 1400 μm^2, and there are not many that are larger. Why is this? There seem to be 3–4 times as many type I cell domains encircled by terminal bars as there are nuclei. Indeed, this observation was made already some hundred years ago by the German pioneer of histology, Albert Kölliker; his interpretation was that part of the alveolar surface was lined by "nonnuclear" cytoplasmic plates ("kernlose Platten") rather than by complete cells. For a modern cell biologist this interpretation cannot be accepted without scrutiny: a "cytoplasmic plate" that is not in a relation of constant exchange with a nucleus is doomed, for it will soon be depleted of the information carriers for protein synthesis, as well as of ribosomes, so that its potential to replace proteins vanishes. It would be similar to erythrocytes or blood platelets which have a limited life span.

It turns out that an alternative explanation is possible. One finds that type I cells are not simple squamous cells but are branched cells with *multiple apical faces*, as shown diagrammatically in Figure

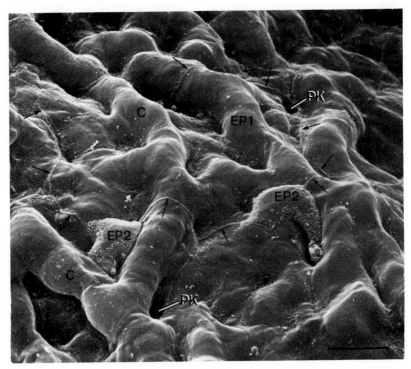

Fig. 9.12 Surface of the alveolar wall in the human lung seen by scanning electron microscopy reveals a mosaic of alveolar epithelium made of type I (EP1) and type II (EP2) cells. Arrows indicate boundary of the cytoplasmic leaflet of the type I cell which extends over many capillaries (C). Note the two interalveolar pores of Kohn (PK). Scale marker: 10 μm. (From Weibel, 1980.)

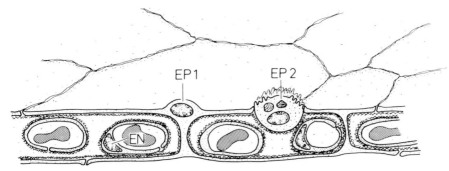

Fig. 9.13 Diagram of the alveolar wall showing the complexity of a type I epithelial cell (EP1) and its relation to a type II cell (EP2) and endothelial cell (EN).

9.13. Thus, what appears as nonnucleated plates are cytoplasmic domains that are connected to the perinuclear cytoplasm by a stalk, spreading out on one side of the alveolar wall or the other; it is evident that several such domains can share a nucleus. This complex shape of type I cells appears like an ingenious solution to the problem of optimizing maintenance pathways within the cell—from the nucleus to the cytoplasm—against the requirement of minimal barrier thickness across the cell in the interest of gas exchange. With the cytoplasmic leaflets arranged in the form of multiple stalked plates, the distance for the transfer of metabolites from the perinuclear region to any point in the periphery becomes shorter than if a single squamous extension simply spreads out more. In fact, by this device the epithelial lining can make do with fewer nuclei, which are comparatively bulky and thus potentially obstruct the diffusion path for O_2.

One may wonder why the same device is not used in the endothelium, where the cells are simple squamous cells with a single apical plate and are, consequently, much more numerous (Table 9.2). The best we can do is speculate along three arguments: (1) it is topologically not as easy to spread branched cells on the surface of a complex capillary network as across a two-sided wall; (2) the epithelium must also accommodate secretory cells, so that the total number of nuclei is nearly the same in epithelium and endothelium (Table 9.2); and (3) the endothelial cells must be simple in shape because they must retain their capacity to divide by mitosis, whereas type I cells have lost this capacity and are replaced from type II cells, as we shall discuss below.

Thus, in spite of some similarity, the two lining cells of the barrier are distinctly different in terms of shape, and this has some important biological consequences, as we shall see.

THE ALVEOLAR SECRETORY CELL: SYNTHESIS OF SURFACTANT

The type II alveolar cell is a conspicuous, but in fact relatively small, cell whose mean volume is less than half that of the type I cell (Table 9.2), although it is often called the "large alveolar cell." Its shape is cuboidal, that is, it is about as high as it is wide and has no cytoplasmic extensions to the side (Figs. 9.12 and 9.14). The apical cell surface bulges toward the lumen and is provided, mostly around its periphery, with a tuft of microvilli, surface specializations usually associated with fluid and solute transport.

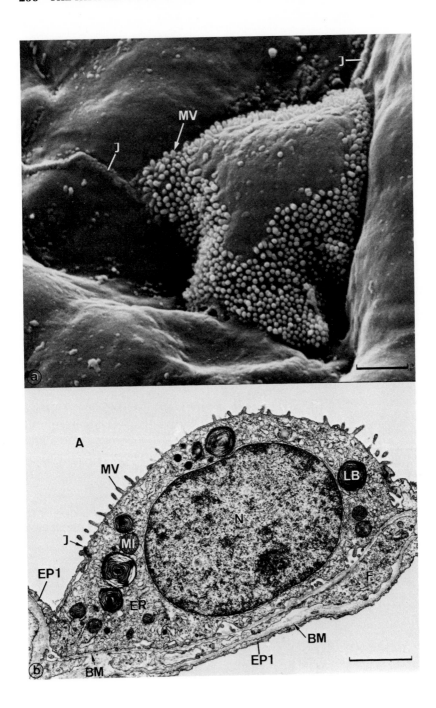

The most conspicuous feature of the type II cell is its wealth in cytoplasmic organelles of all kinds (Fig. 9.14b): mitochondria, a lot of endoplasmic reticulum with ribosomes, and a well-developed Golgi complex surrounded by a set of small lysosomal granules among which so-called multivesicular bodies — membrane-bounded organelles containing a group of small vesicles — stand out. In addition, one finds the characteristic lamellar bodies, larger membrane-bounded organelles that contain a dense stack of phospholipid lamellae which stain black with osmium.

These structural properties are directly related to the type II cell's principal function: the synthesis, storage, and secretion of surfactant, a complex of phospholipids and proteins that spreads in a thin film on the alveolar surface and drastically lowers the surface tension at the air–tissue interface. As we shall see in chapter 11, the curvature of the tiny alveoli is such that the froth-like complex of air chambers in lung parenchyma can only be kept stable if surface tension is very small. In effect, then, the type II cells serve a vital function in view of the goal of maximizing the gas exchange surface.

The main surfactant phospholipid of the lung is dipalmitoylphosphatidylcholine (DPPC), a lecithin whose two fatty acid chains are saturated palmitic acid (Fig. 9.15a); it lowers the surface tension at an air–water interface by spreading on the surface as a monomolecular film with the hydrophilic polar group immersed in the water and the two hydrophobic palmitic acid residues sticking out (Fig. 9.15b). It is well established that the type II cells synthesize DPPC, store it in the lamellar bodies, and secrete it into the thin fluid layer that covers the alveolar epithelium.

In spite of a large number of biochemical studies, it is less certain how the type II cells synthesize DPPC. The problem is that the most common biochemical pathway for the synthesis of lecithins or phos-

---

Fig. 9.14 (a) Higher magnification of a type II cell reveals a "crown" of short microvilli (MV) and a central "bald patch." Note junction lines of type I cells (J) meeting with the type II cell. (b) A type II epithelial cell from the human lung forms junctions (J) with type I epithelial cells (EP1). Its cytoplasm contains osmiophilic lamellar bodies (LB) and a rich complement of organelles: mitochondria (MI), endoplasmic reticulum (ER), and so on. The nucleus (N) is surrounded by a perinuclear cisterna which is perforated by nuclear pores. BM = basement membrane; F = fibroblast; MV = microvilli; A = alveolus. Scale markers: 2 μm. (From Weibel, 1980.)

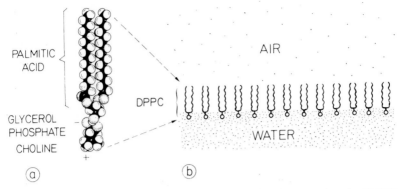

Fig. 9.15 (a) Model of dipalmitoylphosphatidylcholine molecule (DPPC) with polar group which makes the molecule hydrophilic on one end. (b) Monomolecular DPPC film spreads on water surface with the hydrophobic fatty acid ends pointing outwards.

phatidylcholines, the so-called Kennedy pathway (Fig. 9.16), results in phosphatidylcholine where at least one of the two fatty acids, probably the one in the second position, is unsaturated; DPPC, where both fatty acid chains are fully saturated palmitic acids with 16 carbons and no double bonds (16:0), therefore appears like an "unnatural" product which must be made by a two-step procedure.

In the first step the type II cell uses the Kennedy pathway to produce a partially unsaturated phosphatidylcholine. Figure 9.16 shows that various routes are possible, but it appears today that glucose is the preferred starting material for making the backbone of phosphatidic acid through glycerol-3-phosphate. The fatty acid, coupled to coenzyme A, is then added and finally the diacylglycerol is condensed with cytidinediphosphocholine to make a phosphatidylcholine which is unsaturated.

The second step involves remodeling by reacylation where the unsaturated fatty acid in the second position is clipped off by phospholipase A_2 and replaced by palmitic acid, most probably by adding palmitoyl CoA. It appears that the enzymatic equipment of type II cells is such that they will, in this remodeling process, greatly prefer palmitoyl CoA to other acyl CoA substrates. This selectivity is the reason for the abundance or even predominance of dipalmitoyl lecithin among the surfactant phospholipids. There are some species differences, but it seems that, in contrast to other body fluids, up to 75% of the surfactant phospholipids are DPPC. This is why one estimates the maturation state of the pulmonary surfactant system in the human fetus by the ratio of DPPC to unsaturated phospholipids.

The site of DPPC synthesis within the type II cells is not yet precisely localized; possible candidates are the endoplasmic reticulum, parts of the Golgi membranes, the multivesicular bodies, or the lamellar bodies themselves; these organelles are arranged in a kind of complex (Fig. 9.17) and could thus establish a spatial sequence for the intracellular processing of phospholipids. It is possible that all sites are involved at one step or another of the complex pathway leading to DPPC (Fig. 9.16). Thus the initial steps of the Kennedy pathway could be localized somewhere in the endoplasmic reticulum, whereas the remodeling, which involves hydrolytic enzyme action (phospholipase A_2) could occur in elements with lysosomal characteristics; both multivesicular bodies and lamellar bodies have been shown to con-

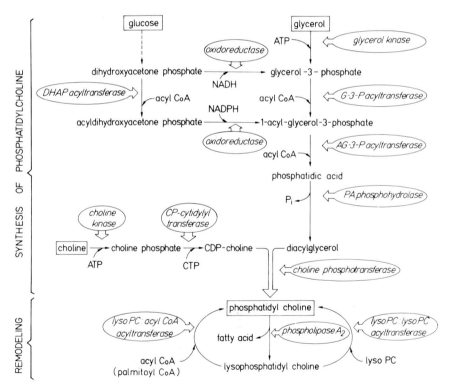

Fig. 9.16 Pathways for the synthesis and remodeling of phosphatidylcholine. (After King, 1979.)

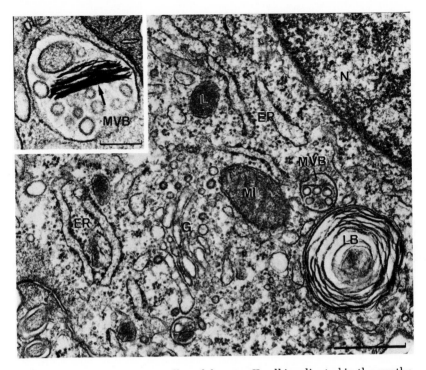

Fig. 9.17 Cytoplasmic organelles of the type II cell implicated in the synthesis of surfactant are the endoplasmic reticulum (ER), Golgi complex (G), lysosomes (L), multivesicular bodies (MVB), and finally lamellar bodies (LB). The inset shows a large multivesicular body with a stack of phospholipid lamellae (arrow). Scale markers: 0.5 μm; (inset) 0.2 μm.

tain hydrolytic enzymes. But much of this still needs to be clarified. One point is beyond doubt, however: the lamellar bodies are the storage sites for "mature," fully saturated DPPC which becomes "crystallized" into a regular layered stack.

The content of lamellar bodies is eventually secreted onto the alveolar surface by exocytosis: the granule membrane fuses with the apical plasma membrane and the content is discharged (Fig. 9.18). In the alveolar lining layer the once densely packed phospholipid lamellae unravel and become associated with an apoprotein which is probably also synthesized by the type II cells by the usual pathway of protein synthesis, involving ribosomes, endoplasmic reticulum, and Golgi complex. Within the lining layer this lipoprotein complex now forms a new pattern of regular array (Fig. 9.19), so-called tubular myelin, and it can spread on its free surface as a monomolecular film.

These structural transformations of the surfactant material are related to the physical properties of DPPC. As shown in Figure 9.15, the DPPC molecule, like all phospholipids, is hydrophilic at its polar choline end, whereas it is strongly hydrophobic (water repellent) at the two fatty-acid chains. In an aqueous medium phospholipids form micelles or bimolecular leaflets with the hydrophobic ends facing each other. In the lamellar bodies such leaflets become densely

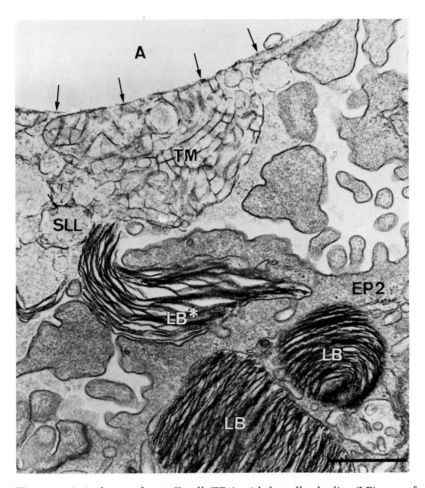

Fig. 9.18 Apical part of type II cell (EP2) with lamellar bodies (LB); one of these (LB*) is seen in the process of being secreted into the surface lining layer (SLL). The free surface of the lining layer is covered by a thin black film of DPPC (arrows) which is connected with tubular myelin (TM) in the hypophase. Scale marker: 0.5 μm. (From Weibel and Gil, 1977.)

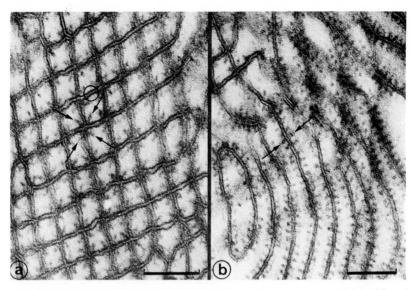

Fig. 9.19   Fine structure of tubular myelin seen on transverse (a) and longitudinal section (b). The lattice is formed by bilayers of DPPC (circle) intersecting according to a square tubular pattern. The surfactant apoproteins appear as particles within the "tubules" (arrows). Scale markers: 0.1 μm. (From Hassett et al., 1980.)

stacked, as shown in Figure 9.20. When the apoprotein is added to the hydrophilic side, the hydrophobic side remains unchanged and will still tend to form bimolecular leaflets, but if they become stacked they will be spaced by the thickness of the apoprotein. This is the picture one observes in the myelin sheaths of nerve fibers. The surfactant lipoprotein has the peculiar, and very characteristic, property of stacking up in the form of square tubules with the apoproteins in the center of the tubule (Fig. 9.19). It seems that this constitutes a reserve form of surfactant which can spread on the free surface directly from tubular myelin as these figures are often continuous with the surface film (Figs. 9.18 and 9.20), but some of this is still open to debate.

Pulmonary surfactant is turned over rather rapidly. Continuous synthesis must therefore be coupled with regulated removal, for which two pathways are known: some of the surfactant leaves the alveolar region over the surface of terminal bronchioles, from where it is removed by the mucociliary escalator; some is engulfed by alveolar macrophages (Fig. 9.20) and broken up in their lysosomes which are known to contain, besides their usual complement of acid hydrolases, phospholipase A_2, the enzyme we have seen to cleave fatty acids from phosphatidylcholine. It is not known whether there are other mechanisms for removing surfactant that has become inactivated, but some recent evidence suggests that part of it may be recycled through the type II cells.

Much of what we have learned on surfactant production and turnover is still speculative to some extent. The question must be asked why, a quarter of a century after the discovery of the phospholipid nature of surfactant, we have not yet solved some of the key issues of surfactant metabolism. One answer is that the topic is difficult to deal with because type II cells are such a small cell population, amounting to less than 10% of alveolar septal tissue and to no more than 4% of lung weight; they are furthermore difficult to separate from macrophages, their functional counterpart. Only very recently has it become possible to isolate type II cells in reasonably pure preparations for thorough biochemical analysis.

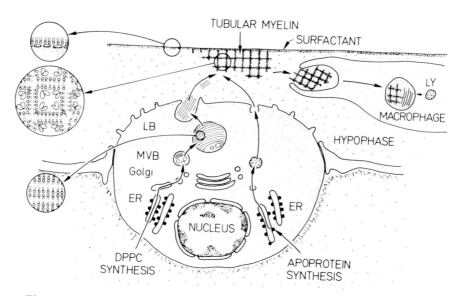

Fig. 9.20 Schematic diagram of pathways for synthesis and secretion of surfactant DPPC and apoproteins by a type II cell, and for their removal by macrophages. Note the arrangement of phospholipids in the lamellar bodies, in tubular myelin, and in the surface film.

A further difficult and only partly understood topic is that of the *regulation* of surfactant synthesis and turnover. One postulates "neurohumoral" pathways, but nothing very precise is as yet known. On the one hand, local regulatory effects must be postulated because one knows that surfactant production becomes stimulated by increased ventilation; this is, of course, sensible because one would expect the demand for surface active material to increase when the alveolar surface becomes more rapidly and more intensely distorted due to augmented ventilatory movements. However, it is possible that this increased surfactant production is the result of neural effects, since it can also be brought about by stimulation of the vagus nerve and by some neurotransmitters, mainly β-adrenergic agonists. The problem with respect to neural control is that the lung parenchyma contains very few nerve fibers and they have not been shown to be related to type II cells.

There is reasonably good evidence that the potential for surfactant synthesis develops under the effect of some hormones, particularly corticosteroids. This plays a major role during fetal lung development. We have seen in chapter 8 that type II cells differentiate at the time of transition from the canalicular to the saccular stage, that is, between the 18th and 25th gestational week in man. Surfactant then begins to be secreted into the lung fluid, where one can observe tubular myelin figures. This is evidently most crucial in view of the fact that, upon the first breath, the newborn baby must be able to instantaneously open up all its alveoli and keep them open. Sufficient quantities of surfactant have usually been produced by the 28th gestational week, although birth normally takes place only at about the 40th week. For this reason premature babies are capable of surviving in a protected environment after the 26th or 28th week. However, in some prematurely born infants this is not the case because the onset of surfactant production shows some variation. Such babies rapidly develop a severe, life-threatening disease called the respiratory distress syndrome of the newborn, because they cannot take up enough O_2 in their ever-collapsing lungs. The tissue becomes damaged and hyaline membranes, a clotted layer of exudate, cover the epithelium, thus worsening the condition. Enormous efforts are required just to give these babies a slim chance of survival. Very often this condition could be avoided if birth could be delayed just long enough for surfactant production to become adequate, which can be promoted by treating the mothers with corticosteroids.

The surfactant content can be monitored because the lung fluid communicates freely with amniotic fluid which can be tapped by amniocentesis: when surfactant production has become adequate one finds the DPPC concentration in amniotic fluid to have risen to a certain level.

Thus, in conclusion, we find that the alveolar secretory or type II cells play a vital role in respiration in that they allow a large surface between air and blood to be maintained from the first breath to the last.

COPING WITH VULNERABILITY

The alveolar epithelium is easily damaged, particularly because each of the very thin type I cells is exposed to air over a much larger surface than any other cell. It is, in fact, astonishing how little seems to happen to this cell which, as we have seen, has only a limited potential for repairing membrane defects, for example. But there is an additional problem: one finds that type I cells are not capable of multiplying by mitosis, neither during lung growth when more cells are needed to coat the expanding alveolar surface, nor upon damage in the adult lung when cells need to be replaced. In both instances new type I cells are made by mitotic division and transformation of type II cells which form squamous extensions and lose their potential for surfactant synthesis, a process which takes about 2–5 days.

This seems to work under normal circumstances. There are, however, conditions where this repair mechanism is too slow to cope with excessive damages, so that a syndrome of severe catastrophic respiratory failure develops which requires intensive care, mechanical ventilation, and supplemental O_2 just to allow the patient to survive. This can happen when the lung becomes diffusely damaged by toxic fumes, and here it is noteworthy that breathing pure O_2 over a prolonged period is highly toxic to lung cells; but it also occurs in shock, for example upon severe blood loss or as a consequence of multiple bone fractures, common effects of traffic accidents. In such patients one finds large parts of the type I cell lining of the alveolar surface to be destroyed; as a consequence, the barrier has become leaky and the alveoli fill with blood plasma, a condition called alveolar edema, so that they can no longer take part in gas exchange.

With proper medical care this alveolar edema can often be resolved within a few days. The alveoli become again filled with air — but in spite of this, gas exchange does not improve. What has happened is that the repair of the severely damaged alveolar epithelium requires a lot of new cells to be made by division of type II cells. These form a rather thick cuboidal lining of the barrier surface, and this thick barrier offers a high resistance to O_2 flow. It takes several weeks until a thin barrier is restored by transformation of the cuboidal cell lining into delicate type I cells. The medical problem is to allow the patient to survive long enough for this to happen. A major difficulty in that respect is that high concentrations of O_2 which would improve oxygenation of the blood might worsen the condition owing to the toxic effects of high O_2 tensions on the lung cells.

To build and maintain a very thin barrier over a large surface is evidently vital, but it results in a design of tissue structure that is highly vulnerable because it may be at the limit of what is feasible. The lung's cell population has evolved mechanisms for coping with this degree of vulnerability, first by establishing a sequence of defense mechanisms from the mucociliary escalator to alveolar macrophages, and then by maintaining a repair potential in the alveolar cells. But this repair potential is greatly limited by the fact that the barrier must be so very thin. When the damage exceeds the normal repair potential, the cells of the barrier must first become considerably bulkier in order to rebuild an integral lining, and this impairs gas exchange.

Summary

The lung's cardinal function, gas exchange, can only be maintained if a number of ancillary functions are performed by cells; among them the maintenance of permeability barriers and of a mechanical support system, the secretion of surfactant to keep the air spaces open and of mucus to cleanse the airways, as well as defense against foreign intruders. To serve all these functions the lung maintains a cell population of some 40 different cell types.

The airways — from the trachea to alveoli — are lined by an uninterrupted epithelial sheet which forms a tight permeability barrier between the interstitial space and the extracellular fluid layer at the epithelial surface. The epithelial cells serve two main functions: lining the surface, and secretion. In conducting airways the lining cells are provided with kinocilia which propel the mucus lining of the epithelium outward; the secretory cells are goblet cells secreting mucus, or, in small bronchioles, Clara cells whose secretory product is not yet clearly identified. In alveoli the lining cells are greatly attenuated squamous cells (type I cells), whereas secretory cells (type II cells) are specialized for the production and secretion of surfactant. The vascular spaces, from the pulmonary artery through capillaries to the pulmonary veins, are lined by a simple endothelial lining which can serve some ancillary functions on the blood, such as the conversion of angiotensin I to angiotensin II. The interstitial space contains a heterogeneous cell population. Fibroblasts are responsible for the synthesis and maintenance of the connective tissue fiber system, but they may also exhibit contractile properties. Smooth muscle cells occur in the wall of conducting blood vessels and airways as regulators of flow resistance, and also in the wall of alveolar ducts.

Defense cells play an important role in the lung. Macrophages are nonspecific defense cells which occur on the airspace surface from alveoli to major bronchi as well as in the interstitial space; they are derived from blood monocytes that originate in the bone marrow and settle in the lung secondarily. Cells of the specific or immune defense system are found throughout the interstitial space. Lymphatic vessels with lymph nodes establish an escape route for defense cells; they originate in the major connective tissue beds near alveoli—not in alveolar septa—and drain into the jugular veins. Some indigestible material—such as carbon particles (soot, smoke) or silica—are permanently deposited in connective tissue, contained in histiocytes.

The cells of the alveolar region are specialized to assist gas exchange; they constitute $\frac{3}{4}$ of all lung cells. The alveolar epithelial lining cells (type I) are very large cells that cover 95% of the alveolar surface by very much attenuated cytoplasmic leaflets. They are complex branched cells that form multiple apical plates and have lost their capacity for proliferation by cell division; when damaged they must be replaced by the proliferation of type II cells, which constitute the stem cell population of the alveolar epithelium. The main function of type II alveolar cells is the synthesis, storage, and secretion of surfactant. They are relatively small cuboidal cells (in spite of their large appearance on sections) richly endowed with cell organelles, particularly with mitochondria and endoplasmic reticulum. Their special features are osmiophilic lamellar granules bounded by a membrane, which are the sites of storage and possibly partial synthesis of surfactant phospholipids. The main surfactant phospholipid is dipalmitoyl-phosphatidylcholine (DPPC), a lecithin whose two fatty acids are saturated palmitic acid. It lowers surface tension at an air–water interface by spreading on the surface as a monomolecular film with the hydrophobic fatty acids pointing outward. The mechanism of DPPC synthesis is not fully established but probably involves two steps: the synthesis of unsaturated phosphatidylcholine followed by reacylation where the unsaturated fatty acids are replaced by palmitic acid. Both steps appear to take place in the type II cells. Surfactant synthesis is regulated partly through hormones, particularly corticosteroids. In the fetal lung surfactant synthesis begins at 18 weeks of gestation; adequate amounts of surfactant should be secreted by 28 weeks when the airways of prematurely born babies should be able to stay open.

Further Reading

GENERAL CELL BIOLOGY

Gabella, G. 1981. Structure of smooth muscle cells. In *Smooth Muscle: An Assessment of Current Knowledge*, ed. E. Bülbring, A. F. Brading, A. W. Jones, and T. Tomita. Austin: University of Texas Press, pp. 1–46.

Loewenstein, W. R. 1981. Junctional intercellular communication: the cell-to-cell membrane channel. *Physiological Reviews* 61:829–913.

Palade, G. E. 1975. Intracellular aspects of the process of protein synthesis. *Science* 189:347–358. (Nobel Lecture.)

LUNG CELLS AND SURFACTANT

Bakhle, Y. S., and J. R. Vane, eds. 1977. *Metabolic Functions of the Lung*. New York: Dekker.

Brain, J. D., D. F. Proctor, and L. M. Reid. 1977. *Respiratory Defense Mechanisms*. New York: Dekker.

Clements, J. A., and R. King. 1976. Composition of surface active material. In *The Biochemical Basis of Pulmonary Function*, ed. R. G. Crystal. New York: Dekker, pp. 363–387.

Crystal, R. G., ed. 1976. *The Biochemical Basis of Pulmonary Function*. New York: Dekker.

Jeffery, P. K., and L. M. Reid. 1977. The respiratory mucous membrane. In *Respiratory Defense Mechanisms*, ed. J. D. Brain, D. F. Proctor, and L. M. Reid. New York: Dekker, pp. 193–245.

Kauffman, S. L. 1980. Cell proliferation in the mammalian lung. *International Review of Experimental Pathology* 22:131–191.

Lauweryns, J. M., and J. H. Baert. 1977. Alveolar clearance and the role of pulmonary lymphatics. *American Review of Respiratory Disease* 115:625–683.

Ryan, U.S., and J. W. Ryan. 1977. Correlations between the fine structure of the alveolar-capillary unit and its metabolic activities. In *Metabolic Functions of the Lung*, ed. Y. S. Bakhle and J. R. Vane. New York: Dekker, pp. 197–232.

Sleigh, M. A. 1977. The nature and action of respiratory tract cilia. In *Respiratory Defense Mechanisms*, pt. I, ed. J. D. Brain, D. F. Proctor, and L. M. Reid. New York: Dekker, pp. 247–288.

Weibel, E. R. 1984. Lung cell biology. In *Handbook of Physiology: Respiration*, vol. 4, ed. A. P. Fishman and A. B. Fisher. Washington: American Physiological Society (in press).

References

CELL BIOLOGY

Adamson, I. Y. R., and D. H. Bowden. 1974. The type 2 cell as progenitor of alveolar epithelial regeneration: a cytodynamic study in mice after exposure to oxygen. *Laboratory Investigation* 30:35–42.

Bachofen, M., and E. R. Weibel. 1977. Alterations of the gas exchange apparatus in adult respiratory insufficiency associated with septicemia. *American Review of Respiratory Disease* 116:589–615.

Bouhuys, A., ed. 1976. *Lung Cells in Disease*. Amsterdam: North-Holland.

Bowden, D. H., and I. Y. Adamson. 1980. Role of monocytes and interstitial cells in the generation of alveolar macrophages. I. Kinetic studies in normal mice. *Laboratory Investigation* 42:511–517.

Bradley, K. H., O. Kawanami, V. J. Ferrans, and R. G. Crystal. 1980. The fibroblast of human lung alveolar structures: a differentiated cell with a major role in lung structure and function. *Methods in Cell Biology* 21A:37–64.

Burri, P. H., and E. R. Weibel. 1973. Funktionelle Aspekte der Lungenmorphologie. In *Röntgendiagnostik der Lunge. Aktuelle Probleme der Röntgendiagnostik 2*, ed. W. A. Fuchs and E. Vögeli. Bern: Huber, pp. 1–17.

Caldwell, P. R. B., and E. R. Weibel. 1980. Pulmonary oxygen toxicity. In *Pulmonary Diseases and Disorders*, ed. A. P. Fishman. New York: McGraw-Hill, pp. 800–805.

Caldwell, P. R. B., B. C. Seegal, K. C. Hsu, M. Das, and R. L. Soffer. 1976. Angiotensin converting enzyme: vascular endothelial localization. *Science* 191:1050–1051.

Crapo, J. D., B. E. Barry, P. Gehr, M. Bachofen, and E. R. Weibel. 1982. Cell number and cell characteristics of the normal human lung. *American Review of Respiratory Diseases* 125:332–337.

Evans, M. J., L. J. Cabral, R. J. Stephens, and G. Freeman. 1975. Transformation of alveolar type 2 cells to type 1 cells following exposure to NO_2. *Experimental Molecular Pathology* 22:142–150.

Fox, B., T. B. Bull, and A. Guz. 1980. Innervation of alveolar walls in the human lung: an electron microscopic study. *Journal of Anatomy* 131:683–692.

Haies, D., J. Gil, and E. R. Weibel. 1981. Morphometric study of rat lung cells. I. Numerical and dimensional characteristics of parenchymal cell population. *American Review of Respiratory Disease* 123:533–541.

Kapanci, Y., A. Assimacopoulos, C. Irle, A. Zwahlen, and G. Gabbiani. 1974. "Contractile interstitial cells" in pulmonary alveolar septa: a possible regulator of ventilation/perfusion ratio? Ultrastructural immunofluorescence and in vitro studies. *Journal of Cell Biology* 60:375–392.

Kapanci, Y., E. R. Weibel, H. P. Kaplan, and F. R. Robinson. 1969. Pathogenesis and reversibility of the pulmonary lesions of oxygen toxicity in monkeys. II. Ultrastructural and morphometric studies. *Laboratory Investigation* 20:101–118.

* Low, F. N. 1953. The pulmonary alveolar epithelium of laboratory animals. *Anatomical Record* 117:241–263.

Ryan, G. B., W. J. Cliff, G. Gabbiani, C. Irle, P. R. Statkov, and G. Majno. 1973. Myofibroblasts in an avascular fibrous tissue. *Laboratory Investigation* 29:197–206.

Stossel, T. P. 1976. The mechanism of phagocytosis. *Journal of the Reticuloendothelial Society* 19:237–245.

Weibel, E. R. 1971. The mystery of "non-nucleated plates" in the alveolar epithelium of the lung explained. *Acta Anatomica* 78:425–443.

——— 1974. On pericytes, particularly their existence on lung capillaries. *Microvascular Research* 8:218–235.

——— 1980. Design and structure of the human lung. In *Pulmonary Diseases and Disorders*, ed. A. P. Fishman. New York: McGraw-Hill, pp. 224–271.

Weibel, E. R., and J. Gil. 1977. Structure–function relationships at the alveolar level. In *Bioengineering Aspects of the Lung*, ed. J. B. West. New York: Dekker, pp. 1–81.

SURFACTANT

Askin, F. B., and C. Kuhn. 1971. The cellular origin of pulmonary surfactant. *Laboratory Investigation* 25:260–268.

* Buckingham, S., and M. E. Avery. 1962. Time of appearance of lung surfactant in the fetal mouse. *Nature* 193:688–689.

Buckingham, S., H. O. Heinemann, S. C. Sommers, and W. F. McNary. 1966. Phospholipid synthesis in the large pulmonary alveolar cells. *American Journal of Pathology* 48:1027–1041.

Clements, J. A. 1970. Pulmonary surfactant. *American Review of Respiratory Disease* 101:984–990.

* Gil, J., and O. K. Reiss. 1973. Isolation and characterization of lamellar bodies and tubular myelin from rat lung homogenates. *Journal of Cell Biology* 58:152–171.

Gluck, L., M. V. Kulovich, A. I. Eidelman, L. Cordero, and A. F. Khazin. 1972. Biochemical development of surface activity in mammalian lung. IV. Pulmonary lecithin synthesis in the human fetus and newborn and etiology of the respiratory distress syndrome. *Pediatric Research* 6:81–99.

Hassett, R. J., W. Engelman, and C. Kuhn. 1980. Extramembranous particles in tubular myelin from rat lung. *Journal of Ultrastructure Research* 71:60–67.

Hitchcock, K. R. 1980. Lung development and the pulmonary surfactant system: hormonal influences. *Anatomical Record* 198:13–34.

Jacobs, H., A. Jobe, M. Ikegami, and D. Conaway. 1983. The significance of reutilization of surfactant phospholipids. *Journal of Biological Chemistry* 258:4156–4165.

King, R. J. 1979. Utilization of alveolar epithelial type II cells for the study of pulmonary surfactant. *Federation Proceedings* 38:2637–2643.

King, R. J., H. Martin, D. Mitts, and F. M. Holmstrom. 1977. Metabolism of the apoproteins in pulmonary surfactant. *Journal of Applied Physiology* 42:483–491.

10

AIRWAYS AND BLOOD VESSELS

A MAJOR PROBLEM in designing a pulmonary gas exchanger is to set up routes for efficient renewal of air and blood on the large gas exchanging surface. The basic design principle is to build three interdigitating trees, one each for airways, arteries, and veins, and to arrange the gas exchange units about their end twigs. Evidently, this can only function if the design of these three trees is well matched. In this chapter we shall examine the design properties of the airway and vascular trees as they affect ventilation and blood flow.

The Airway Tree

The lung's airways originate in a single tube, the trachea, penetrate into each lung with a main-stem bronchus, and then continue to branch by dichotomy like a tree, progressively reducing their diameters (Fig. 10.1). The airways begin as simple branched tubes whose surface is lined by a mucous membrane, as we saw in chapter 9. As we approach the periphery their structure changes in that more and more alveoli, containing a gas exchange surface, are formed as outpocketings of their wall until, in the last few generations, the circumference of the alveolar ducts and sacs is totally occupied by alveoli (Fig. 10.2).

On the basis of these design features one assigns the airways to different classes or functional zones (Fig. 10.3): bronchi and bron-

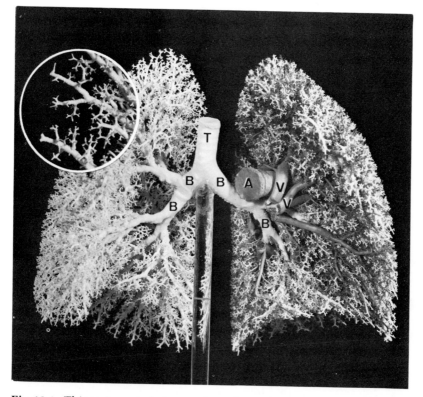

Fig. 10.1 This resin cast of a human lung shows the branching pattern of the bronchial tree (B) which originates from the trachea (T). In the left lung the pulmonary arteries (A) and veins (V) are filled as well. The inset shows the peripheral airway branching at higher power.

chioles are purely conducting structures whose main function is to distribute the air into the peripheral units; respiratory bronchioles and alveolar ducts are transitional elements as they distribute the air into the respiratory zone, the alveoli with which they are intimately associated.

This structural hierarchy of the airways is of great importance for understanding many of the functional events that are related to ventilation and to gas exchange. In that respect I should like to point out that one of the units of lung structure is defined through the hierarchic properties of the airways: the *acinus* is the complex of all airways distal to the terminal bronchiole and thus served by a first order respiratory bronchiole (Fig. 10.3), that is, the largest unit in

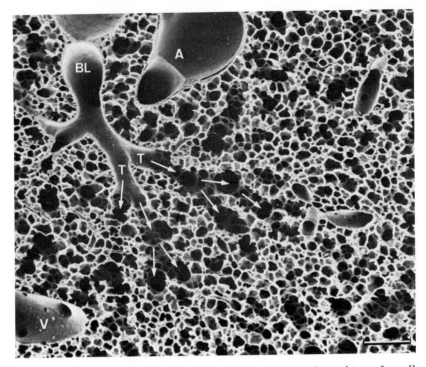

Fig. 10.2 Scanning electron micrograph of lung shows branching of small peripheral bronchiole (BL) into terminal bronchioles (T) from where the airways continue into respiratory bronchioles and alveolar ducts (arrows). Note the location of the pulmonary artery (A) and vein (V). Scale marker: 200 μm.

which all airways participate, to a greater or lesser extent, in gas exchange. It is intuitively plausible that different conditions will have to prevail in acinar as compared with conducting airways.

If we now look at the pattern of airway branching, we observe that each parent branch gives rise to two smaller daughter branches — the same pattern that we saw in the growth of the airway tree during lung development (Figs. 8.3 to 8.6). In the mature lung we observe that the two daughter branches from the same parent branch often differ in diameter and length (Fig. 10.1). This pattern is called *irregular dichotomy*, in contrast to regular dichotomy where all branches in one generation are of the same size (Fig. 10.4). Nonetheless, the morphometric analysis of such trees reveals that the progression of airway dimensions from the trachea to the periphery follows strict laws which are functionally relevant.

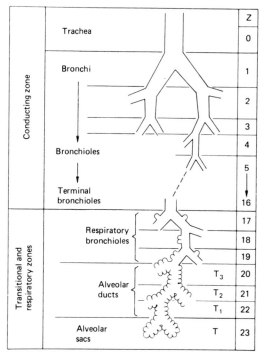

Fig. 10.3 Organization of the airway tree by functional zones in relation to generations (z) of dichotomous branching. (From Weibel, 1963).

There are two basic ways for classifying branches in a tree, and I should mention them briefly in order to explain certain concepts. The first approach is to number the branches progressively by generation as one goes down the (inverted) tree, starting with generation

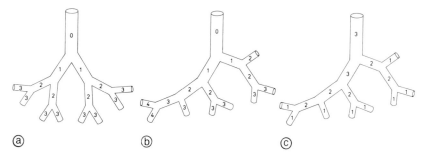

Fig. 10.4 Patterns of airway branching: (a) regular dichotomy; (b) irregular dichotomy numbered by "generations down"; (c) irregular dichotomy numbered by "orders up." (From Weibel, 1980.)

$z = 0$ at the trachea (Fig. 10.4a). I would like to call this the morpho-genetic approach because it simply follows the pattern of branching as it occurred during lung morphogenesis. Note that the number of branches in any generation z is twice that in the parent generation $(z - 1)$:

$$N(z) = 2 \cdot N(z - 1), \tag{10.1}$$

an obvious consequence of dichotomy. From this we can now imme-diately derive the total number of branches in generation z to be

$$N(z) = 2^z, \tag{10.2}$$

a very simple relation that is, in fact, quite useful. Note that this approach also holds in trees that branch by irregular dichotomy (Fig. 10.4b) with the limitation that end twigs will appear in various generations; accordingly, $N(z)$ will be smaller than 2^z in any genera-tion beyond that where the first termination occurred.

The alternative approach is to start numbering at the end twig which is designated as "order 1" (Fig. 10.4c). As we go up the tree the order is increased by 1 when two branches of the same order come together, but it remains unchanged when, for example, an order 2 branch meets an order 3 branch. In this so-called Strahler method one considers the airways as a system of tubes converging from the periphery toward the center, an approach used with success in describing river systems. It also makes sense in the lung if we consider, for example, the acini as the fundamental ventilatory units which are connected to the trachea by a system of bronchi of varying pathway length. One of the fundamental descriptors of this model is the branching ratio, that is, the ratio of the total number of branches in one order to that in the next higher order. For the human airway tree this branching ratio is found to be about 1.4 on the average, whereas it is, by definition, 2 in the dichotomy model.

The two models are conceptually different. In a way the Strahler model has some appeal because it naturally takes the irregularity of airway branching into account. Indeed, one can show that the diame-ter of any branch is proportional to the number or volume of periph-eral units into which it leads. The Strahler model accounts for this to a certain extent so that the variability of airway dimensions per Strahler order is less than that per dichotomy generation. However, the Strahler model seems to pose some analytical difficulties, so that the vast majority of physiological studies on air flow in the airways has so far been based on the dichotomy model. On the other hand, this does not really introduce major difficulties because both approaches lead to the same conclusions, in principle. I shall therefore base the following descriptions on the dichotomy model.

Let us first try to assign the various generations to the different types of airways (Fig. 10.3). By counting the number of alveolar sacs, the terminal airway elements, one can estimate that, in an adult human lung, the airways must branch over approximately 23 dichotomous generations, on the average, before they eventually end in a blind sac. This means that the total number of end branches is about $2^{23} \sim 8 \cdot 10^6$. By similar arguments one finds that terminal bronchioles, the last purely conducting airways, are located in about generation 16. Beyond the 16th generation all airways have alveoli in their wall and can hence participate in gas exchange. Evidently, these are average numbers; we disregard, for the time being, the fact that, in the real lung, terminal alveolar sacs may appear anywhere from about the 18th to the 30th generation of irregular dichotomy.

Let us now consider the reduction of airway diameters with progressive branching. In a first step we again simplify the model by "regularizing" the dichotomy, that is, we consider the mean diameter of all branches in a given generation to be the characteristic diameter d(z) for that generation. Figure 10.5 shows that, on a semilogarithmic plot, d(z) falls approximately along a straight line following the simple law

$$d(z) = d_0 \cdot 2^{-z/3} = d_0 \cdot \left[\sqrt[3]{\frac{1}{2}} \right]^z \tag{10.3}$$

where d_0 is the "ideal" diameter of the trachea. This relation shows that with each generation the airway diameter is reduced by the cube root of the branching ratio 2, a law that is well known in hydrodynamics, as it describes an optimal design of a branched system of tubes through which air or fluids can flow with a minimal loss of energy. By the way, performing this analysis on the Strahler model leads to the same result. It therefore appears that, from an engineering point of view, the airways of the lung are well designed to assure optimal conditions of air flow.

Figure 10.5 shows that the diameters of the acinar airways (generations 17 to 23) do not follow the law of reduction by $2^{-1/3}$; the diameters of respiratory bronchioles and alveolar ducts change very little

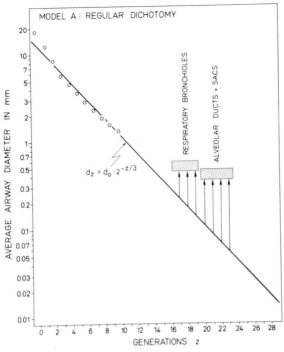

Fig. 10.5 The average diameter of airways in the human lung plotted semilogarithmically by generations of regularized dichotomous branching. The intra-acinar airways (generations 17–23) are comparatively larger than the conducting airways. (After Weibel, 1963.)

with each generation, as can easily be verified on real specimens (Fig. 10.2). Does this imply less than an optimal design at the periphery of the airways? No, on the contrary. The cube-root-of-2 law relates to optimizing mass flow of a liquid or of air. In the most peripheral airways mass flow is only part, and even a small part, of the means to bring O_2 toward the gas exchange surface. Since the airways are blind ending tubes, and since a sizable amount of residual air remains in the alveolar region after expiration (see below), O_2 molecules must penetrate through residual air by diffusion (Fig. 10.6). But O_2 diffusion is best served by as large a cross section of the airways as possible. Since in the respiratory zone the airway diameter remains nearly unchanged as branching progresses, the total airway cross section nearly doubles with each generation.

Thus, on the whole, the design of the pulmonary airway system appears to be governed by strict engineering rules, striving to optimize the conditions for convective O_2 transport in the purely conducting bronchi and bronchioles, and those for diffusive O_2 transport within the acinus.

We can now consider the irregularity of dichotomous branching of the airways by estimating the distribution of airways of a given diameter over a range of generations; we find, for example, 2 mm bronchi to be located in generations 4 to 13, with a mean of 8. The reasoning behind this analysis is that the diameter of an airway is somehow proportional to the volume of lung parenchyma into which it leads; since a human lung contains about 400 such bronchi, the units they supply must have a volume of about 12 ml. But since these bronchi occur over a range of generations, their distance to the

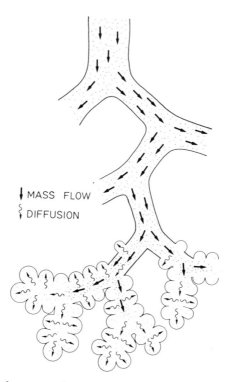

MASS FLOW

DIFFUSION

Fig. 10.6 In the lung periphery O_2 molecules reach alveoli by combined mass air flow (convection) and by molecular diffusion within the air phase. (From Weibel, 1980.)

trachea, called the bronchial pathway length, will show a certain distribution; as shown in Figure 10.7 it varies from 18 to 31 cm from the root of the trachea at the larynx, with an average of 23 cm. Some of the units served by these 2 mm bronchi are therefore much further away from the entrance to the airways than others.

There is one unit of this kind which merits our special attention: the acinus as the ventilatory unit fed by first-order respiratory bronchioles and in which all airways participate in gas exchange. In the human lung the acinus measures about 5 mm in length and has a mean volume of $30 - 40$ mm³; one estimates that there are some 150,000 acini. The first-order respiratory bronchioles have a mean diameter of 0.54 mm and were found to fall into the 17th generation in the regular dichotomy model; 2^{17} is about 130,000. One now finds that the average of nine generations that lead from 2 mm bronchi to first-order respiratory bronchioles covers an average pathway length of approximately 5 cm. Making a number of assumptions about the statistical distribution of such pathway lengths, one can now derive a distribution function which locates the entrances to acini with respect to the root of the trachea (Fig. 10.7): the total bronchial pathway length to acini averages 30 cm but covers the range of 23–38 cm. Note that this is the distance from the larynx; about 15 cm should be added to account for the total pathway length from the nostrils through nose and throat to the lung.

The morphometric analysis of airway dimensions furthermore permits some calculations about the distribution of air volume to the

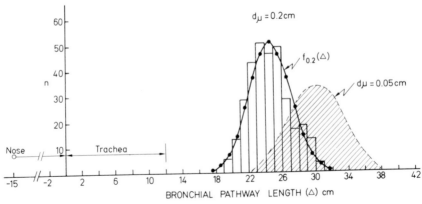

Fig. 10.7 Distribution of airways of diameter 0.2 cm and 0.05 cm with respect to bronchial pathway length (distance from larynx or nose).

TABLE 10.1 APPROXIMATE DISTRIBUTION OF TOTAL LUNG VOLUME IN ML FOR ADULT HUMAN LUNG INFLATED TO $\frac{3}{4}$ TOTAL LUNG CAPACITY.

	Compartments		
Zones	Airways	Tissue	Blood
Conducting	Bronchi 170	Walls Septa	Arteries 150 / Veins 150
Transition	Respiratory bronchioles	Fibers Lymph	Arterioles 60 / Venules 60
	Alveolar ducts 1,500	Pleura 200	
Respiratory	Alveoli 3,150	Barrier 150	Capillaries 140
Total	4,820	350	560
		5,730	
Maximal inflation	TLC 6,400	350	650
		7,400	

various functional zones of the lung. This is done in Table 10.1 for an adult human lung inflated to about $\frac{3}{4}$ of its total lung capacity or maximal lung volume. We note that over 80% of the total lung volume is air, of which the bulk is found in the acini. Only some 170 ml of air is contained in the bronchi and bronchioles of the conducting zone; this is called the *anatomic dead space* because the air entering this part of the airway tree on inspiration cannot contribute to gas exchange but is exhaled unaltered on expiration. The anatomic dead space can also be estimated by physiological methods; it comes out at the same value. In Table 10.1 we have subdivided the air contained in the acini into two compartments: the alveoli where gas exchange with blood occurs, and the transitional bronchioles and ducts which are part of the airway tree. This subdivision is not of great functional importance, however, because the gas in alveoli and ducts must be well equilibrated; the term "alveolar gas volume" used in physiology actually comprises all elements of the acini, alveoli as well as ducts. As we have seen above (Fig. 10.6), O_2 moves mostly by diffusion through these acinar airways; but, clearly, expansion of the lung on inspiration and shrinkage on expiration lead to considerable volume changes primarily in this part of the airway system.

Ventilation

If we now look at the physiology of the airway system, we first note that various static volumes of the lung can be defined. By letting a subject breathe normally into a spirometer, as shown in Figure 10.8, we can estimate the *tidal volume* (V_T), that is, the volume of air he moves back and forth between inspiration and expiration. At rest the tidal volume measures about 500 ml, but it can increase to several liters in exercise. If we ask the subject to take as deep a breath as he can take and to then exhale as completely as possible, we obtain the *vital capacity* (VC), the maximal volume of air that he can move into and out of the lung, which amounts to about 5 – 6 liters. But at the end of maximal expiration there is still about 1.5 liters of air left in the lung; we call this the *residual volume* (RV). Two further lung volumes are of importance: the *total lung capacity* (TLC) is the sum of vital capacity and residual volume, whereas the *functional residual*

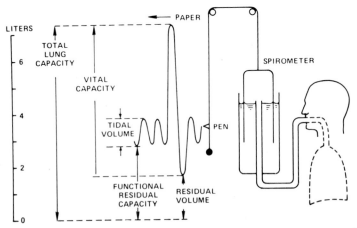

Fig. 10.8 Definition of the various physiological lung volumes in man. Note that the functional residual capacity, residual volume, and total lung capacity cannot be measured with the spirometer directly. (From West, 1974.)

capacity (FRC) is the volume of gas left in the lung after a normal expiration.

Neither the residual volume nor TLC and FRC can be measured directly by spirometry. However, one can estimate FRC by a dilution technique: the subject is connected to a spirometer of volume V_s that contains a known concentration C_1 of an inert tracer gas, for example helium. After several breaths the gases in the lung and in the spirometer become equilibrated, and the helium concentration falls to C_2 in proportion to the dilution that occurred as FRC was mixed in with the gas in the spirometer. FRC is calculated from these two concentrations:

$$FRC = V_s \cdot (C_1 - C_2)/C_2. \tag{10.4}$$

From this one can evidently calculate TLC and RV by using the direct spirometry data (Fig. 10.8).

Ventilation is the process by which air in the lung is renewed. We calculate its rate, the so-called minute volume or total ventilation, as the product of tidal volume times respiratory frequency (f).

$$\dot{V}_E = f \cdot V_T. \tag{10.5}$$

Minute volume is commonly given the subscript E because it is measured on expiration. Thus, if the tidal volume is 500 ml and the breathing frequency 15 per minute, total ventilation amounts to 7,500 ml·min^{-1}. However, only part of this will reach the respiratory part of the lung; with each breath about 150 ml will stay behind in the anatomic dead space in order to be exhaled without having contributed to gas exchange. The ventilation of the acini ($\dot{V}_A$), called "alveolar" ventilation in physiology, is obtained by subtracting the dead-space volume from each tidal volume

$$\dot{V}_A = f \cdot (V_T - V_D) = \dot{V}_E - \dot{V}_D \tag{10.6}$$

where $\dot{V}_D$ is called dead-space ventilation. In the case of the normal resting subject mentioned above, alveolar ventilation amounts to 5,250 ml·min^{-1}. It is worth noting that this level of alveolar ventilation operates against an FRC of approximately 2,500 ml, which is hence turned over about twice every minute.

An important part of the scope of this book is to search out the functional capacities of the respiratory system by identifying limiting conditions. We should therefore examine the changes in ventilation that occur in heavy exercise. Table 10.2 shows a set of data obtained by a group of Swedish physiologists on healthy young men exercising on a bicycle for 50 minutes; the level of exercise was rather strenuous as evidenced by the high heart rate and the 8.6 fold increase in O_2 consumption. We note that total ventilation increased by a factor of 9.6, but that alveolar ventilation was increased 11 fold. The reason for this is that tidal volume increases more than breathing rate, so that inspired air can penetrate deeper into the acinar air spaces. Accordingly, dead-space ventilation increases less, although the dead space becomes enlarged when we breathe at higher lung volumes because the greater tension on the tissue fibers causes the bronchi and bronchioles to widen somewhat.

The dimensions of the airway tree influence the ventilatory flow of air in a number of ways. First of all, air flow velocity falls along the airway tree because the total cross-sectional area of the airways

TABLE 10.2. EFFECTS OF HEAVY EXERCISE ON VENTILATION AND CIRCULATION IN YOUNG HEALTHY MEN.

Variable	Symbol [units]	Rest	Exercise	Exercise/ Rest
O_2 consumption	$\dot{V}_{O_2}[ml \cdot min^{-1}]$	270	2,420	8.6
	$\dot{V}_{O_2}[mMol \cdot min^{-1}]$	12.5	108	
Ventilation				
Total ventilation	$\dot{V}_E[ml \cdot min^{-1}]$	7,100	68,100	9.6
Alveolar ventilation	$\dot{V}_A[ml \cdot min^{-1}]$	4,600	51,700	11.2
Respiratory rate	$f_R[min^{-1}]$	15	30	2.0
Tidal volume	$V_T[ml]$	475	2,270	4.8
Dead space	$V_D[ml]$	170	550	3.2
Circulation				
Blood flow	$\dot{Q}[ml \cdot min^{-1}]$	6,300	15,800	2.5
Heart rate	$f_H[min^{-1}]$	76	166	2.2
Stroke volume	$[ml]$	83	95	1.15
Ventilation/perfusion ratio	$\dot{V}_A/\dot{Q}$	0.73	3.27	4.5

Data adapted from Dejours (1981) and Ekelund and Holmgren (1964).

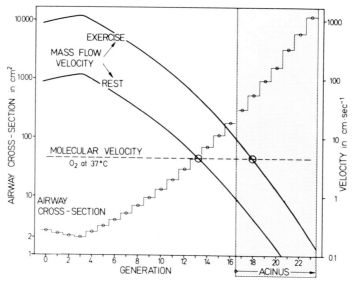

Fig. 10.9 As total airway cross section increases with the generations of airway branching, the mass flow velocity of inspired air decreases rapidly, falling below the molecular velocity of O_2 diffusion in air as we enter the acinus.

increases with every generation (Fig. 10.9); whereas the cross-sectional area of the trachea is about 2.5 cm², that of the 1024 airways in the 10th generation taken together is 13 cm², and as we approach the acinar airways the total cross section reaches 300 cm². But since the same air volume flows through all generations, the flow velocity falls by more than 100 fold from the trachea to the acini: at rest the mean flow velocity on inspiration is about 1 m·sec⁻¹ in the trachea and less than 1 cm·sec⁻¹ in the first-order respiratory bronchioles. This shows that in the small airways the transport of O_2 by mass air flow is slower than that by diffusion, since O_2 molecules move through air at a velocity of about 5 cm·sec⁻¹. In exercise the flow velocities are up to ten times greater, in proportion to the increased ventilation (Table 10.2), and, accordingly, mass flow velocity is somewhat greater than molecular velocity at the entrance into the acini (Fig. 10.9).

The size of airways also determines the resistance to air flow. The overall resistance is, however, rather small; it is given by the reciprocal of the ratio of ventilatory air flow to the pressure difference between the mouth and alveoli, which is normally no greater than about 1 cm H_2O (mbar) or less than 1 mm Hg. It is large enough, however, to potentially affect the distribution of ventilation to the many gas exchange units. The resistance offered by a tube of radius r and length l is given by Poiseuille's law

$$R = k \cdot l / r^4 \tag{10.7}$$

which means that a doubling of the airway diameter reduces resistance by 16 fold. Thus a slight size difference between two airways will affect the distribution of air flow in favor of the wider branch. In the normal lung the size of airways appears well adjusted to ensure rather even distribution of air flow to the peripheral units. In diseased lungs, however, this may be greatly disturbed for various reasons. One such case is asthma, where contraction of the smooth muscle sleeve of bronchioles, together with inflammation, increases airway resistance, requiring greater work to ventilate the lung; uneven narrowing of the airways may then also cause ventilation of acini to be uneven. This example also demonstrates that regulation of airway caliber by smooth muscle activity plays an important role in ensuring even distribution of ventilatory air flow in the normal lung.

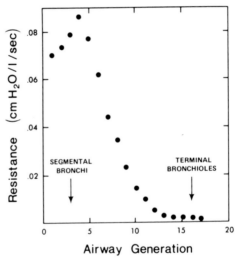

Fig. 10.10 Airway resistance to mass air flow is located mostly in the conducting airways and falls rapidly toward the periphery. (Redrawn after Pedley et al., 1970.)

Since the diameter of airways decreases as they branch (Fig. 10.5), one would suspect that their resistance increases toward the periphery. Apparently this is not the case, as the major pressure drop along the airways occurs in medium-sized bronchi; mainly because the flow velocity falls so rapidly as airways branch, the small airways have a low resistance (Fig. 10.10). This is further accentuated by the fact that the thin-walled bronchioles become widened as the lung expands on inspiration because they are subject to the tissue tensions in the coarse fiber system of the lung. Airway resistance is therefore seen to fall as lung volume increases. When this effect of tissue tension is disturbed, such as in emphysema, small bronchioles may collapse. This causes ventilation of the peripheral lung units to become highly uneven.

The Vascular Trees

The pulmonary arteries form a tree which is almost congruent with that of the airways. The main pulmonary artery arises from the right ventricle of the heart, lies to the left of the ascending aorta, and splits into its right and left branch under the aortic arch (Fig. 10.11). These branches join the bronchi while still in the mediastinum and remain in this close association all along the branching airway tree. Characteristically, each bronchus is associated with one branch of the pulmonary artery, and this relationship is strictly maintained to the periphery, that is, to the respiratory bronchioles in the acinus (Fig. 10.12).

In contrast, the pulmonary veins follow a course independent of the airways; rather they lie about midway between two pairs of airways and arteries. The detail of a resin cast shown in Figure 10.12 demonstrates that the structural lung units, that is, acini or lobules, have the airways and the arteries in their axis whereas the veins are at their periphery. Accordingly, the lung units are supplied by one artery, the one accompanying the airway, whereas their blood is drained into several veins; and thus, evidently, each vein collects blood from several units. The units of lung parenchyma are therefore bronchoarterial units which share their venous drainage with neighboring units. This intermediate or peripheral position of the pulmonary veins is also maintained throughout their course, right to the hilus where one finds, on each side, two main veins to lead into the left atrium located at the back of the heart (Fig. 10.11).

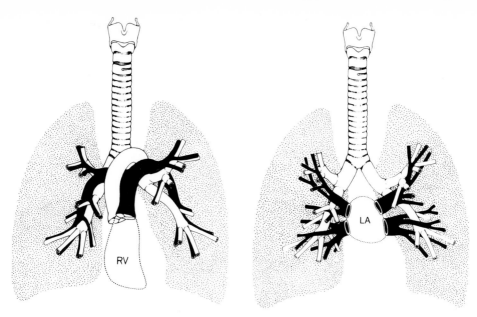

Fig. 10.11 Arrangement of the main pulmonary vessels: (left) the pulmonary arteries arise from the right ventricle (RV) and penetrate into the lung along the bronchi, whereas (right) two main stems of the pulmonary veins leave the lung on each side to lead into the left atrium (LA). (From Weibel, 1980.)

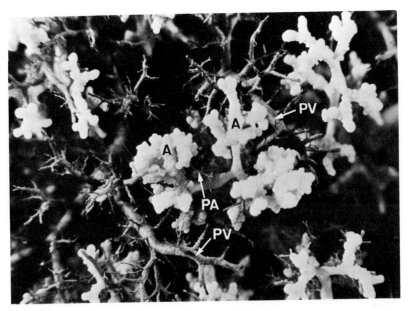

Fig. 10.12 Detail of cast of airways and blood vessels of human lung shows how pulmonary artery (PA) closely follows the airways (A) to the periphery, whereas the pulmonary vein branches (PV) lie between the units.

Since the arterial and the bronchial trees follow each other very closely, we can also analyze the dimensions of the pulmonary arteries by the model of a dichotomous tree (Fig. 10.4). However, at the periphery the arteries branch over a greater number of generations so that their terminal branches, the arterioles, are found in the 28th generation on the average. We shall see below that this is due to the fact that the microvascular unit of the lung is considerably smaller than the ventilatory unit.

The diameter of each pulmonary artery branch approximates closely that of its accompanying conducting airway (Figs. 10.1 and 10.12). Therefore, it is evident that the average diameter of the pulmonary artery branches also falls in proportion to $2^{-z/3}$ along the branching tree (Fig. 10.13). The terminal arteries, called arterioles or precapillaries, have a diameter of 20 to 50 μm. If this range of diameters is plotted at about generation 28 into the semilogarithmic plot of Figure 10.13, we find that it falls very nicely onto the extended line with slope $2^{-z/3}$. Thus it appears that the size reduction of pulmonary

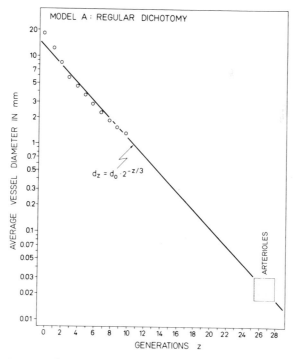

Fig. 10.13 Average diameter of pulmonary arteries follows the law of optimized mass flow of blood out to the most peripheral arterioles.

arteries abides to the cube-root-of-2 law from beginning to end. Evidently, blood is transported to the capillary bed by mass flow only, and we must therefore conclude that the pulmonary arteries optimize their dimensions to minimize the loss of energy due to blood flow. By the way, this design principle seems to hold also for arterial trees in the systemic circulation.

The alveolar capillary network of the lung is very different from that of the systemic circulation. Whereas in muscle, for example, we had found long capillaries to be joined in a loose network (Figs. 7.3 and 7.4), the capillaries of the alveolar walls form dense meshworks made of very short segments (Fig. 10.14). The meshes are so dense that some people believe blood flows through the alveolar walls like a

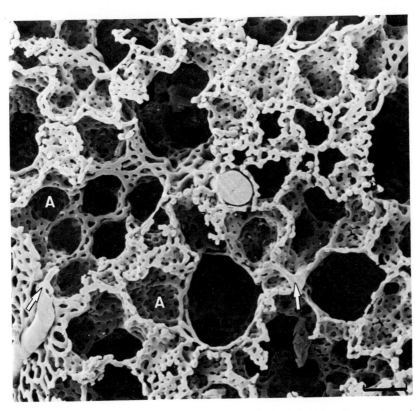

Fig. 10.14 Alveolar capillary network in walls of alveoli (A) demonstrated by a casting technique. Note larger vessel which leads into network (arrow). Scale marker: 50 μm. (Scanning electron micrograph courtesy Drs. L. Fischer and P. Burri.)

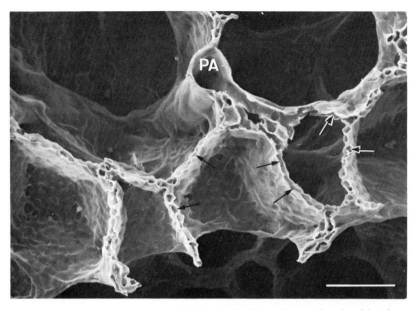

Fig. 10.15 Scanning electron micrograph of perfusion-fixed rabbit lung shows small pulmonary arteriole (PA) connecting to (empty) capillaries in alveolar walls (arrows). Scale marker: 50 μm.

sheet rather than through a system of interconnected tubes. In this sheet-flow concept the sheet is bounded by two flat membranes, the air–blood barrier, connected by numerous "posts." When blood flows through this sheet it is not channeled in a given direction but has freedom to move in a tortuous way between the posts. Although this concept oversimplifies the actual structural conditions, it does provide a useful description of the pattern of blood flow through the alveolar walls and explains why blood flow is not interrupted when some parts of the capillary bed become squashed flat at high inflation levels, as we shall discuss in the next chapter; the capillaries which remain open are simply some channels of this broad sheet. It is furthermore important to note that the capillary network or sheet is continuous through many alveolar walls, probably at least through-out the entire acinus, if not for greater distances. It is hence not possible to isolate microvascular units. One finds, rather, that arterial end branches simply feed into this broad sheet at more or less even distances, and that the veins drain these sheets in a similar pattern (Fig. 10.15). But now we must remember that the arteries reach the acinus along the airways whereas the veins are in a peripheral location (Fig. 10.12). In principle, therefore, blood flows through the acinar capillary sheet from the center to the periphery.

Pulmonary Blood Flow

Let us first remember that the pulmonary circulation is perfused with the total cardiac output, pumped by the right ventricle, and that the mean arterial pressure is 15 mm Hg in the pulmonary artery, as compared to 100 mm Hg in the systemic circulation (chapter 6). When the blood returns to the atria its pressure has fallen to a few mm Hg.

It is a well-known physical principle that blood flow ($\dot{Q}$) is determined by the pressure difference between the arterial and venous ends and by the resistance (R) offered by the vascular bed:

$$\dot{Q} = (P_a - P_v)/R. \tag{10.8}$$

Thus, evidently, the overall vascular resistance of the pulmonary vascular bed must be five times lower than that of systemic circulation, since blood flow is the same in spite of a smaller pressure difference. Pulmonary circulation is therefore described as a low pressure and low resistance system.

It is also well known that the resistance to blood flow is essentially determined by the size of the vessels; Poiseuille's law (equation 10.7) tells us that a small change in radius will have a large effect on resistance because the radius enters as its fourth power. Although blood flow does not obey Poiseuille's law in every respect, particularly in small vessels because of the presence of blood corpuscles, the general principle is still valid. It is therefore important for vessels to carefully regulate their size because, in a branched system of vessels, the distribution of blood flow to peripheral units greatly depends on the distribution of resistances in the vascular tree: if the resistance in one segment increases, blood flow to the unit served by that segment will be reduced.

The caliber of an artery is the result of two forces in balance: the distending force of blood pressure and the tension of the wall, regulated through the tone in the smooth muscle sleeve (Fig. 6.11). It is interesting to note that the thickness of the muscle sleeve is five times smaller in pulmonary than in systemic arteries, in keeping with the difference in blood pressure. But the tone of smooth muscle is variable and can be increased or lowered by vasoactive substances that are liberated through the sympathetic and parasympathetic nervous system. One of these substances is serotonin, which increases muscle tone and hence may cause the resistance to rise, because increased muscle tone leads to narrowing of the arterial cross section, unless blood pressure is increased as well.

The pressure drop that one observes to occur in a vascular system from the entrance to the arteries to the exit from the veins is the result of the serial arrangement of a large number of relatively small resistances; since they are in series, they are additive. The crucial question is where the main pressure drop occurs. In the systemic circulation arterial pressure falls from a mean of 100 mm Hg in the aorta to less than 30 mm Hg before the blood reaches the thin walled capillaries; this is an important factor in preventing fluid from leaking into the tissues. The resistance is therefore mainly in the arteries, specifically in their last branches, the arterioles, which are provided with a strong smooth muscle sleeve relative to their small diameter (Fig. 6.9). By this device the systemic circulation can efficiently regulate the distribution of blood flow to the many organs by simply varying local resistance in their arteries.

In the pulmonary arteries the pressure is low to begin with, and accordingly the pressure drop is small; starting with a mean pressure of 15 mm Hg in the main pulmonary artery, one still finds a pressure of about 12 mm Hg at the entrance to the capillary bed; consequently the wall of pulmonary arteries is relatively thin. Much of the pressure drop in the pulmonary circulation occurs in the capillaries.

There is an additional important difference: whereas systemic vessels are embedded in the tissues, pulmonary vessels are surrounded by air and are suspended on the fibrous tension system we shall describe in chapter 11. This introduces complications because the pressure gradient across the vessel wall, the so-called transmural pressure which influences flow conditions, may be quite variable. We shall see that the capillary bed will be shaped in part under the influence of surface tension and tissue forces: in a highly inflated lung many capillaries are squashed flat, offering high resistance, whereas they are wide at lower lung volumes. Pulmonary arteries and veins are much less affected by surface forces, but they do increase their cross section when the fiber system is extended; this is due to the fact that arteries and veins are embedded in connective tissue sheaths which are part of the fiber continuum and are therefore subject to tensions on lung inflation. Thus, as the lung is distended we should expect the arteries and veins to widen somehow which should reduce resistance. But as the lung is inflated, total pulmonary resistance increases. The only way to explain this is to assume that the major resistance is, indeed, in the capillary network. As the lung is deflated to very low lung volumes, resistance also increases; this is commonly explained by narrowing of arteries or veins because their wall is not pulled open by fiber tension.

Pulmonary vascular resistance is also found to fall when arterial or venous pressure is increased. This is often discussed in terms of recruitment of collapsed capillaries versus homogeneous dilation of the entire capillary network or sheet. Such discussions are, in a way, based on too simplistic models of the mechanical properties of capillaries, which we shall examine critically in the next chapter.

We should finally ask what happens to blood flow when a person goes from rest to strenuous exercise (Table 10.2). We observe that blood flow increases by a factor of 2.5 on exercise, hence much less than O_2 consumption and ventilation. From the Fick principle (equation 6.11) we must conclude that arteriovenous O_2 concentration difference must increase by about a factor of 3.5 in exercise which is due to a greater O_2 extraction in the tissues, particularly in the working muscles where venous P_{O_2} can fall to about 15 mm Hg.

Blood flow is the product of heart rate and stroke volume, the volume of blood ejected by the right (or left) ventricle in one beat. We observe that the stroke volume increases relatively little on exercise so that blood flow is essentially elevated by stepping up the heart beat. We should mention, however, that long-term vigorous training for strenuous exercise leads to enlargement of the heart chambers and of the stroke volume; this is why the heart of well-trained endurance athletes — cyclists or long-distance runners, for example — beats at a rather low frequency.

Ventilation – Perfusion Matching

In man at rest one finds the lung to be perfused and ventilated at about the same rates — roughly at 5 $l \cdot min^{-1}$. On exercise, however, ventilation increases four times more than perfusion (Table 10.2).

This global ventilation–perfusion "mismatch" is of little consequence, however, since O_2 extraction from the air increases, partly because of the greater O_2 concentration or partial pressure difference between arterial and venous blood, noted above.

It is more important, however, that the lung assure good matching of ventilation and perfusion in each of its functional units. But here there are a number of effects which can lead to considerable mismatch, and this, in turn, will tend to make gas exchange less efficient.

The first point is that ventilation of the acini is not even throughout the lung. We shall see in the next chapter that on inspiration the chest is widened mostly in its lower parts, because the diaphragm elongates the chest cavity, and because the additive effect of contraction of the external intercostals leads to a greater deflection of the lower ribs. As a consequence the lower parts of the lung are inflated to a somewhat greater extent than the upper parts (Fig. 10.16); the lung attempts to minimize this difference by allowing its bulk to shift downward along the slippery pleural surface, but this does not even out the unequal ventilation altogether.

Regional perfusion of the lung is also uneven in the sense that the lower parts are better perfused. This can be explained by hydrostatic pressure differences in the column of blood in the pulmonary arterial

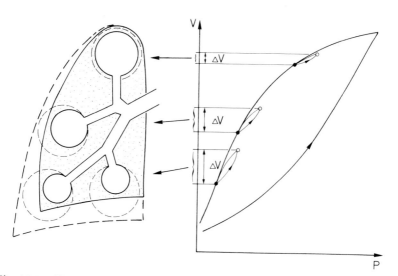

Fig. 10.16 During quiet breathing the lower parts of the lung show greater volume changes (ventilation) than the upper parts.

system. If the lung measures about 30 cm from apex to base, the weight of the column of blood will cause a pressure difference of about 30 cm H_2O or 23 mm Hg to exist between apical and basal blood vessels. Taking the outflow tract of the heart to be at about mid-height of the lung, this means that the right ventricle must pump the blood to the apex against a pressure head of about 12 mm Hg, which is very nearly equal to the mean pulmonary arterial pressure, and even slightly above diastolic pressure. There is, hence, an extremely small pressure available to drive blood through capillaries in the apical region. At the bottom of the lung the opposite is the case: hydrostatic pressure is added to hemodynamic pressure on both arterial and venous side, so that all vessels are widened.

The uneven distribution of blood flow in the lung is commonly described in terms of three zones and the relations between alveolar, arterial, and venous pressure (Fig. 10.17). Alveolar pressure, P_A, is close to atmospheric and, evidently, equal in all parts of the lung. As we have seen, local arterial and venous pressures, P_a and P_v, respectively, depend on the addition (or difference) of hemodynamic and hydrostatic pressures. In zone 1 at the top of the lung P_a may be smaller than P_A if hydrostatic pressure exceeds hemodynamic pressure; the alveolar capillaries cannot be opened and there is no blood

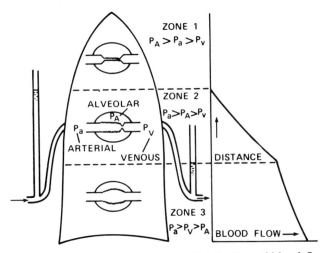

Fig. 10.17 Model to explain the uneven distribution of blood flow in the lung, depending on the distribution of alveolar (P_A), arterial (P_a) and venous (P_v) pressures affecting the capillaries. (From West et al., 1964.)

flow. In the normal lung, zone 1 conditions do not exist. In zone 2 $P_a > P_A$ because hemodynamic pressure now exceeds hydrostatic pressure; however in the veins the pressure is below atmospheric. Blood flow through the capillaries is said to be similar to that over a waterfall: it is not governed by the arterial – venous pressure gradient but by the pressure difference between pulmonary artery and alveoli. This may cause parts of the capillaries to collapse. In zone 3 finally $P_v > P_A$; the capillaries become distended and flow is proportional to the arteriovenous pressure difference.

As one moves down the lung through these zones, one finds blood flow to increase gradually. In zone 2 this is possibly due to recruitment, that is, opening up of capillaries closed by the waterfall effect, whereas in zone 3 resistance falls because the capillaries and small arteries widen under the effect of the positive total pressure in the blood vessels, positive with respect to alveolar air.

It turns out that the gradients in regional ventilation and perfusion go in the same direction, both increasing from apex to base, with the result that, in the normal lung, the inhomogeneities in ventilation – perfusion ratio are less than expected. Nevertheless, variations in the ventilation – perfusion ratio seem to be responsible for most of the deficiencies in gas exchange, particularly in diseased lungs. In the healthy lung, however, their effects are relatively small, particularly because it turns out that the drastic increase in ventilation and perfusion observed to occur in exercise (Table 10.2) tends to even out inhomogeneities.

From the foregoing it might appear that the ventilation – perfusion ratio depends essentially on passive effects. There is at least one active process, however, that contributes to matching perfusion to ventilation. This is hypoxic vasoconstriction. It can be shown that branches of the pulmonary artery constrict when they are exposed to hypoxic air in alveoli, an effect that does not seem to be dependent on the nervous system. It is evident that hypoxic vasoconstriction is an important device for matching perfusion to ventilation: in poorly ventilated acini the alveolar P_{O_2} falls rapidly; this causes the arterial branches in this underventilated unit to constrict, with the result that the increased vascular resistance shifts blood flow away from this unit. Hypoxic vasoconstriction occurs also when P_{O_2} in inspired air falls, such as at high altitude. But now all vessels contract and increase pulmonary vascular resistance; pulmonary arterial pressure must become elevated to maintain blood flow. This is the basis for high altitude pulmonary hypertension with its sequel of hypertrophy of the right ventricle.

Finally, it has recently been realized that ventilation and perfusion are poorly matched within the acinus. The reason for this is that the ventilatory unit of lung parenchyma is much larger than the perfusion unit. In fact, we have said that the acinus must be taken as the ventilatory unit, and that within the acinus O_2 reaches the gas exchanging surfaces by molecular diffusion through the air. The perfusion units, on the other hand, are about the size of alveoli. It is now important to note that a very large number of such perfusion units are aligned serially along the alveolar duct pathway (Fig. 10.18), built into the wall of alveoli, and that these perfusion units are perfused in parallel, all receiving blood of identical P_{O_2}. But the alveoli are "ventilated" serially by O_2 diffusion, so that in the periphery of the acinus they are probably less well replenished with O_2 than in the center. The result is an inhomogeneity of ventilation–perfusion matching at the microscale. We shall discuss later that this may have an effect on the efficiency of gas exchange.

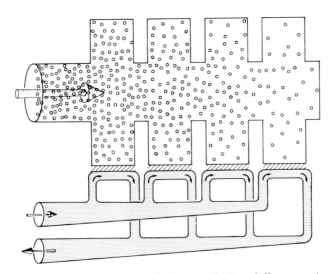

Fig. 10.18 Model to explain ventilation–perfusion differences in the gas exchange units within an acinus, since they are perfused in parallel but ventilated in series. (From Weibel, 1981.)

Summary

The airways branch by dichotomy. Starting with a single tube (the trachea), they thus form some 8 million end branches in the human lung. Depending on their differentiation the airways are assigned to three functional zones: the bronchi and bronchioles, their wall lined by columnar epithelium, belong to the conducting zone, whereas the alveoli form the respiratory zone; the alveolar ducts and respiratory bronchioles are transitional elements. Gas exchange takes place in the respiratory and transitional zones, whereas the conducting zone distributes air to the peripheral gas exchange units; it does not participate in gas exchange and constitutes the dead space.

In spite of some irregularity the branching pattern of airways is conveniently analyzed by a model of dichotomy in which the number of branches is doubled with each generation. In this model purely conducting airways of the human lung extend, on the average, to generation 16, followed by three generations of respiratory bronchioles and then by four generations of alveolar ducts. The human airway tree therefore branches over an average of 23 generations; the irregularity of branching causes terminal alveolar ducts or sacs to occur from about generations 18 to 30.

As airways branch, their diameter becomes reduced by a constant factor of cube root of $\frac{1}{2}$. Comparison with laws of hydrodynamics reveals that this conforms with optimal design principles that minimize the loss of energy in the mass flow of fluids through branched tubes. In the respiratory zone the diameter of alveolar ducts remains nearly constant, which optimizes design with respect to the diffusion of O_2 in the gas phase along the branched alveolar ducts.

Ventilation of the lung through the airways is described in terms of different volumes. The volume moved in and out in a breath is called the tidal volume (about 500 ml in man at rest), the maximal volume that can be inhaled after deep expiration is the vital capacity (5–6 liters in man). The volume that remains in the air after normal expiration is the functional residual capacity FRC (2.5 liters), that which remains after deep expiration the residual volume (1.5 liters). Residual volume and vital capacity together are the total lung capacity, TLC, the maximal amount of air the lung can contain. The rate of ventilation —called minute volume or total ventilation —is the product of tidal volume times breathing frequency. At rest we breathe at a frequency of about 15 per minute, so that total ventilation is about

7,500 ml·min⁻¹. Only part of this reaches alveoli; about 150 ml of each tidal volume of 500 ml remains in the anatomic dead space (conducting airways). In exercise, breathing frequency and tidal volume are increased so that total ventilation can be augmented tenfold, alveolar ventilation even more because the dead space volume remains constant. The dimensions of the airway tree influence ventilation. Air flow velocity falls along the airway tree because the total airway cross-section enlarges with progressive branching. The size of airways determines resistance to air flow; resistance falls toward the periphery. Differences in airway dimensions (for example due to contraction of smooth muscle) affect the distribution of air to the gas exchange units.

The pulmonary arteries form a tree which is nearly congruent with that of the airways which they follow very closely, but they branch over a total of 28 generations, on the average. The pulmonary veins form a similar tree, but they follow a course independent of the airways, being located between bronchoarterial units. In the acini blood therefore flows from the center outward. The diameter of pulmonary artery branches decreases with progressive branching according to the same law as bronchi, but it maintains this cube-root-of-$\frac{1}{2}$ law out to the last branches which lead into the capillary network: blood is transported by mass flow throughout its path. The alveolar capillaries form a very dense network through which blood flows as a sheet.

The pulmonary circulation is perfused by the entire cardiac output. Blood flow is determined by the pressure difference between pulmonary arteries and veins (about 15 mm Hg) and by the vascular resistance. Pulmonary circulation is a low-pressure low-resistance system. The distribution of blood flow to the gas exchange units depends on the distribution of resistances which is affected by contraction of the smooth muscle wall of arteries. In hypoxia (low O_2 content of air) resistance increases. On exercise total blood flow through the lung increases, mostly owing to an increase in heart rate.

If the lung is to function well as a gas exchanger, ventilation and perfusion of the gas exchange area must be well matched. There are notable regional differences, however. The lower parts of the lung are better ventilated than the rest, but these regions are also better perfused. Hypoxic vasoconstriction shunts the blood away from poorly ventilated acini. All this helps to improve ventilation–perfusion matching.

Further Reading

Fung, Y. B., and S. S. Sobin. 1977. Pulmonary alveolar blood flow. In *Bioengineering Aspects of the Lung*, ed. J. B. West. New York: Dekker, pp. 267–359.

Pedley, T. J., R. C. Schroter, and M. F. Sudlow. 1977. Gas flow and mixing in the airways. In *Bioengineering Aspects of the Lung*, ed. J. B. West. New York: Dekker, pp. 163–265.

West, J. B. 1974. *Respiration Physiology: The Essentials*. Baltimore: Williams & Wilkins.

———, ed. 1977. *Bioengineering Aspects of the Lung*. New York: Dekker.

References

Fung, Y. C., and S. S. Sobin. 1969. Theory of sheet flow in lung alveoli. *Journal of Applied Physiology* 26:472–488.

Glazier, J. B., J. M. B. Hughes, J. E. Maloney, and J. B. West. 1967. Vertical gradient of alveolar size in lungs of dogs frozen intact. *Journal of Applied Physiology* 23:694–705.

——— 1969. Measurements of capillary dimensions and blood volume in rapidly frozen lungs. *Journal of Applied Physiology* 26:65–76.

Guntheroth, W. G., D. L. Luchtel, and I. Kawabori. 1982. Pulmonary microcirculation: tubules rather than sheet and post. *Journal of Applied Physiology* 53:510–515.

Horsfield, K., G. Dart, D. E. Olson, G. F. Filley, and G. Cumming. 1971. Models of the human bronchial tree. *Journal of Applied Physiology* 31:207–217.

Pedley, T. J., R. C. Schroter, and M. F. Sudlow. 1970. The prediction of pressure drop and variation of resistance within the human bronchial airways. *Respiration Physiology* 9:387–405.

Weibel, E. R. 1963. *Morphometry of the Human Lung*. Heidelberg: Springer. New York: Academic.

——— 1980. Design and structure of the human lung. In *Pulmonary Diseases and Disorders*, ed. A. P. Fishman. New York: McGraw-Hill, pp. 224–271.

——— 1981. Morphological basis for $\dot{V}_A/\dot{Q}$ distribution. In *Proceedings of the 28th International Congress of Physiological Sciences*, ed. I. Hutas and L. A. Debreczeni. Budapest: Akademia Kiado, pp. 179–189.

West, J. B. 1974. *Respiration Physiology: The Essentials*. Baltimore: Williams & Wilkins.

* West, J. B., C. T. Dollery, and A. Naimark. 1964. Distribution of blood flow in isolated lung: relation to vascular and alveolar pressures. *Journal of Applied Physiology* 19:713–724.

11

THE LUNG'S MECHANICAL SUPPORT

THE LUNG with its millions of alveoli connected to outside air via the airways behaves like a balloon which is kept expanded in a closed box, the thorax: if its surface membrane ruptures it will immediately collapse and the chest cavity will fill with air. The mechanical key problem, reflected in this pathological incidence, is this: the lung must be built as an elastic bag so as to allow the air volume it contains to be ventilated, that is, renewed with outside air by rhythmic expansions and contractions. This bag is mounted within the pump, the chest cavity, but it must be able to move freely so as to allow homogeneous expansion of all parts; the lung is therefore not fixed to the chest wall but totally separated from it by a narrow fluid-filled gap, the pleural space. The interior of the bag must be finely partitioned so as to build the large surface required to accommodate the blood capillaries in close contact with air; this results in a foam-like structure where surface tension will tend to collapse the tiny bubbles. And finally, the tissue used to build this interior scaffold for the gas exchange units must be kept minimal; this will require a clever disposition of the connective tissue fibers so as to obtain maximal mechanical strength with a minimal amount of material.

External Support and Motive Force

The thoracic cage is made of twelve pairs of ribs that extend in an arc from the thoracic part of the spine to the sternum in the anterior mid-line. The ribs are attached to the spine by two joints: one between the rib's head and the vertebral body, and one between the tubercle and the vertebral transverse process, with the rib's head being more anterior and medial than the tubercle (Fig. 11.1). In a resting state the ribs slope downward.

The motive force for the chest wall is primarily provided by the *intercostal muscles* whose muscle fibers course from the lower edge of one rib to the upper edge of the next. The external intercostal muscles slope downward and forward; since the lower attachment point is forward, the ribs are pulled upward by contraction of these muscles. The internal intercostal muscles take an opposite course so that their contraction pulls the ribs downward.

To understand the effects of contracting intercostal muscles we must note that, in a resting state, the ribs droop forward and to the side, and also that the line connecting the two rib joints forms an angle of 45° to the mid-plane (Fig. 11.1). For these reasons, lifting the ribs by contraction of the external intercostals deflects them to the side and also moves the sternum upward; in consequence this causes both the lateral and the anteroposterior diameter of the chest to become enlarged. Evidently, contracting the internal intercostals reverses the process and can reduce the chest diameters even beyond the resting state. Through these effects the external intercostals are inspiratory muscles, causing air to flow through the airways into the enlarged lung, whereas the internal intercostals are expiratory muscles. In forced inspiration these muscles are assisted by the scalene muscles that arise from the cervical spine and attach to the first two ribs, and by the sternomastoid muscle that lifts the sternum upward. Similarly, the muscles of the abdominal wall, particularly the rectus muscles, are auxiliary expirators, pulling the chest wall downward on forced expiration; this is one reason why the abdominal wall muscles contract on coughing.

The most important inspiratory muscle is, however, the *diaphragm*, which can be described as a flat ring of radial muscle fibers that arise at the lower edge of the rib cage and converge toward a central strong connective tissue membrane (Fig. 11.1). As the muscle fibers contract, the dome-like diaphragm flattens and the chest cavity is enlarged in the vertical direction. The contraction of the diaphragm is counteracted by the muscle membranes of the abdominal wall that push the abdominal content toward the chest.

Thus, to and fro respiration requires alternating and coupled con-

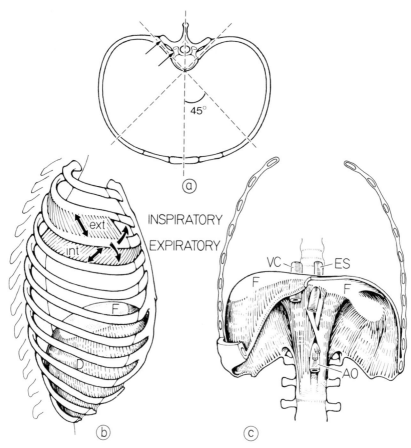

Fig. 11.1 Anatomy of the chest wall. (a) The ribs are fixed to the vertebrae by two joints (arrows) that form an angle of 45° to the mid-plane. (b) Because of their oblique course the external (ext) and internal (int) intercostal muscles act as inspiratory and expiratory muscles respectively. Note the dome-like shape of the diaphragm (D). (c) Sheet-like muscle of diaphragm that arises from lower edge of rib cage forms the diaphragmatic dome, whereas the tracts that arise from the vertebral column form a complex system of crura that permit the esophagus (ES) and aorta (AO) to penetrate into the abdominal cavity. The inferior vena cava traverses the fibrous plate (F) of the diaphragm.

traction and relaxation of inspiratory and expiratory muscles. These are controlled by different nerves: segmental spinal nerves supply the intercostal and the abdominal wall muscles, whereas the diaphragm receives its innervation through the phrenic nerve, a nerve arising in the cervical plexus.

The basic structure of the chest and its muscles is the same in all mammals, but there are differences in shape. In man, with his erect posture, the chest is broad and the spine extends deep into the chest so that a good part of the lung lies to the side and even behind the spine. In quadrupeds the chest is narrow, elongated toward the sternum.

The Pleural Cavity

In the mid-plane the chest houses the mediastinum with the pericardium which contains the heart. These structures separate the original coelomic cavity into two pleural cavities, one for the left and one for the right lung, as we saw in chapter 8. We should remember that this space is bounded by the somatopleura, an epithelial or rather mesothelial sheet that now forms the *parietal pleura*, a complete lining of the interior surface of chest wall, diaphragm, and mediastinum toward the pleural cavities. We had also seen that the lung anlage is bounded by a similar mesothelial lining, the *visceral pleura*, that is continuous with the parietal pleura at the hilum where the main bronchus as well as the pulmonary artery and veins enter the lung from the mediastinum (Fig. 11.2). Thus the lung remains separated from the chest wall by a narrow cleft, the pleural space, which is bounded by epithelial linings and contains a small amount of serosal fluid. This gives the lung some freedom to move within the pleural cavity since the visceral pleura can glide on the parietal pleura, the serosal fluid serving as a lubricant.

When we take as deep a breath as we can take, the lung fills the pleural cavity almost completely. As it becomes deflated its lower edges retract upward; the pleural cavity is now larger than the lung and the parietal pleura of the diaphragm becomes apposed to that of the chest wall; pleural recesses are formed, narrow clefts containing some serosal fluid (Fig. 11.2). Similarly, the forward edges of the lung retract sideways and pleural recesses appear between the pericardium and the anterior chest wall. These pleural recesses allow the lung to reexpand on inspiration into an enlarging pleural cavity. Because the diaphragm is the most important inspiratory muscle, its contraction will cause the pleural cavity to expand mostly downward: flattening the diaphragmatic dome opens up the costodiaphragmatic recess (Fig. 11.2), and this will pull down the lower surface of the lung. However, in order to allow all air-space units to

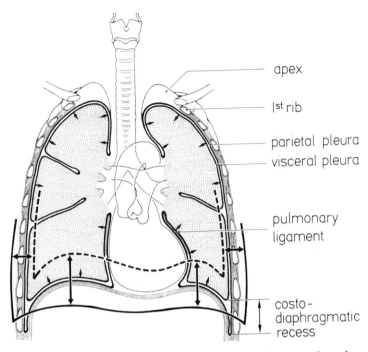

apex

1st rib

parietal pleura
visceral pleura

pulmonary
ligament

costo-
diaphragmatic
recess

Fig. 11.2 Frontal section of human chest and lung showing pleural space. Single arrows indicate retractile force of lung. Double arrows show the excursion of the lung bases and periphery between deep inspiration and expiration. Note the costodiaphragmatic recess as a reserve space for lung expansion. (From Weibel, 1980.)

expand more or less homogeneously, all parts of the lung will have to follow this downward movement to some extent, so that much of the visceral pleura will have to glide along the parietal pleura lining the chest wall. It is therefore most important that the pleural space be well lubricated over its entire surface. Pleural adhesions, the consequence of inflammatory events such as pneumonia or pleurisy, can disturb the freedom of this movement and cause uneven ventilation. We have seen, however, that even in the normal lung its lower parts are more intensely expanded than the upper parts, causing ventilation to be somewhat inhomogeneous (see chapter 10).

The retractive or *recoil force* of the lung, generated by surface tension and, to a lesser degree, by connective tissue fiber tension, exerts a concentric pull on the visceral pleura which is counteracted by the chest wall and the muscle tone of diaphragm and intercostal muscles. As a consequence the pressure in the pleural space is negative. Because of the weight of lung tissue and blood, the negative intrapleural pressure shows a gradient from top to bottom, ranging, in the human lung, from about -10 cm H_2O (mbar) at the apex to about -2.5 cm H_2O at the base. The existence and importance of this negative intrapleural pressure become immediately apparent when, for some reason, the visceral pleura of the lung ruptures; air can then escape from the airways into the pleural cavity and the lung collapses by retracting toward the hilum, a condition called pneumothorax.

The Lung's Fiber Skeleton

THE FIBER CONTINUUM

The principal structural "backbone" of the lung is a continuous system of fibers that are anchored at the hilum and are put under tension by the negative intrapleural pressure that tugs on the visceral pleura. The general construction principle follows from the formation of the mesenchymal sheath of the airway units in the developing lung, which we had seen to derive from the splanchnopleura (Fig. 8.3). As the airway tree grows, its branches remain separated by layers of mesenchyme within which blood vessels form (Fig. 8.5). When fiber networks develop within this mesenchyme they will enwrap all airway units and extend from the hilum right to the visceral pleura. The *pulmonary fiber system* hence forms a three-dimensional fibrous continuum that is structured by the airway system and is closely related to the blood vessels. By virtue of the design of this fibrous continuum the lung becomes, in fact, subdivided into millions of little bellows that are connected to the airway tree, as represented schematically in Figure 11.3; they expand with expansion of the chest because the tension exerted on the visceral pleura by the negative intrapleural pressure becomes transmitted to the bellows' walls through that fiber system.

To try to put some order into this fiber system we can first single out two major components that one can easily identify (Fig. 11.3). First we find that all airways, from the main stem bronchus that enters the lung at the hilum out to the terminal bronchioles and beyond, are enwrapped by a strong sheath of fibers. We shall call these fibers the *axial fiber system*; they form the "bark" of the tree

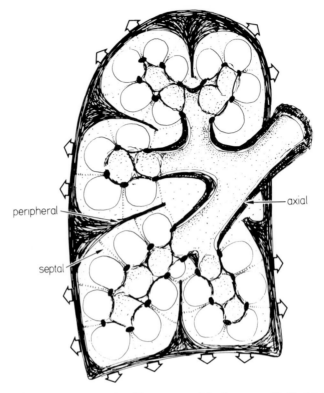

Fig. 11.3 The major connective fiber tracts of the lung are divided into *axial* fibers along the airways and *peripheral* fibers connected to the pleura. They are connected by fibers in the *alveolar* septa. (From Weibel and Gil, 1977.)

whose roots are at the hilum and whose branches penetrate deep into lung parenchyma, following the course of the airways. A second major fiber system is related to the visceral pleura which is made of strong fiber bags that enwrap all lobes, reaching the margin of the hilum where they are connected to the fibers of the parietal pleura. We then find connective tissue septa to penetrate from the visceral pleura into lung parenchyma, separating units of the airway tree. We shall call these fibers the *peripheral fiber system* because they make the boundaries between the units of respiratory lung tissue. Of the major pulmonary blood vessels, the veins follow the peripheral fiber system whereas the arteries course along the airways, closely apposed to the axial fiber system.

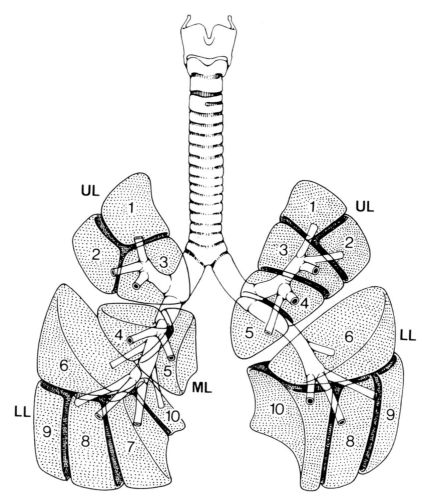

Fig. 11.4 Organization of human lung into lobes and bronchopulmonary segments. The left upper lobe (UL) consists of (1) apical, (2) posterior, (3) anterior, (4) superior lingular, and (5) inferior lingular segments. The right upper lobe has segments (1 – 3), with middle lobe (ML) made of (4) lateral and (5) medial segments as a separate unit. Lower lobes (LL) consist of (6) superior (apical), (7) medial-basal, (8) anterior-basal, (9) lateral-basal, and (10) posterior-basal segments. The medial-basal segment (7) is absent in the left lung. (From Weibel, 1980.)

The peripheral fiber system subdivides the lung into a number of units that are not simple to define because they form a continuous hierarchy in accordance with the pattern of airway tree branching. Two such units appear to be natural, however: the *lobes*, which are demarcated by a more or less complete lining by visceral pleura with a serosal cleft interposed (Fig. 11.2); and the *acinus* which is defined as that portion of lung parenchyma that is supplied by a first-order respiratory bronchiole, that is, a parenchymal unit in which all airways participate in gas exchange (see chapter 10). To indicate orders of magnitude, an acinus has a diameter of a few millimeters in the human lung. Lobes are, however, gross structures; in the human lung we find two lobes on the left, an upper and a lower lobe, and three on the right, an upper, middle, and lower lobe (Fig. 11.4). There is some interspecies variation with respect to lobes; as we have seen, most animals have a fourth lobe on the right, the cardiac lobe, whereas in some smaller mammals, such as rats or mice, there is only a single lobe on the left.

All other lung units are somewhat arbitrarily defined, so that I shall not discuss them at length. The *lung segments*, the first subdivisions of the lobes (Fig. 11.4), have some practical importance because they are often bounded by sufficiently massive connective tissue septa to allow their surgical separation. A frequently used unit at the other end of the spectrum is the *secondary lobule* which, in the human lung, comprises about a dozen acini and measures roughly 1 cm³; the secondary lobule is often bounded by a conspicuous septum (Fig. 11.5) which is incomplete in man but can be rather strong in some species, such as the goat, cow, pig, or horse.

We should have a closer look at the construction of the acinus, the functional unit of lung parenchyma. The airway that leads into the acinus, the first order respiratory bronchiole (see chapter 10), continues branching within the acinus for about 6–10 additional generations (Figs. 10.3 and 11.6). These intra-acinar airways, called respiratory bronchioles and alveolar ducts, also carry in their wall relatively strong fibers of the axial fiber system that extend to the end of the duct system. But since the wall of intra-acinar air ducts is densely settled with alveoli, these fibers form a kind of network whose meshes encircle the alveolar mouths (Figs. 11.6 and 11.7). These fiber rings serve as a scaffold for a network of finer fibers that spread within the alveolar septa (Fig. 11.7). But now we must note that in a

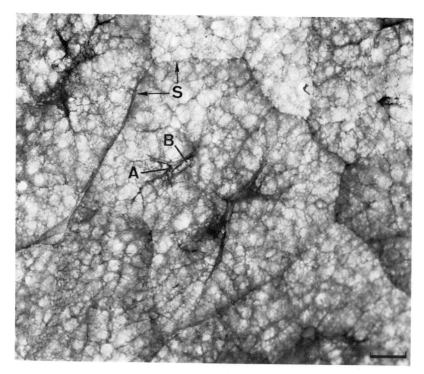

Fig. 11.5 Lobule of human lung is demarcated by connective tissue septa (S) that are part of the peripheral fiber system. Note the bronchiole (B) and accompanying pulmonary artery (A) in center. Dried lung specimen. Scale marker: 2,000 μm.

fiber system there may be no loose ends: the ropes of a suspension bridge must be firmly anchored at both ends in order to support the roadway. In that sense, the *septal fiber system* must also be anchored at both ends: on the network of axial fibers around the alveolar ducts, and on extensions of the peripheral fibers that penetrate into the acinus from interlobular septa. Thus the fiber system of the lung becomes a continuum that spans the entire space of the lung, from the hilum to the visceral pleura (Fig. 11.3). It is put under varying tension as the pleura is expanded by the chest wall and diaphragm.

The continuous nature of a well-ordered fiber system is an essential design feature of the lung. This becomes evident in certain diseases when some of the fibers become disrupted. As they cannot be kept under tension, they will retract and larger air spaces form in the process of rearranging the fiber system in the surroundings of the damage, a condition called emphysema. Small foci of emphysema form in most lungs in the course of time. If they become widespread and expand progressively, they will eventually cause severe respiratory troubles. On the one hand, a good part of the gas exchanging surface is lost, and, on the other hand, ventilation of the alveoli becomes difficult because of the widened and irregular air spaces. The compliance of the lung is increased, that is, less force is required to ventilate it, but this does not help the patient because large quantities of air remain trapped in the lung, partly because of reduced recoil forces and partly because of deformation or destruction of small airways.

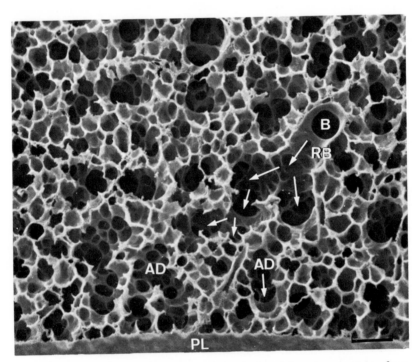

Fig. 11.6 Branching of peripheral airways (arrows) in acinus, arising from terminal bronchiole (B) as respiratory bronchioles (RB) and continuing as alveolar ducts (AD), ending, in this instance, at the pleura (PL). Scale marker: 200 μm. (From Weibel, 1980.)

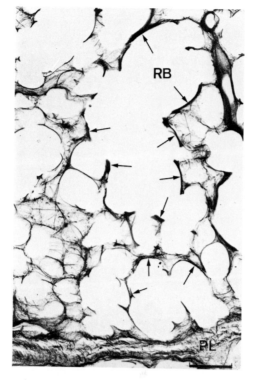

Fig. 11.7 Connective tissue stain reveals the strong fiber rings that demarcate the alveolar ducts (arrows). Scale marker: 200 μm.

The opposite can also occur. If the lung responds to a damage by overproduction of connective tissue, the lung becomes stiff, a condition called fibrosis. It results in respiratory troubles largely because the stiffness prevents adequate ventilation.

THE SUPPORT OF BLOOD VESSELS

The fiber system serves mainly as a mechanical support for the blood vessels with which it is intimately associated in an orderly fashion. We have seen in chapter 10 that the pulmonary artery branches in parallel with the airway tree and penetrates into the acinus along the axial fiber system; the pulmonary veins are associated with the peripheral fiber system and are thus located between the airway units, as can be seen in Figure 10.12. In the alveolar septa the

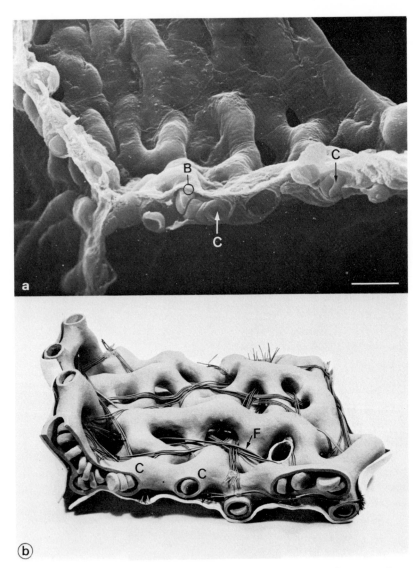

Fig. 11.8 In the alveolar wall, shown in (a) in a scanning electron micrograph from a human lung, the capillary blood (C) is separated from the air by a very thin tissue barrier (B). The model (b) shows the capillary network (C) to be interwoven with the meshwork of septal fibers (F). Scale marker: 10 µm.

capillary network spreads out as a broad sheet of vessels whose paths are continuous throughout the system of interconnected alveolar walls of the acinus (Fig. 10.14).

The problem of supporting the capillaries on the septal fibers with as little tissue as possible has been solved ingeniously: we find that the fiber network is interlaced with the capillary network; Figure 11.8 shows that, when the fibers are taut, the capillaries weave from one side of the septum to the other. This arrangement has a three-fold advantage: (1) it allows the capillaries to be supported unit by unit directly on the fiber strands without the need of additional "binders"; (2) it causes the capillaries to become spread out on the alveolar surface when the fibers are stretched; and (3) it optimizes the gas exchange conditions by limiting the presence of fibers — which must interfere with O_2 flow — to half the capillary surface. The thin section of a capillary shown in Figure 11.9 reveals that an interstitial space with fibers and fibroblasts exists only on one side of the capillary, whereas on the other the two lining cells, endothelium and epithelium, become closely joined with only a single, common basement membrane interposed. Over half the surface the capillary blood can therefore be separated from the air merely by the minimal tissue barrier which we have discussed in relation to Figure 9.12.

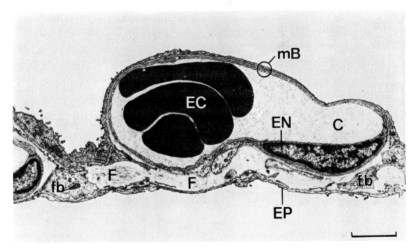

Fig. 11.9 Thin section of alveolar wall from human lung shows capillary (C) with erythrocytes (EC); it is separated from air by a minimal barrier (mB) on the upper side, whereas the thicker barrier on the lower side contains connective tissue fibers (F) and fibroblasts (fb) between epithelium (EP) and endothelium (EN). Scale marker: 1 μm.

MECHANICAL PROPERTIES OF THE FIBERS

We should finally address the question of the mechanical properties of the lung's fiber system. As in all connective tissue the fibers of the lung are composed of collagen and elastic fibers. The collagen fibers are bundles of fibrils bound together by proteoglycans; they are practically inextensible (less than 2%) and have a very high tensile strength so that they rupture only at loads of 50–70 dyn·cm^{-2} which means that a collagen fiber of 1 mm diameter can support a weight of over 500 g. In contrast, elastic fibers have a much lower tensile strength but a high extensibility: they can be stretched to about 130% of their relaxed length before rupturing.

In the fiber system of lung parenchyma, collagen and elastic fibers occur in a volume ratio of about 2.5 : 1, whereas this ratio is 10 : 1 for the visceral pleura. In a relaxed state one will find the collagen fibers to be longer than the accompanying elastic fibers so that they appear wavy. Because of the association between "rubber-like" elastic and "twine-like" collagen fibers, the connective tissue strands behave like an elastic band: they are easy to stretch up to the point where the collagen fibers are taut, but from there on they resist stretching very strongly.

The elastic properties of the lung's fiber system can be studied by filling the airways with fluid so as to eliminate the effects of surface tension. Figure 11.10 shows that pressures up to about 6 cm H$_2$O (6 mbar) are sufficient to increase the lung volume to 90% of total lung capacity by fluid filling. A further increase in inflation pressure leads to small volume increments; if one goes beyond 20 cm H$_2$O the lung volume does not further increase until the pleura begins to rupture. As the pressure is released, the lung volume falls again. The deflation curve is only slightly displaced to the left, which means that very little work has to be done to extend the fiber system on inflation; note that work is proportional to the area of the hysteresis loop of the inflation-deflation curves. The notable insight derived from such studies is that the lung's fiber system has a high compliance until high levels of inflation are reached, and that the retractive or recoil force generated by the fiber system amounts to no more than a few mbar at physiological inflation levels. The actual recoil force in the air-filled lung, reflected by the negative pressure in the pleural space, is appreciably higher, but this is due to surface tension rather than to the retractive force of the fibers.

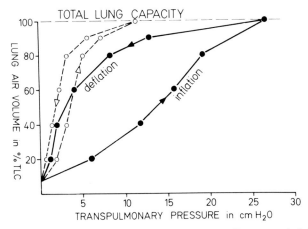

Fig. 11.10 Pressure-volume curves recorded on inflation and deflation on rabbit lungs inflated with air (solid line) and with saline (broken line). (Data from Gil et al., 1979.)

Surface Tension

The recognition that surface forces play a dominant role in lung mechanics was one of the major breakthroughs in lung physiology. The Swiss physician Kurt von Neergaard was the first to note, in 1929, that lungs were easier to distend with saline than with air; he correctly concluded that the retractive force of the lung which opposed inflation was to a large extent due to surface tension at the alveolar surface. This discovery remained unnoticed until the 1950s when Jere Mead and his collaborators at Harvard began to study the physics of lung mechanics and — independently — rediscovered the same phenomenon. But they also made another striking observation, namely the large hysteresis of the air inflation-deflation curve (Fig. 11.10), which meant that the retractive force due to surface tension was much smaller on deflation than on inflation, a discovery of great importance as we shall see.

Surface tension arises at any gas–liquid interface because the forces between the molecules of the liquid are much stronger than those between the liquid and the gas. As a result the liquid surface will tend to become as small as possible. Thus the surface of fluid in a trough is flat, whereas an unrestrained bubble of gas in water will be spherical, since the sphere offers the smallest surface for a given volume of gas. A curved surface, such as that of the bubble, generates a pressure which is proportional to the curvature and to the surface tension coefficient γ. The general formula of Gibbs relates this pressure, P_s, to the mean curvature, $\overline{K}$:

$$P_s = 2\gamma \cdot \overline{K}. \tag{11.1}$$

In a sphere the curvature is simply the reciprocal of the radius r, so that one can write the formula of Laplace as

$$P_s = 2\gamma/r. \tag{11.2}$$

Note that in a soap bubble the surface force acts on both sides of the film so that a coefficient of 4 rather than 2 is used in these formulas.

Surface forces of this kind are generated in the lung because the fluid lined alveoli have a curved, "nearly spherical" surface (Fig. 11.11). If we block the airways, this force can be measured as a pressure, but in the normal lung with open airways the force exerts a pull on the pleura which causes the intrapleural pressure to be negative; the "recoil pressure" then is the difference between ambient and intrapleural pressure which is of the order of 10 mbar in the normal human lung.

But the most critical effect of surface tension is that it endangers air space stability. Let us look at a simple model made of two soap bubbles blown at the end of a Y-tube (Fig. 11.11b); invariably one bubble, the smaller one, shrinks and empties into the other, which becomes larger. The reason is evidently that the smaller bubble generates a larger pressure due to its larger curvature. A set of connected bubbles is therefore inherently unstable: all of them will eventually collapse except the largest one which becomes larger by collecting the gas content of all others. Since the 300 million alveoli are all connected with each other through the airways, the lung is inherently unstable: why do the alveoli not all collapse and empty into one large bubble? There are two principal reasons.

The first reason is one of tissue structure. The alveoli are not simply soap bubbles in a froth, but their walls contain an intricate fiber system, as we have seen. Thus, when an alveolus tends to shrink (Fig. 11.11c), the fibers in the wall of adjoining alveoli are stretched and this will prevent the alveolus from collapsing. It is said that alveoli are *mechanically interdependent* and that this stabilizes them.

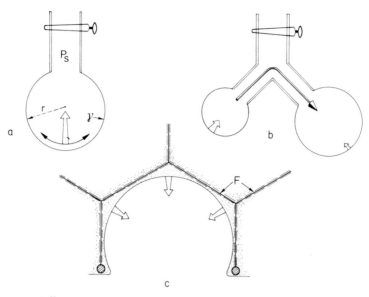

Fig. 11.11 Effect of surface tension in bubbles. (a) The pressure recorded in a soap bubble at the open end of a closed glass tube is due to the curvature $(1/r)$ and the surface tension γ of the fluid film. (b) The pressure generated by surface forces in a small bubble is greater than that in one of greater diameter so that the system is unstable. (c) In a pulmonary alveolus, part of the surface force that tends to collapse the alveolus is supported by fiber (F) tension.

The second reason is related to the fact that the alveolar surface is not simply water exposed to air, but that it is lined by surfactant, a material that has peculiar surface properties. In 1955 a British physicochemist, R. E. Pattle, observed what had been seen before him thousands of times, namely that froth which exudes from a cut surface of lung tissue is unusually stable: the bubbles would stay for hours, whereas soap froths or bubble baths will collapse after a much shorter time. In contrast to all the others who had seen this effect without really taking notice — or who did not have the patience to see how long a "lung bubble" could stay alive — Pattle interpreted his observation to mean that surface tension in lung fluids must be unusually low, and that this contributed to stabilizing alveoli. This finding is a milestone in pulmonary physiology; it was a most important breakthrough, based — as is so often the case — on very inexpensive simple experiments but good observation and sharp reasoning. Pattle's work was soon followed by another series of now classical studies, those by John Clements, who showed that the lung's peculiar surface properties were due to a phospholipid coat, and who also demonstrated that surface tension was variable.

If we look at Figure 11.10 we will note that the pressure-volume curves of inflation and deflation are quite different: to maintain a lung volume of 60% TLC on deflation requires a pressure of no more than 5 cm H_2O, in contrast to the 15 cm H_2O needed to expand the lung to that volume on inflation. We must conclude that on deflation the surface tension γ is very low; in fact it falls to nearly zero at 60% TLC, whereas it is clearly positive on inflation. This suggests that surface tension of pulmonary surfactant is not constant. Indeed, from a large volume of evidence it is now established that surface tension falls as the alveolar surface becomes smaller, and that it rises when the surface expands. Because of this feature, alveoli do not behave like soap bubbles whose surface tension remains constant. When an alveolus begins to shrink, the surface tension of its lining layer falls and the retractive force generated at the surface is reduced or even abolished. Combined with interdependence, this property of surfactant allows the complex of alveoli to remain stable.

That this is a peculiar property of pulmonary surfactant related to its phospholipid nature can be shown by *in vitro* experiments. One can extract pulmonary surfactant by washing the air spaces with saline, and study its surface tension properties on a surface balance (Fig. 11.12). This instrument consists of a trough filled with saline to the edge. If a small amount of surfactant is spread on the saline, its surface tension can be measured by the force exerted on a platinum strip that is submersed just beneath the surface. The trough is also provided with a barrier by which one can change the area of the film. If this barrier is moved back and forth, we find that surface tension changes in the form of a loop, reaching very low values on compression. This is quite different from detergents; although these can also reduce surface tension relative to water, no change occurs in compression of this film. Note that, although detergents have surface tensions corresponding to the average surface tension of surfactant, they can never reach the very low values observed in a compressed phospholipid film.

By rather ingenious experiments it has been shown that surface tension of pulmonary surfactant is also variable *in situ* as a function of expansion and compression of alveolar surface. Local surface tension in individual alveoli has been measured by depositing mi-

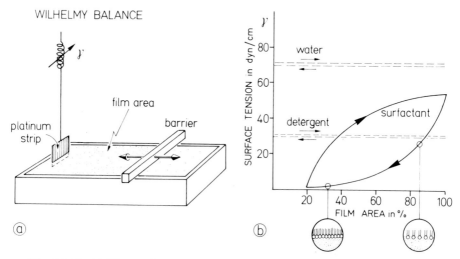

Fig. 11.12 (a) The surface tension of a surface film on a water surface is measured in a Wilhelmy balance as a function of film compression by a barrier. (b) On compression of the film, surfactant shows a hysteresis loop whereas the surface tension of a detergent and of water are unaffected.

crodroplets of test fluids with different surface tensions on the alveolar surface and by observing with a microscope their shape changes during inflation and deflation. One can conclude that surface tension falls to nearly zero when the lung is deflated to about $\frac{1}{2}$ TLC, and that it increases on inflation.

The variable surface tension of surfactant seems to be related to its phospholipid nature, since one gets the same effect by studying films of pure dipalmitoyl lecithin (DPPC) on the surface balance. As the film is compressed, the molecules of the monolayer of dipalmitoyl lecithin are pushed together; on expansion they are pulled apart (Fig. 11.12). A densely compressed film shields the subjacent water molecules from contact with air, and surface tension becomes very low. There is only one, perhaps minor, problem with this simple and plausible model — namely, that it does not account for the fact that in surfactant, dipalmitoyl lecithin is actually bound to apoprotein (Fig. 9.20). It is possible that this will cause the expanding surfactant film to disrupt into small islands rather than spread out homogeneously, but physical arguments indicate that this should have much the same effect on surface tension.

Which of the two factors for stabilizing lung structure is now the most important: interdependence or surfactant properties? It turns out that both are essential. If we deplete the lung of its surfactant lining by washing with a detergent, the pressure-volume curve changes dramatically (Fig. 11.13): on deflation lung volume falls rapidly. If we look at samples from lungs fixed at the same volume (60% TLC) but derived from either normal or detergent-rinsed lungs, we find that surfactant depletion causes the alveoli to collapse (Fig. 11.14). This causes, however, the alveolar ducts to enlarge, stretching the strong fiber nets at the mouths of the collapsed alveoli. The ducts do not collapse because of interdependence between adjacent units.

In the normal air-filled lung, surfactant properties and interdependence due to fiber tension both contribute to stabilizing the complex of alveoli and alveolar ducts. To understand this, let us examine Figure 11.15, which shows a highly simplified diagram of a parenchymal unit. Interdependence is established by the continuum of axial, septal, and peripheral fibers. Surface tension exerts an inward pull in the hollow alveoli where curvature is negative. However, over the free edge of the alveolar septa, along the outline of the duct,

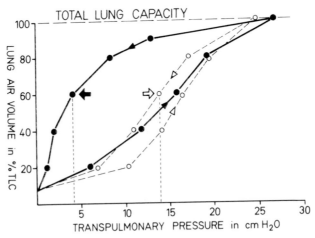

Fig. 11.13 Comparison of pressure-volume curve of a normal air-filled rabbit lung (compare Fig. 11.10) with that of a surfactant depleted lung (broken line). The arrows indicate the points at which the lungs shown in Figure 11.14 have been fixed by vascular perfusion. (Data from Bachofen et al., 1979.)

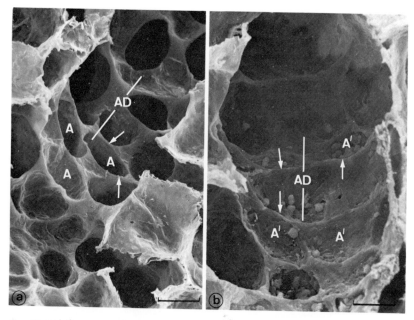

Fig. 11.14 Scanning electron micrographs of normal air-filled (a) and surfactant-depleted (b) rabbit lungs fixed at 60% TLC on the deflation curve (Fig. 11.13) show alveoli to be open (A) in (a), collapsed (A′) in (b). The alveolar duct (AD) is widened in the surfactant-depleted lung, resulting in a stretching of the fiber strands around the alveolar mouths (arrows). Scale markers: 50 μm. (From Wilson and Bachofen, 1982.)

the surface tension must pull outward because the curvature is positive. The latter force must be rather strong because the radius of curvature is very small on the septal edge; but this force is counteracted by the strong fiber strands, usually provided with some smooth muscle cells, that we find in the free edge of the alveolar septum (Figs. 11.6 and 11.7). Thus interdependence is an important factor in preventing the complex hollow of the lung, where negative and positive curvatures coexist, from collapsing. But its capacity to do so is limited and requires low surface tensions, particularly on deflation when the fibers tend to slack. If surface tension becomes too high, the lung's foam-like structure will partly collapse in spite of fiber interdependence (Fig. 11.14).

The one particularly striking disease where the inadequate provision of surfactant leads to a life-threatening condition is the respira-

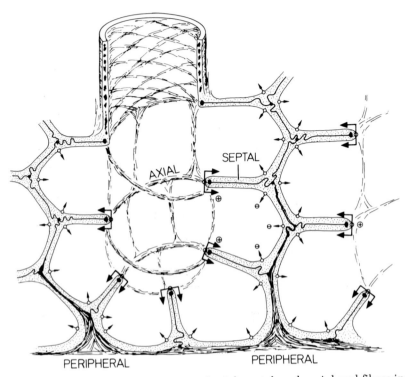

Fig. 11.15 Model of the disposition of axial, septal, and peripheral fibers in an acinus showing the effect of surface forces (arrows).

tory distress syndrome of the newborn, mentioned already in chapter 9. If an infant is prematurely born, the type II cells may not have developed their full potential for the synthesis of dipalmitoyl lecithin. The surface tension of lung fluids is high and the baby needs to use rather high forces to open up its airways during the first breaths. Although this is often possible, the airways cannot be kept air-filled because the stabilizing effect of surfactant is missing: large areas of atelectasis, regions of collapsed alveoli, develop and the lung is hard to ventilate. The infant affected by this condition cannot take up sufficient oxygen and is therefore in severe respiratory distress. As the disease persists it becomes aggravated by transudation of blood plasma into the air spaces, again an effect of the lack of surfactant because the strong retractive force due to high surface tension sucks fluid into the air spaces. The management of this disease is most difficult; the best measure is therefore prevention which has become possible to some extent since one can estimate the level of surfactant production from samples of amniotic fluid obtained through amnio-centesis.

Micromechanics and the Configuration of the Alveolar Septum

Let us now look at the mechanical factors which shape the alveolar septum in an air-filled lung. As we have seen, the alveolar septum is made of a single capillary network that is interlaced with fibers (Fig. 11.8). When the fibers are stretched, the capillaries bulge alter-natingly to one side or the other and this will cause pits and crevices to occur in the meshes of the capillary network, leading to a highly corrugated surface texture on both sides of the septum.

This irregular surface is to some extent evened out by the presence of an extracellular layer of lining fluid which is rather thin over the capillaries but forms little pools in the intercapillary pits (Fig. 11.16). This alveolar surface lining consists of two basic components: an aqueous layer of variable thickness called the hypophase, and sur-factant which forms a film on the surface of the hypophase. The nature of the hypophase is as yet poorly understood. It seems to contain proteins and mucopolysaccharides, but also considerable amounts of reserve surfactant material. The latter is complete sur-factant, that is, DPPC bound to the apoprotein, and occurs in a very characteristic configuration called "tubular myelin" (Fig. 9.20). Be-cause some of the leaflets of tubular myelin are continuous with the surfactant film at the surface of the hypophase, one assumes that tubular myelin is folded-up surfactant which can be unraveled when the area of the air–fluid interface expands. Thus, in principle, the alveolar lining layer always contains an excess amount of surfactant which can be spread on the surface when the need arises.

In the alveolar septum the tissue structures are extremely delicate, as we have seen; its configuration is therefore not exclusively deter-mined by structural features but results from the molding effect of various forces that must be kept in balance. Figure 11.17 shows how the three principal mechanical forces — tissue tension, surface ten-sion, and capillary distending pressure — interact in the septum. The fibers of the alveolar septum are under a tension whose magnitude depends on the level of lung inflation. This tends to straighten out the fibers so that a force (pressure) normal to the fiber axis results which is responsible for shifting the capillaries to one side of the septum or the other (Figs. 11.8 and 11.17). The wall of the capillaries is exposed to the luminal pressure, which is the result of blood pressure in pulmonary arteries and veins but also depends on gravity, for one finds wider capillaries at the bottom of the lung than at the top. If this distending pressure acts homogeneously over the circumference of the capillary, it will push against the fibers on one side but will cause

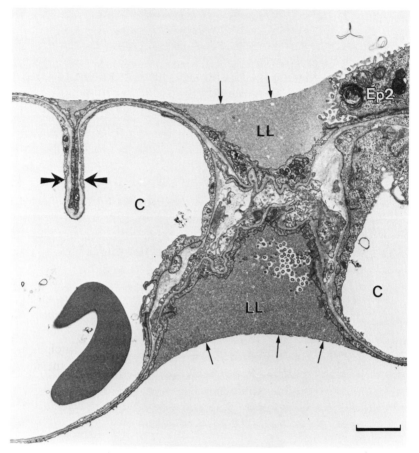

Fig. 11.16 Alveolar septum of human lung fixed by perfusion through blood vessels shows alveolar lining layer (LL) in crevices between capillaries (C) topped by surfactant film which appears as a fine black line (arrows). Note the type II cell with lamellar bodies and the fold in thin tissue barrier (bold arrows). Scale marker: 2 μm. (From Weibel, 1979.)

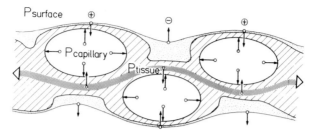

Fig. 11.17 Model showing the micromechanical forces of surface tension, tissue tension, and capillary distending pressure that shape the alveolar septum.

the thin barrier on the opposite side to bulge outward. This effect is to some extent counteracted by surface tension which arises at the air–tissue interface and exerts a force normal to the surface (Fig. 11.17). This force depends on two factors: its direction depends on the orientation of curvature, acting toward the alveolar space over concave regions (negative curvature) and toward the tissue over convexities (positive curvature); its magnitude depends on the degree of curvature and on the value of the surface tension coefficient γ.

The alveolar septum achieves a stable configuration when all these interacting forces are in balance. In principle we can say that the capillary is intercalated between the fibers and the air–tissue interface whose combined forces tend to squash the capillary flat. This happens, indeed, at high levels of lung inflation when the fibers are under high tension and the surface tension coefficient of surfactant reaches its highest value due to expansion of the surface (Fig. 11.12). On deflation the fibers are relaxed and surface tension falls drastically. The capillary distending pressure now exceeds both the tissue and the surface forces, with the result that the slack fibers are bent, weaving through the capillary network, whereas the capillaries bulge slightly toward the air space. Surface tension is apparently so low as to permit a considerable degree of surface "crumpling" to persist (Fig. 11.18).

The importance of the balance between the forces that act on the septum is also shown in Figure 11.19, where we have modified the pressure in the capillaries. Remember that, in relation to Figure 10.17, we have seen that the blood pressure in the pulmonary vessels increases from top to bottom due to hydrostatic pressure. Only in zone 3 (Fig. 10.17) can we expect the capillaries to be fully perfused because capillary pressure is larger than "alveolar pressure"; on the basis of the model shown in Figure 11.17, "alveolar pressure" must evidently be interpreted as the combined effect of fiber tension and surface forces. The specimen of Figure 11.19b was fixed under zone 3 perfusion conditions and all the capillaries are wide, partly bulging toward the air space, as in Figure 11.18. This is different in Figure 11.19a, which was fixed under zone 2 conditions: in the flat part of the septum the capillaries are squashed flat, because the surface and tissue forces now exceed the vascular distending pressure. It is interesting, however, that the capillaries in the corners remain wide, a point we shall clarify in a moment.

In the air-filled lung the alveolar septa always appear as flat walls between the air spaces. This is interesting because the fibers are taut only at the highest inflation levels, whereas at 50% TLC they must be about 25% too long. What happens is that the surface forces tuck some excess fibers into the "alveolar corners" (Fig. 11.20), that is, into the region where three septa come together (Fig. 11.15). The fibers

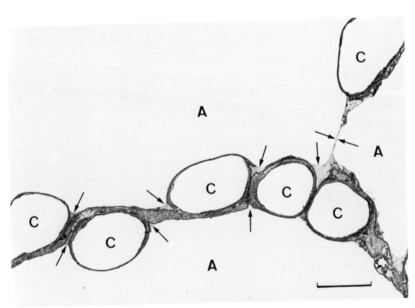

Fig. 11.18 Alveolar septum of air-filled rabbit lung perfusion-fixed at 60% TLC shows empty capillaries (C) which bulge toward the alveolar air space (A). Note pools of surface lining layer in the crevices between capillaries (arrows) and film spanning across alveolar pore (double arrows). Scale marker: 5 μm. (From Gil et al., 1979.)

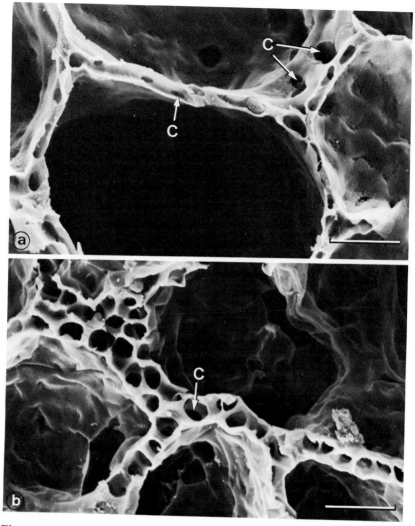

Fig. 11.19 Scanning electron micrographs of alveolar walls of rabbit lungs fixed under (a) zone 2 and (b) zone 3 conditions of perfusion. Note that capillaries (C) are wide in zone 3 and slit-like in zone 2, except "corner capillaries," which are wide in either case. Scale markers: 20 μm. (From Bachofen et al., 1983.)

remaining in the flat part of the septum are sufficiently tensed to support the capillary network. This tucking away of fibers into the alveolar corners is an intriguing finding. But we must remember that alveolar corners form where three septa meet along a so-called triple

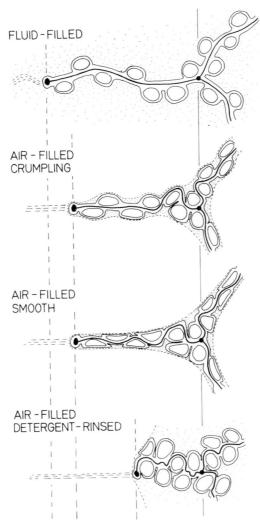

FLUID-FILLED

AIR-FILLED
CRUMPLING

AIR-FILLED
SMOOTH

AIR-FILLED
DETERGENT-RINSED

Fig. 11.20 The alveolar septum assumes different configurations depending on the interaction of micromechanical forces.

line (Fig. 11.15); here surface tension must exert a particularly strong outward pull on the tissue because the curvature is highly negative on three sides of the triple line, with the result that the pressure in the tissue is negative in this region. Besides pulling in fibers, this has the additional effects of allowing the capillaries in the corners to remain wide in all conditions (Fig. 11.19), even at high inflations, and of sucking interstitial fluid from the septum toward the triple line.

Thus, in summary, the stable configuration of the alveolar septum is the result of balancing the three forces that act on the tissue. Since surface tension decreases as tissue tension relaxes on deflation, the overall effect is to allow a maximal and nearly constant surface of contact between air and blood to be maintained over a wide range of airspace distension.

Keeping the Barrier Dry and Thin

The need to keep the air–blood barrier thin meets with a number of problems because two of the mechanical forces acting on the septum have a tendency to drive fluid into the tissue: the capillary pressure should cause plasma to filter through the endothelium, whereas the surface forces should draw fluid toward the alveolus. Why does this not lead to progressive thickening of the tissue barrier and eventually to flooding of the alveoli?

The flow of fluid between a capillary and its surrounding tissue is customarily described by Starling's law:

$$\dot{V}_{net} = K_f(P_c - P_i) - K_r(\pi_c - \pi_i) \tag{11.3}$$

where P_c and P_i are hydrostatic pressures, π_c and π_i colloid osmotic pressures in capillaries and interstitium, respectively; the permeability factors K_f and K_r are called filtration and reflection coefficients, respectively, and are essentially determined by the properties of the barrier.

Although Starling's law must hold in principle, the conditions are not quite as simple in the lung for a number of reasons. First, we are really dealing with a three-compartment system (Fig. 11.21) where two cellular barriers, endothelium and epithelium, separate three extracellular fluid spaces: blood plasma, interstitial fluid (lymph), and alveolar lining layer. This introduces complications because, in fact, we would have to consider two fluid flow rates, one into the tissue and one from the tissue to the alveolar lining layer. And for this we would need three hydrostatic and three colloid osmotic pressures, as well as two sets of permeability coefficients. But we shall also see that the hydrostatic pressures prevailing outside the capillary are quite variable from place to place on the alveolar septum.

The permeability of the two cellular barriers is different. We have seen that the alveolar epithelium forms a tight barrier. In contrast,

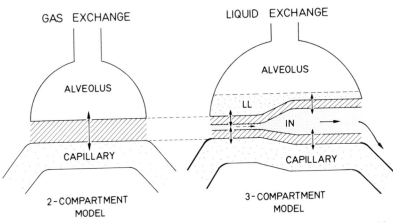

Fig. 11.21 Gas exchange and liquid exchange in the lung are described by two-compartment and three-compartment models, respectively. (From Weibel and Bachofen, 1979.)

the endothelium is rather leaky, as its loose tight junctions (see chapter 9) allow electrolytes and even smaller macromolecules such as albumin to pass. There is hence rather free exchange between plasma and interstitial space, whereas the transfer of matter between the interstitium and alveolar lining layer is more selective.

Colloid osmotic or oncotic pressure is determined mostly by the protein concentration, which is rather constant in plasma but variable in the interstitial fluid and in the alveolar lining layer. On the whole it appears, however, that plasma oncotic pressure exceeds that of tissue so that it tends to draw fluid back into the plasma. It has been shown that a transient increase in plasma colloid osmotic pressure extracts water from the lung cells as one would predict because of the semipermeability of cell membranes. Water is also extracted from the alveolar lining layer because of the very tight junctions between epithelial cells, whereas the interstitial space remains unchanged due to the free solute exchange through the endothelium. The lung reacts very rapidly to such changes and reverts to normal dimensions as soon as the composition of plasma is normalized.

The hydrostatic pressure gradients show considerable local variations in the alveolar septum. If we consult Figure 11.17 we note that the capillary pressure is opposed by surface pressure in the thin barrier region where the surface tends to have positive curvature; the pressure gradient from plasma to tissue is therefore small. This is quite different in the region of intercapillary pits, where the negative curvature causes the surface force to be directed outward; the pressure in the pool of lining layer must be relatively low, if not negative. In the depth of the septum such pits are surrounded by capillaries and the hydrostatic pressure gradient from plasma to lining layer is therefore appreciable. Note that this gradient is greatly influenced by surface tension; surfactant has therefore an important protective effect in that it reduces the suction exerted by the surface force over the pits.

The distribution of pressure gradients over the septum is important for keeping the barrier thin (Fig. 11.17). It will cause the structurally thin part of the barrier to remain thin and dry under nearly all conditions: not only does the positive surface pressure reduce the depth of the lining layer to a minimum by driving its hypophase into the intercapillary pits, but the two opposing pressures also prevent plasma from accumulating in the tissue space. Note, however, that, in the thin barrier portion, there is no real interstitial space which could accommodate appreciable fluid masses, because here the two basement membranes of endothelium and epithelium are fused (Fig. 11.9).

There is a real interstitial space, however, in the thick barrier parts which are found between capillaries and pits. Considering the leakiness of the endothelium and the hydrostatic pressure gradient caused by positive capillary and negative surface pressures (Fig. 11.17), we must wonder why fluid does not progressively accumulate in this region. There are a number of reasons. One of them is that interstitial fluid is rapidly drained away from the alveolar septa. The interstitial spaces of the septum are associated with the septal fibers and thus form a system of interconnected channels which find an outlet in the larger structures of the peripheral fiber system. Remember that the fiber system forms a continuum so that the system of channels is also continuous. The overall distribution of surface forces in an acinus (Fig. 11.15) causes the interstitial pressure to become progressively more negative as we move from the axial fibers through the septa and triple lines to the peripheral connective tissue, and this drives the fluid from the septa to the larger connective tissue masses at the periphery of the acini. Here one also finds the lymphatics which collect the fluid in order to drain it back to the blood via the lymph system.

It is furthermore possible that the septal interstitium is actively prevented from accepting larger quantities of fluid. In chapter 9 we have seen that most of the fibroblasts of the alveolar septum are contractile myofibroblasts. Their bundles of actomyosin filaments are contained in cytoplasmic branches that connect the epithelial and endothelial basement membranes (Fig. 9.6) and thus span the interstitial space. These conspicuous structures are still "in search of a function." It has been postulated that they could restrict the expansion of the capillary network under the effect of luminal pressure. But one could also imagine that they could restrict, and perhaps even actively regulate, the compliance of the interstitial space to fluid accumulation. If this were so, they could contribute importantly to keeping the barrier dry.

In summary, the barrier is kept dry and thin by the interaction of multiple factors. Design features of the tissue, namely the restriction of spaces and the establishment of drainage channels, are just as important as a proper balance between the various forces that affect fluid movements. That this is so becomes strikingly evident in certain diseases. In heart failure the hydrostatic capillary pressure may rise because the outflow of blood into the left atrium is inhibited: fluid becomes extruded from the congested capillaries at such a rate that the drainage system cannot cope with it. This fluid first builds up in the large connective tissue masses surrounding blood vessels and bronchi, a condition called interstitial edema. At some point in time the fluid may also penetrate across the epithelium and flood alveoli one by one. This so-called hemodynamic pulmonary edema causes severe respiratory troubles because the flooded alveoli cannot be ventilated; a good part of the blood passes through the lung without picking up oxygen. As another example, the respiratory distress syndrome of the premature newborn is due to inadequate surfactant production; surface tension is so high that fluid is drawn into the alveolar spaces, thus exacerbating the respiratory troubles that are already bad enough.

Summary

The lung is built as a complex of elastic bags kept expanded within the chest cavity in order to allow ventilation of the gas exchange units. The motive force for ventilation is provided by the intercostal muscles of which the external part is an inspiratory muscle because it lifts the ribs; the internal intercostals are expiratory muscles. The most important inspiratory muscle is the diaphragm, a dome-like flat ring of radial muscle fibers that insert at the lower edge of the rib cage and converge toward a central connective tissue membrane. Contraction of the diaphragm flattens the dome and enlarges the chest cavity downward. The lung is separated from the chest wall and the diaphragm by the pleural space which contains some serosal fluid. If air penetrates into the pleural space the lung collapses (pneumothorax); the pressure in the pleural space is negative (-2.5 to -10 cm H_2O) because of the recoil force of the lung. At expiration the lung does not fill the chest cavity completely; pleural recesses form which can be opened on inspiration to allow the lung to expand into the now enlarged chest cavity.

The structural backbone of the lung is a continuous system of fibers that are anchored at the hilum and are kept under tension by the negative intrapleural pressure that tugs on the visceral pleura. The system can be described in terms of three parts: the axial fiber system begins at the hilum and enwraps all airways out to alveolar ducts; the peripheral fiber system is related to the visceral pleura and extends into the lung in the form of septa that incompletely separate parenchymal lung units such as segments, lobules, or acini; within the acinus (the lung unit where all airways are devoted to gas exchange) a system of fine septal fibers extends from the axial fibers of the alveolar ducts to the peripheral fiber strands. The continuous nature of the three-dimensional fiber system of the lung is an essential feature; the septal fibers are thus indirectly subjected to the pull of the visceral pleura. This is important because the gas exchange units are supported by the septal fibers which are interlaced with the capillary network. The fiber system is composed of collagen and elastic fibers that have different mechanical properties: elastic fibers are extensible (to 130% of relaxed length) whereas the inextensible collagen fibers have very high tensile strength; the system can be compared to an elastic band made of a mixture of rubber bands and twine. In order to study the mechanical properties of the lung's fiber system the airways must be filled with saline to eliminate surface tension effects.

The major part of the lung's recoil force results from surface tension at the air–fluid interface of the alveoli. The pressure generated by surface tension in a hollow body is the product of the mean curvature times the surface tension coefficient. Since the curvature of a small alveolus is greater than that of a large one, surface tension should make the lung unstable because smaller alveoli would collapse and empty into larger ones. Two mechanisms can prevent this from happening. (1) The fiber system makes the alveoli interdependent; when an alveolus tends to collapse this may be counteracted by the increasing fiber tension in surrounding alveolar walls. (2) The surfactant lining of alveoli can vary its surface tension: as the alveolus begins to shrink its surface becomes smaller and the ensuing compression of the phospholipid film (the DPPC molecules are pushed closer together) leads to a fall in surface tension, down to nearly zero. As a result of this feature, alveoli (small bubbles $\frac{1}{4}$ mm in diameter) do not behave like soap bubbles; the alveolar complex is astonishingly stable. In the normal lung, both fiber interdependence and variable surfactant properties are important for the stabilization of respiratory air spaces; the interplay between these two features allows the gas exchange surface to remain adequately expanded.

Fiber tension and surface forces also affect the configuration of capillaries in the alveolar septa. The capillary network is expanded in the septal plane due to the extension of the septal fibers with which it is interlaced. Capillary blood pressure pushes the capillary wall outward, away from the (stretched) fibers. This causes the surface of the alveolar septum to be corrugated. The thin alveolar surface lining layer smooths this surface texture to some extent but residual local curvatures (convexities over bulging capillaries) tend to be further evened out by surface tension. The configuration of the alveolar septum is the result of balancing the various micromechanical forces that act on the thin air–blood tissue barrier: tissue tension, blood pressure, and surface tension.

Keeping the air–blood barrier dry and thin is a further mechanical problem, important to ensure adequate conditions for efficient gas exchange. It is solved by giving the two cellular linings of epithelium and endothelium different permeability properties, and by providing the septal interstitial space with features that allow rapid drainage of lymph fluid. An important feature is that the epithelial and endothelial basement membranes are fused over half the barrier surface, thus eliminating an interstitial space in these regions.

Further Reading

Agostoni, E. 1972. Mechanics of the pleural space. *Physiological Reviews* 52:57–128.

Hance, A. J., and R. G. Crystal. 1976. Collagen. In *The Biochemical Basis of Pulmonary Function*, ed. R. G. Crystal. New York: Dekker, pp. 215–271.

Hoppin, F. G., and H. Hildebrandt. 1977. Mechanical properties of the lung. In *Bioengineering Aspects of the Lung*, ed. J. B. West. New York: Dekker, pp. 83–162.

Mead, J. 1961. Mechanical properties of lungs. *Physiological Reviews* 41:281–330.

Pattle, R. E. 1965. Surface lining of lung alveoli. *Physiological Reviews* 45:48–79.

Staub, N. C. 1974. Pulmonary edema. *Physiological Reviews* 54:678–811.

Weibel, E. R. 1984. Functional morphology of lung parenchyma. In *Handbook of Physiology: Mechanics of Breathing*, ed. P. Macklem and J. Mead. Washington: American Physiological Society (in press).

Weibel, E. R., and J. Gil. 1977. Structure–function relationships at the alveolar level. In *Bioengineering Aspects of the Lung*, ed. J. B. West. New York: Dekker, pp. 1–81.

West, J. B. 1977. Stresses. In *Regional Differences in the Lung*, ed. J. B. West. New York: Academic, pp. 281–322.

Wilson, T. A. 1979. Parenchymal mechanics at the alveolar level. *Federation Proceedings* 38:7–10.

References

* Avery, M. E., and J. Mead. 1959. Surface properties in relation to atelectasis and hyaline membrane disease. *American Journal of Diseases of Children* 97:517–523.

Bachofen, H., P. Gehr, and E. R. Weibel. 1979. Alterations of mechanical properties and morphology in excised rabbit lungs rinsed with a detergent. *Journal of Applied Physiology* 47:1002–1010.

Bachofen, H., J. Weber, D. Wangensteen, and E. R. Weibel. 1983. Morphometric estimates of diffusing capacity in lungs fixed under zone II and zone III conditions. *Respiration Physiology* 52:41–52.

* Clements, J. A., R. F. Hustead, R. P. Johnson, and I. Bribetz. 1961. Pulmonary surface tension and alveolar stability. *Journal of Applied Physiology* 16:444–450.

Gil, J., H. Bachofen, P. Gehr, and E. R. Weibel. 1979. Alveolar volume–surface area relation in air- and saline-filled lungs fixed by vascular perfusion. *Journal of Applied Physiology* 47:990–1001.

Macklem, P., and J. Mead, eds. 1984. *Handbook of Physiology: Mechanics of Breathing*. Washington: American Physiological Society (in press).

Mead, J., T. Takishima, and D. Leith. 1970. Stress distribution in lungs: a model of pulmonary elasticity. *Journal of Applied Physiology* 28:596–608.

* Mead, J., J. L. Whittenberger, and E. P. Radford, Jr. 1957. Surface tension as a factor in pulmonary volume-pressure hysteresis. *Journal of Applied Physiology* 10:191–196.

* Neergaard, K. von. 1929. Neue Auffassungen über einen Grundbegriff der Atemmechanik. Die Retraktionskraft der Lunge, abhängig von der Oberflächenspannung in den Alveolen. *Zeitschrift Gesamte Experimentelle Medizin* 66:373–394.

* Orsós, F. 1936. Die Gerüstsysteme der Lunge und deren physiologische und pathologische Bedeutung. I. Normal-anatomische Verhältnisse. *Beiträge Klinische Tuberkulose* 87:568–609.

* Pattle, R. E. 1955. Properties, function and origin of the alveolar lining layer. *Nature* 175:1125–1126.

Schneeberger, E. E., and M. J. Karnovsky. 1968. The ultrastructural basis of alveolar-capillary membrane permeability to peroxidase used as a tracer. *Journal of Cell Biology* 37:781–793.

Schürch, S., J. Goerke, and J. A. Clements. 1978. Direct determination of volume and time dependence of alveolar surface tension in excised lungs. *Proceedings of the National Academy of Sciences USA* 75:3417–3421.

Wangensteen, D., H. Bachofen, and E. R. Weibel. 1981. Lung tissue volume changes induced by hypertonic NaCl: morphometric evaluation. *Journal of Applied Physiology* 51:1443–1450.

Wangensteen, O. D., E. Lysaker, and P. Savaryn. 1977. Pulmonary capillary filtration and reflection coefficients in the adult rabbit. *Microvascular Research* 14:81–97.

Weibel, E. R. 1979. Looking into the lung: what can it tell us? *American Journal of Roentgenology* 133:1021–1031.

——— 1980. Design and structure of the human lung. In *Pulmonary Diseases and Disorders*, ed. A. P. Fishman. New York: McGraw-Hill, pp. 224–271.

Weibel, E. R., and H. Bachofen. 1979. Structural design of the alveolar septum and fluid exchange. In *Pulmonary Edema*, ed. A. P. Fishman and E. M. Renkin. Washington: American Physiological Society, pp. 1–20.

Weibel, E. R., and J. Gil. 1968. Electron microscopic demonstration of an extracellular duplex lining layer of alveoli. *Respiration Physiology* 4:42–57.

——— 1977. Structure–function relationships at the alveolar level. In *Bioengineering Aspects of the Lung*, ed. J. B. West. New York: Dekker, pp. 1–81.

Wilson, T. A., and H. Bachofen. 1982. A model for mechanical structure of the alveolar duct. *Journal of Applied Physiology* 52:1064–1070.

12

THE LUNG AS GAS EXCHANGER

IN THE PRECEDING CHAPTERS we have seen how airways and blood vessels of the lung, by successive branching, set up a large number of units in which air and blood come into intimate contact. These units must be ventilated with air and perfused with blood; but they must also be stabilized mechanically, so that the large surface of air–blood contact can be maintained. Ventilation and perfusion, as well as mechanical stability, are evidently important determinants of gas exchange. In this chapter we now concentrate on the gas exchange units of lung parenchyma and ask how their structural and functional properties may affect the flow of O_2 from air to blood, or the discharge of CO_2 in the opposite direction.

Design of the Gas Exchanger

We have now seen repeatedly that the gas exchange units of the lung are found in the alveoli, whose walls are densely populated by blood capillaries. Alveoli are cup-like chambers formed in the walls of the last airway generations (Figs. 10.2, 10.3, and 11.5); they are thus all widely open to the air in the acinar air ducts. In the human lung alveoli measure about $\frac{1}{4}$ mm in diameter (Fig. 12.1) and are thus just visible to the bare eye. Their number is about 300 million in the adult lung, so that each acinus contains some 2000 alveoli attached to its air ducts. During the last stages of lung development (see chapter 8) the tissue separating lung units becomes so greatly reduced that

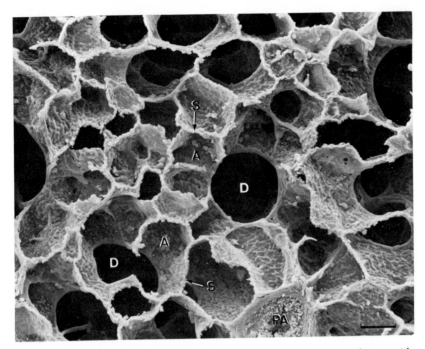

Fig. 12.1 Scanning electron micrograph of human lung parenchyma. Alveolar ducts (D) are surrounded by alveoli (A) which are separated by thin septa (S). Note the small branch of pulmonary artery (PA). Scale marker: 100 μm. (From Weibel, 1980.)

alveoli of adjacent units come to lie very close to each other. As a consequence the gas exchanging lung parenchyma has the appearance of a thin-walled froth with the important difference that each "bubble" is connected to outside air through the duct system and can thus be ventilated. The result of this design is that the lung has a very large internal surface, well over 100 m² in man, or nearly the size of a tennis court. But this large surface is arranged in a systematic manner around the last generations of the airway tree in the acini so that the distance between this surface and outside air is no more than about 40–50 cm (Fig. 10.7).

As a further result of tissue reduction during lung development (see chapter 8), the alveolar walls of the mature lung contain only a single dense capillary network and a minimal amount of tissue to ensure complete separation of air and blood (Fig. 12.2). One of the important design properties of the pulmonary gas exchanger is therefore that each unit of the capillary network is exposed to at least two alveoli which may or may not appertain to the same air-duct system. Furthermore, the surface of the capillary network is nearly equal to that of the alveoli.

The capillary network contains approximately 200 ml of blood that is spread out in a film so thin that it appears like a single layer of erythrocytes, with the result that each red cell is exposed to air on all sides (Fig. 12.2). We should now remember that this capillary network is tapped by about 300 million arterial end branches and by the same number of veins. It is therefore subdivided into a number of microvascular units that are about the size of a single alveolus, athough individual capillary units are not directly related to individual alveoli.

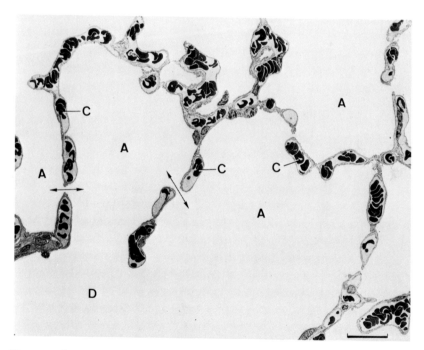

Fig. 12.2 Low power electron micrograph of dog lung parenchyma showing several alveoli (A), two of which open on an alveolar duct (D). The alveolar walls are densely populated by capillaries (C) whose blood is separated from air by a very thin tissue barrier. Note that the alveolar walls are perforated by pores of Kohn (double arrows). Scale marker: 20 µm. (From Weibel, 1973.)

The third consequence of tissue reduction is the extraordinary thinness of the air–blood barrier in the gas exchange region (Fig. 12.3); its thinnest parts make up about half the barrier surface and measure no more than 0.2 μm in man, but can be even less than 0.1 μm thick in very small mammals. It is interesting to note that the barrier is considerably thicker in amphibian and reptilian lungs but that it may be as thin or even thinner in bird lungs. Remember that the barrier is completely lined by epithelial and endothelial cells even in its thinnest parts (Fig. 9.12).

We should also not forget that the tissue barrier is covered by the alveolar lining layer which is, however, extremely thin over the thinnest barrier portions (Figs. 11.16 and 11.18). On the other hand we have noted in chapter 11 that the lining layer contributes importantly to molding the alveolar septum in the air-filled lung. As a result some parts of the air–blood barrier may be shifted into crevices between capillaries and therefore not be available for gas ex-

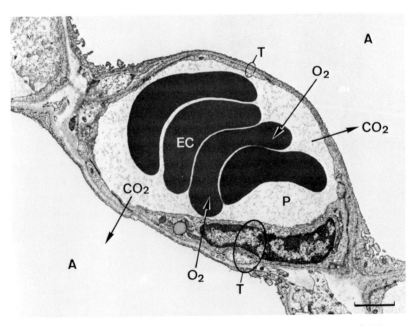

Fig. 12.3 Alveolar capillary from human lung showing how O_2 and CO_2 are exchanged between alveolar air (A) and capillary blood with erythrocytes (EC) in plasma (P), across a tissue barrier (T) of variable thickness. Scale marker: 2μm.

change. In discussing the design of the pulmonary gas exchanger we will therefore have to account for the micromechanical forces interacting in the alveolar walls (see chapter 11).

Physiological Basis for Gas Exchange

Gas exchange between air and blood occurs by diffusion across the air–blood barrier. We have learned before (chapter 4) that O_2 flow by diffusion depends on the product of a conductance and a partial pressure gradient as driving force. Let us first consider the driving force which must be the O_2 partial pressure difference between alveolar air and capillary blood (Fig. 12.4). How is this gradient established and maintained? *

The alveolar O_2 partial pressure, PA_{O_2}, is the result of O_2 extraction by the blood and O_2 replenishment through ventilation. When we take a breath of fresh air, it first becomes warmed up to body temperature and completely saturated with water vapor while passing through the conducting airways. The P_{O_2} of air that reaches the acini therefore is

$$PI_{O_2} = (P_B - 47) \cdot 0.2095 \text{ mm Hg} \tag{12.1}$$

where P_B is ambient barometric pressure, 47 mm Hg is the partial pressure of water vapor at 37° C, and 0.2095 is the fractional O_2 concentration in fresh air. Thus at sea level ($P_B = 760$ mm Hg) we find $PI_{O_2} = 150$ mm Hg. With each breath one tidal volume minus the dead space is introduced into the air that remained in the lung at the end of expiration and which has been depleted of some of its O_2. The P_{O_2} of this residual air, measured by exhaling very deeply down to residual volume, is found to be about 100 mm Hg. With a tidal volume of 500 ml, a dead space of 150 ml, and a FRC of 3000 ml (Fig. 10.8), the average P_{O_2} in the acini rises by no more than 5 mm Hg on

---

*In this chapter there is a slight formal inconsistency in the symbolism resulting from different customs in the physiologic and morphometric literature. In morphometry phase identifiers are given either in parentheses or as a subscript to the parameter symbol, for example S_A for alveolar surface area. In respiration physiology the phase identifier is written on the line of the parameter symbol, for example PA_{O_2} for alveolar P_{O_2}.

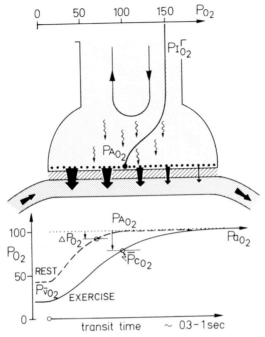

Fig. 12.4 Change of P_{O_2} in alveolar air and in capillary blood along the path from pulmonary artery (venous blood) to pulmonary vein (arterial blood).

inspiration. Thus, at rest, the alveolar P_{O_2} varies very little around 100 mm Hg.

In exercise the tidal volume increases up to five times (Table 10.2) and FRC is reduced, but O_2 extraction rises considerably with the result that $P_{A_{O_2}}$ remains around 100 mm Hg.

The inflow of fresh air on inspiration establishes, at first, a rather steep P_{O_2} gradient across the cushion of residual air, from the center of the acinus to the actual alveolar surface. But since the distances are very short, one usually assumes mixing by diffusion to be instantaneous. In recent years, however, the evidence is growing that a certain gradient persists in the acinar air, a phenomenon called stratification. I shall discuss this point in greater detail below.

What really counts for gas exchange between air and blood is the P_{O_2} in the layer of air that is immediately adjacent to the air–blood barrier, which we shall call alveolar P_{O_2} or $P_{A_{O_2}}$ in the narrow sense (Fig. 12.4). This value is usually taken to be equal to the P_{O_2} of arterial blood, Pa_{O_2}, under the assumption that the blood which leaves the alveolar capillaries is completely equilibrated with alveolar air; it is again found to be about 100 mm Hg.

Let us now look at the P_{O_2} in capillary blood by considering a rather simple model where the microvascular unit is represented by a single "tube" that passes along the air–blood barrier (Fig. 12.4). Venous blood enters this unit from the pulmonary artery at a P_{O_2} of about 40 mm Hg in a healthy human at rest. When the blood reaches the end of the capillary unit, to be drained as arterial blood into the pulmonary vein, it will have completely equilibrated with alveolar air. Thus the alveolar–capillary P_{O_2} gradient ranges from 60 mm Hg at the entrance to 0 mm Hg at the end, with the result that the flow rate of O_2 across the barrier must decrease as capillary P_{O_2} rises. But the P_{O_2} profile in the capillary is not a simple affair; it depends on the blood flow velocity, on the diffusion properties of the barrier, and on the O_2 binding properties of blood, specifically on the O_2-hemoglobin equilibrium curve discussed in chapter 6.

One estimates that in man *at rest* an erythrocyte spends less than 1 second in the alveolar capillary. Under the effect of the large gradients in the first parts of its path along the alveolus, O_2 inflow is very rapid so that the P_{O_2} of blood has nearly reached that in alveolar air after the first third of the capillary path (Fig. 12.4). This is different *in exercise* where blood flow velocity is higher so that the red cells leave the microvascular unit after about 0.3 seconds. And since in exercise venous blood has a lower P_{O_2}, the entire capillary path length may be required to load O_2 onto the blood. At rest our lung evidently has a considerable diffusion reserve, but it may exploit it completely when the gas exchanger is stressed to the limit in strenuous exercise. This becomes strikingly evident when we breathe air of low O_2 content, such as at high altitude. Under these circumstances we need most of the capillary path length for saturating blood even at rest; there is less reserve for increasing O_2 uptake and our capacity to work strenuously at high altitude is severely limited.

For several reasons it would be interesting to know how the capillary P_{O_2} increases along the capillary; most importantly we should be able to calculate the mean capillary P_{O_2} for, as we shall see below, this is an important determinant of total O_2 flow from air to blood. All we know a priori is that the capillary P_{O_2} should increase nonlinearly from mixed venous to end-capillary P_{O_2} because the driving force for O_2 inflow into blood should gradually decrease as Pc_{O_2} increases, eventually becoming vanishingly small as Pc_{O_2} approaches PA_{O_2}. Christian Bohr, the prominent Danish physiologist who discovered the Bohr effect (see chapter 6), has calculated the first Pc_{O_2} profile in 1909 by assuming O_2 flow from air to blood to be proportional to the P_{O_2} gradient across the barrier; the procedure is still known as Bohr integration between the P_{O_2} of mixed venous and end capillary blood. In the course of time some of the original assumptions had to be revised to account for the effects of the nonlinear O_2-hemoglobin equilibrium curve (Fig. 6.4): at low saturation levels, that is, in the first part of the capillary path the blood can bind large quantities of O_2 without changing P_{O_2} a lot, whereas above 80% saturation the P_{O_2} increases rapidly. As a consequence a relatively large P_{O_2} gradient is maintained in the initial part of the capillary and O_2 loading onto blood is more rapid than previously expected.

In fact, the gas exchange conditions are better still because of the Bohr effect. Figure 6.7 shows that the O_2-Hb equilibrium curve of venous blood is shifted to the right primarily because of the pH of 7.2 due to the high CO_2 content. As CO_2 is discharged in the lung the dissociation curve shifts back to the left, reaching a higher saturation at the end-capillary P_{O_2}. We have seen in Figure 6.7 that the "physiological" dissociation curve of blood in the lung is steeper than the physicochemical curve; the Bohr effect therefore helps to maintain a large P_{O_2} gradient from air to blood while O_2 is being taken up.

This is a good place to say a few words about CO_2 discharge in the lung. In chapter 6 we have seen that venous blood contains CO_2 in three forms: as dissolved CO_2, as bicarbonate, and as carbamino compounds. The reactions that generate bicarbonate and carbamino compounds are reversible. As dissolved CO_2 is released by diffusion into alveolar air the carbonic anhydrase of erythrocytes converts bicarbonate into CO_2. This maintains a high P_{CO_2} in alveolar capillary blood in spite of the high diffusivity of CO_2, which is about 20 times larger than that of O_2 owing to greater solubility. Note in this respect that the P_{CO_2} difference between arterial and mixed venous blood is much smaller than is the P_{O_2} difference: P_{CO_2} falls only from 50 to 40 mm Hg while blood passes through the lung. Alveolar air also has a P_{CO_2} of about 40 mm Hg so that the P_{CO_2} gradient across the barrier is rather small. We have seen that this is important for regulating acid–base balance in blood and tissue (chapter 6): if we hyperventilate, our lung alveolar P_{CO_2} falls and allows an excessive amount of CO_2 to be discharged from the blood, causing alkalosis to develop.

It is not quite known how CO_2 discharge is related to O_2 uptake along the capillary path. Because of the chemical reactions required to liberate CO_2 from bicarbonate or carbamino compounds, diffusive transfer of CO_2 across the barrier probably takes place over most of the path. In first approximation we can therefore assume the local O_2 and CO_2 exchanges to be roughly proportional. As P_{CO_2} falls, pH rises and the O_2-hemoglobin dissociation curve shifts gradually to the left. But the situation is more complex still because the CO_2 binding properties of blood are also affected by P_{O_2} through the Haldane effect (Fig. 6.7).

The calculation of a precise and accurate P_{O_2} profile along the hypothetical capillary path is, evidently, complex and loaded with partly untested assumptions. It is made even worse by the fact that capillaries are not simple straight tubes along which blood flows at even speed. Rather, the capillaries form dense networks through which blood flows more or less like a sheet, spreading in all directions from the point of inflow at the pulmonary artery to several outflow points at the venous end. The blood flow path through the capillaries is definitely not streamlined but may be quite tortuous. For all those reasons it is hard to calculate with a reasonable safety margin the pattern of P_{CO_2} change as a "typical" red cell moves through the lung. We must therefore be content with approximate indications of possible P_{O_2} profiles which are different in exercise and at rest.

Pulmonary Diffusing Capacity: Physiology

Bohr proposed, in 1909, to estimate the functional potential of the lung as gas exchanger by its diffusing capacity for O_2, DL_{O_2}. This factor relates O_2 flow rate, $\dot{V}_{O_2}$, to the partial pressure difference from alveolar air to blood:

$$\dot{V}_{O_2} = DL_{O_2} \cdot (PA_{O_2} - \overline{P}_{CO_2}).\tag{12.2}$$

It is a measure of the O_2 flow that arises from a P_{O_2} gradient of 1 mm Hg and hence estimates the global conductance of the lung for O_2 transfer to the blood by diffusion. From Figure 12.4 it is evident that estimating the P_{O_2} gradient may be tricky. It is perhaps easy enough to say that PA_{O_2} must be the P_{O_2} in the layer of alveolar air immediately adjacent to the barrier—although even this may be questionable;

but then we are still faced with the problem of how to estimate it. It is, however, definitely problematic to estimate, from the measurable quantities $P\bar{v}_{O_2}$ and Pa_{O_2}, a relevant mean value for capillary blood P_{O_2} as long as the P_{O_2} profile along the capillary path is not better characterized. These difficulties are very critical, particularly because PA_{O_2} and $\bar{P}c_{O_2}$ are rather close to each other so that their difference is very small; this is because the end-capillary blood is equilibrated with alveolar air and because the P_{O_2} profile rises steeply in its initial part. A small error in either P_{O_2} estimate may lead to a large error in their difference.

To overcome these problems one has used a number of tricks. One is to have the subject breathe a hypoxic gas mixture, for example, 12% O_2 in N_2. Alveolar P_{O_2} then falls to about 50 mm Hg and the gradient is much smaller at the venous end of the capillary; in addition the rise of P_{O_2} as O_2 content of blood increases is less because of the shape of the dissociation curve (Fig. 6.4). For both reasons the capillary P_{O_2} profile is less steep and a larger part of the capillary path is used to load O_2 onto the blood, with the result that mean Pc_{O_2} is lower relative to PA_{O_2}. It is also possible that end-capillary P_{O_2} does not reach PA_{O_2}, particularly in exercise. The alveolar-capillary gradient becomes measurable.

Another approach is to estimate D_L by means of a tracer gas which also binds to hemoglobin, namely carbon monoxide, CO. It is found that CO binds to hemoglobin with such avidity that the CO partial pressure of blood remains so low that it can be neglected. One can therefore estimate DL_{CO} by simplifying the general relation

$$DL_{CO} = \dot{V}_{CO}/(PA_{CO} - Pb_{CO}) \approx \dot{V}_{CO}/PA_{CO}. \tag{12.3}$$

One therefore only needs two measurements which are relatively easy to obtain: CO uptake and alveolar P_{CO}. One way of obtaining them is the so-called single breath method: the subject makes a deep inspiration of a dilute mixture of CO in air and holds the breath for 10 seconds; one then calculates both CO uptake and alveolar P_{CO} from the measurement of CO concentrations in inspired and expired air. Another approach is to allow the subject to breathe a low concentration of CO until a steady state is achieved, after which CO uptake and alveolar P_{CO} are measured.

Measurement of DL_{CO} is evidently an indirect approach to estimating DL_{O_2}, the parameter which is functionally relevant. However, one

can assume that the diffusion of CO from alveolar air to the erythrocytes is basically governed by the same factors which apply for O_2.
But because of differences in solubility and diffusivity of the two
molecules in water, one assumes that the diffusion of O_2 should be
faster by a factor of 1.23, so that one can approximately derive DL_{O_2} by

$$DL_{O_2} \approx 1.23 \cdot DL_{CO}. \tag{12.4}$$

Physiological estimates of pulmonary diffusing capacity in man at
rest usually yield values of DL_{O_2} of about 20–30 ml $O_2 \cdot min^{-1} \cdot mm$
Hg^{-1} (or $25–37 \cdot 10^{-2}$ ml $O_2 \cdot sec^{-1} \cdot mbar^{-1}$). On exercise one finds
DL_{O_2} to increase by about a factor of four to approximately 100 ml
$O_2 \cdot min^{-1} \cdot mm\ Hg^{-1}$ (or 1.25 ml $O_2 \cdot sec^{-1} \cdot mbar^{-1}$). This is not astonishing if we consider that, at rest, the capillary P_{O_2} reaches PA_{O_2}
already after about a third of the capillary path so that the remaining
$\frac{2}{3}$ do not contribute to gas exchange at all (Fig. 12.4). In strenuous
exercise, however, where the demand on the lung as gas exchanger is
maximally stressed, capillary blood equilibrates with alveolar air
only near the end of the path. It is hence evident that the "true"
diffusing capacity of the lung must be closer to the value estimated in
exercise than to that obtained at rest.

The discussion of the nonlinear increase in capillary P_{O_2} has already indicated that the O_2 binding properties of blood must have an
important effect on DL_{O_2}. In fact, one finds DL_{O_2} to be considerably
below the normal value in anemic patients whose blood has a reduced capacity to bind O_2 because of lower red cell content. As
shown in Figure 12.5 one can therefore split D_L into two sequential
components. In the first part, called the membrane diffusing capacity
D_M, O_2 diffuses through the tissue barrier and blood plasma to the red
cell; in the second part O_2 disperses within the red cells and binds to
hemoglobin. The second part is a rather complex process but it is
dominated by the reaction kinetics of O_2-Hb binding; it is therefore
customary to express it as the product of capillary blood volume, V_c,
and a coefficient θ which describes the rate at which O_2 is bound to a
unit volume of blood. Since θ is given as ml $O_2 \cdot min^{-1} \cdot mm\ Hg^{-1}$ per
ml of blood, the product $\theta \cdot V_c$ has the same units as the diffusing
capacity.

It follows from equation 12.2 that D_L is the overall conductance for
O_2 diffusion, or the reciprocal of the diffusion resistance. If D_L is split
into two components in series, D_M and $\theta \cdot V_c$, then we must add their

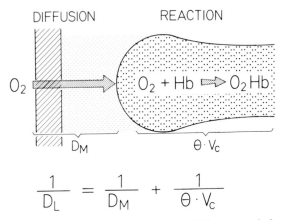

$$\frac{1}{D_L} = \frac{1}{D_M} + \frac{1}{\theta \cdot V_c}$$

Fig. 12.5 Oxygen uptake in the lung involves diffusion and chemical reaction between O_2 and hemoglobin.

respective resistances to obtain the overall resistance, so that

$$\frac{1}{D_L} = \frac{1}{D_M} + \frac{1}{\theta \cdot V_c}, \qquad (12.5)$$

the relation introduced in 1957 by F. J. W. Roughton and R. E. Forster, who did the pioneering work that clarified the role of blood reactions on pulmonary gas exchange.

The practical usefulness of this relation is that it should allow us to calculate capillary blood volume if an independent estimate of D_M is obtained and if θ is known. Estimating the reaction of O_2 with erythrocytes turns out to be a rather difficult undertaking; the values that have been obtained in different laboratories differ by as much as a factor of three. I shall discuss this further in the next section.

Before leaving this topic I should indicate that the lung's gas exchange function is also affected by blood flow: one of the reasons why $D_{L_{O_2}}$ is larger in exercise than at rest is that blood flow is increased about three-fold (Table 10.2), so that capillary blood is turned over at a faster rate. Ventilation is clearly also important because this affects alveolar P_{O_2}. Here again we must remember that alveolar ventilation is increased on exercise (Table 10.2). It is furthermore important that ventilation and perfusion are well matched in all lung units, otherwise the overall efficiency of gas exchange is impaired, in spite of a large diffusing capacity.

Pulmonary Diffusing Capacity: Morphometry

In the last section it was assumed that the diffusive transfer of O_2 from alveolar air to blood meets with some resistance, although it is presumably small. The diffusing capacity DL_{O_2} is, in fact, nothing else than an estimate of the global conductance or the reciprocal of the total resistance to diffusion of O_2 offered by the gas exchanger. It is evident that this resistance must somehow depend on the design and on the dimensions of the pulmonary gas exchanger; in chapter 3 we found that O_2 flow by diffusion from compartment A to B is governed by Fick's law:

$$\dot{V}_{O_2}(A-B) = K \cdot \frac{S}{\tau}\left(P_{O_2}(A) - P_{O_2}(B) \right) \qquad (12.6)$$

where K is a permeability coefficient, S the surface, and τ the thickness of the barrier separating A and B (Fig. 12.6). In many respiratory physiology texts this relation is taken as equivalent to equation 12.2 with the obvious conclusion that

$$DL_{O_2} = K \cdot S / \tau \qquad (12.7)$$

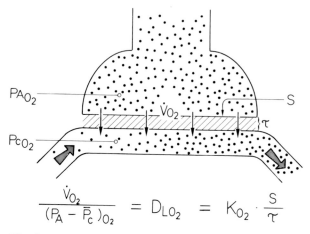

Fig. 12.6 The lung's conductance for diffusion of O_2 from air to blood is called pulmonary diffusing capacity, DL_{O_2}; it is estimated from functional (left) or structural variables (right).

where S would be the alveolar (or capillary) surface area and τ the thickness of the tissue barrier (Fig. 12.6). Since the alveolar surface of a human lung is so immense and the barrier so extraordinarily thin, it is understandable why the diffusing capacity is so large, or the resistance so immeasurably low.

However, this model is really too simple. In fact, we have already seen in the last section (Fig. 12.5) that the gas exchange path for O_2 consists of several segments in which different conditions prevail; diffusion through the barrier must be matched by O_2 binding to hemoglobin.

The electron micrograph shown in Figure 12.3 forms the basis for developing a better model for diffusing capacity based on the lung's design features. Imagine this picture to reflect a snapshot of red cells passing through the capillary at high velocity; indeed, the average time that a red cell is exposed to a given point on the air–blood barrier is of the order of 10–30 msec! So, at least two separate parts of this gas exchanger must be distinguished: the tissue barrier that is quite stable with respect to time, and the blood flowing by rapidly. But within the blood, plasma and red cells offer different conditions to diffusing O_2 molecules: whereas plasma is traversed essentially by passive molecular diffusion, O_2 molecules that penetrate into the red cell enter a complicated milieu in which their movement is greatly influenced by the high concentration of hemoglobin they encounter; not only is the binding of O_2 to hemoglobin a decisive factor in gas exchange, but hemoglobin can also facilitate diffusion, a phenomenon addressed in chapter 6.

To account for these differences we can subdivide the O_2 path from alveolar air to its hemoglobin binding site into three parts (Fig. 12.7): (1) the air–blood barrier made of tissue; (2) the plasma layer that separates the erythocyte from the tissue; and (3) the path within the erythrocyte.

These three segments of the O_2 path offer three distinct resistances to O_2 diffusion, and since they are in series the total resistance is their sum. For convenience I shall develop below expressions for the conductance (D) in the tissue barrier (t), in blood plasma (p), and in the erythrocyte (e); since the resistance is simply 1/D we obtain for the total diffusion resistance in the lung:

$$\frac{1}{D_L} = \frac{1}{D_t} + \frac{1}{D_p} + \frac{1}{D_e}. \tag{12.8}$$

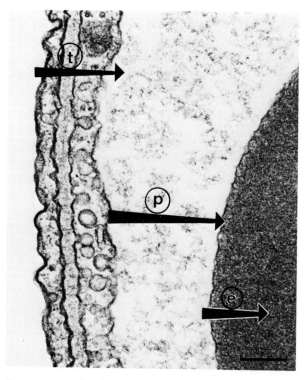

Fig. 12.7 Oxygen transfer from air to hemoglobin involves three steps: diffusion through the tissue barrier (t), diffusion through plasma (p), and diffusion and binding reaction within the red cells (e). Scale marker: 0.2 μm.

It is easily seen that the reciprocal of this sum is the pulmonary diffusing capacity, the lung's global conductance for O_2 diffusion.

Let us now try to find for each of the partial conductances an expression that accounts for the morphometric features of the system. The tissue barrier is a sheet of thickness τ which separates two compartments, alveolar air and plasma, over an area S; thus Fick's law determines O_2 flow according to equation 12.6 and, therefore, the conductance given by equation 12.7 applies to this case. The lung, however, is not a model as simple as that shown in Figure 12.6; the tissue barrier is so refined a structure that we have, in fact, devoted three whole chapters to describing its structural and functional complexity. Its two bounding surfaces are formed by independent cell layers, epithelium and endothelium, and they are related to two independent functional spaces, alveoli and capillaries. As a result of all this the two surfaces are not perfectly matched and the thickness of the barrier varies considerably (Fig. 12.3). How does this affect the diffusion conductance of the barrier?

First the barrier surfaces: O_2 enters the barrier on its alveolar and leaves it through its capillary surface, so that it is reasonable to use the mean of these two surface areas, $(S_A + S_c)/2$, as an estimate of the effective area of the tissue barrier. The effect of varying barrier thickness is that the conductance for O_2 will be variable from point to point, in fact, inversely proportional to the local thickness. If we imagine the barrier built of a set of units of equal area but varying thickness τ (Fig. 12.8), we find the overall conductance of the barrier as the mean of the unit conductances, because they are all in parallel. The only variable being the thickness — whose reciprocal determines the conductance, as we saw — we find that the relevant estimate of barrier thickness is its harmonic mean, τ_{ht}, that is, the mean of the reciprocal local thicknesses. This turns out to be quite important for we find that the value of the harmonic mean thickness of the pulmonary air–blood barrier is consistently about three times smaller than the arithmetic mean thickness $\bar{\tau}_t$; in man, for example, τ_{ht} is about 0.6 μm as compared to 2.2 μm for $\bar{\tau}_t$, whereas in the rat we find 0.5 μm versus 1.5 μm. This difference is the result of design features which must optimize various functional requirements. Thus we need fibers to support the capillaries; but it suffices to have them in only half of the barrier, keeping the other half very thin (Figs. 11.8 and 11.9). Or, the barrier needs cell bodies with bulky nuclei to maintain the cell linings alive; but these can be tucked away into the meshes of the capillary network (Fig. 9.11) where the tissue is already relatively thick because this is where the fiber tracts cross the capillary sheet from one side to the other. Thus the barrier needs to maintain a certain minimal mass to ensure its integrity, and this is reflected in the arithmetic mean barrier thickness; but it disposes of it in such a fashion as to interfere as little as possible with gas exchange. Barrier thickness becomes highly irregular, but this turns out to be an advantage in that it allows the diffusion-effective mean thickness to be three times smaller than if a barrier of the same total mass were made of even thickness — a remarkable finding!

On the basis of these arguments we find the conductance of the tissue barrier to be

$$D_t = K_t \cdot (S_A + S_c)/(2\tau_{ht}). \tag{12.9}$$

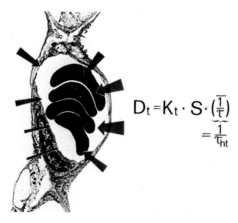

$$D_t = K_t \cdot S \cdot \left(\frac{\bar{1}}{\tau}\right)$$
$$= \frac{1}{\bar{\tau}_{ht}}$$

Fig. 12.8 The flow rate of O_2 by diffusion across the tissue barrier is inversely proportional to local barrier thickness.

The morphometric variables, S_A, S_c, and τ_{ht}, can all be measured on electron micrographs of lung sections using stereological methods (see chapter 4), provided the micrographs are obtained by proper statistical random sampling. The coefficient K_t — Krogh's permeation coefficient — is the product of solubility and diffusivity coefficients for a gas, be it O_2 or CO, in lung tissue; values for these coefficients are listed in Table 12.1.

If we look at the conductance of blood plasma we note that it also is that of a sheet, highly irregular in thickness, that separates the inner surface of the tissue barrier from the surface of the red cells (Fig. 12.3). Accordingly, the conductance of the plasma barrier is

$$D_p = K_p \cdot S_c / \tau_{hp}. \tag{12.10}$$

Note that we take the capillary surface, S_c, as an estimator of the effective area of the plasma barrier and do not consider the erythrocyte surface as a counterpart; the reason is that part of the erythrocyte surface is, in fact, "hidden" from the capillary surface by neighboring erythrocytes (Fig. 12.3) so that the "accessible" erythrocyte surface is found to be similar to S_c. The values for K_p are quite similar to those of K_t, as seen in Table 12.1.

The third conductance, that of erythrocytes, D_e, is of a different nature in that it involves two coupled events: facilitated diffusion

TABLE 12.1.   COEFFICIENTS FOR CALCULATING PULMONARY DIFFUSING CAPACITY FROM MORPHOMETRIC DATA.

Coefficient	O_2	CO	Units
$K_t = K_p$	$3.3 \cdot 10^{-8}$	$2.68 \cdot 10^{-8}$	$cm^2 \cdot min^{-1} \cdot mm\ Hg^{-1}$
	$4.1 \cdot 10^{-10}$	$3.33 \cdot 10^{-10}$	$cm^2 \cdot sec^{-1} \cdot mbar^{-1}$
θ^a	1.5	0.8	$ml \cdot ml^{-1} \cdot min^{-1} \cdot mm\ Hg^{-1}$
	$1.87 \cdot 10^{-2}$	0.01	$ml \cdot ml^{-1} \cdot sec^{-1} \cdot mbar^{-1}$

a.   The θ values refer to desaturated blood.

through the concentrated hemoglobin solution within the cell, as well as the reaction of the gas, O_2 or CO, with hemoglobin (see chapter 6). Following the suggestion of Roughton and Forster discussed in the last section (see equation 12.5) we can write

$$D_e = \theta \cdot V_c \qquad (12.11)$$

where V_c is the total capillary volume which can again be estimated on sections by stereological methods (see chapter 4). The coefficient θ is the rate at which O_2 (or CO) is bound to whole blood; because one tries to account for a rather complex set of events in a single factor, this turns out to be somewhat problematic. Not only is its estimation through in vitro experiments so difficult that values differing by as much as a factor of three have been obtained; it is furthermore uncertain what the real or effective value of θ is in the alveolar capillary blood. Let me just mention one of the problems (Fig. 12.9). If one measures θ_{O_2} on desaturated blood, one finds a value of 1.5 ml $O_2 \cdot min^{-1} \cdot mm\ Hg^{-1} \cdot ml^{-1}$. This value remains fairly constant up to saturation levels of about 70% and then falls off; indeed it is plausible that θ_{O_2} should go to zero when hemoglobin is fully saturated because then no sites for O_2 binding are available. The problem now is that venous blood enters the alveolar capillaries at a saturation of just about 70% (perhaps down to 40% in heavy exercise), and leaves them nearly fully saturated. We must therefore suspect that θ_{O_2} will vary along the capillary path from 1.5 to nearly zero as O_2 is loaded onto hemoglobin, that is, as the P_{O_2} rises from the mixed venous to the end-capillary level (Fig. 12.4). What is then the effective or mean value of θ_{O_2} in the total capillary blood, from venous to arterial end? To calculate such a value we lack essential information, such as the precise pattern of θ_{O_2} reduction as saturation increases, or even the pattern of saturation rise along the capillary path, as discussed in the last section.

Because this problem is very critical for our purpose, I have nevertheless made an attempt in Figure 12.10 to approximate the θ_{O_2} profile along the capillary path using the best available data. Since we are looking for limiting conditions I have considered the case of strenuous exercise, where mixed venous P_{O_2} is about 20 mm Hg and mean transit time is about 0.3 sec. The P_{O_2} profile results from Bohr integration and O_2-hemoglobin saturation from the "physiological" O_2-Hb equilibrium curve (Fig. 6.7). The most recent data estimate θ_{O_2} at 1.5 ml $O_2 \cdot min^{-1} \cdot mm\ Hg^{-1} \cdot ml^{-1}$ in desaturated blood; as a consequence of rising saturation, θ_{O_2} falls to around 0.25 in end-capillary blood, resulting in a weighted mean $\bar{\theta}_{O_2} \approx 0.85$. Admittedly, there is a lot of speculation and uncertainty in this, but it demonstrates that the effective θ_{O_2} is probably quite a bit lower than the values obtained in vitro for desaturated blood.

The rate of O_2 binding θ_{O_2} is different in different species since it is affected by the size of the red cells (Table 6.2): the smaller the red cells the higher θ_{O_2}. It is found further that θ_{O_2} depends on hematocrit, the volume fraction of red cells in the blood. Note that the hematocrit also varies somehow between species (Table 6.2); in the goat with its very small red cells it is only 33%, for example. In

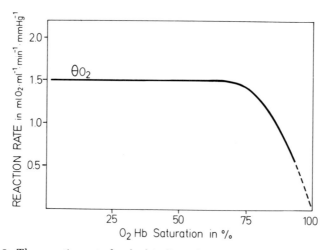

Fig. 12.9 The reaction rate for the binding of O_2 to whole blood, θ_{O_2}, depends on O_2-hemoglobin saturation.

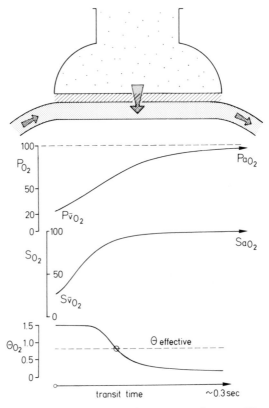

Fig. 12.10 Oxygen saturation of blood increases along capillary path so that θ_{O_2} must fall.

anemic patients where the erythrocyte content of blood is greatly reduced one finds the rate at which whole blood binds O_2 to be reduced. In equation 12.11 one should correctly consider the capillary erythrocyte volume; but since θ_{O_2} is estimated for whole blood at a standard hematocrit, H_c^*, one can take this into consideration by introducing the ratio of actual measured hematocrit, H_c, to standard hematocrit as a correction term:

$$D_e = \theta_{O_2} \cdot V_c \cdot (H_c / H_c^*). \tag{12.12}$$

We have thus assembled an approach for estimating the total conductance of the lung for gas exchange from morphometric data.

In principle and by definition, DL_{O_2} estimated in this way by equations 12.8 to 12.12 should be the same as that obtained from physiological data, as described in the last section. We can also use the morphometric data to calculate what the physiologist calls the "membrane" diffusing capacity, D_M; comparing equations 12.8 and 12.5, we note that in the morphometric model D_M comprises the barrier from the alveolar surface to the surface of the erythrocytes, so that we obtain it by

$$\frac{1}{D_M} = \frac{1}{D_t} + \frac{1}{D_p}. \tag{12.13}$$

This then offers a direct approach for quantitative structure–function correlation in pulmonary gas exchange. The morphometric data describe the system independently of the gas that is being exchanged. Thus by using the appropriate physical coefficients listed in Table 12.1 we can calculate D_L and D_M as well for O_2 as for CO.

Structure and Function Compared

I would now like to attempt to put lung structure into a functional perspective by means of the diffusing capacity models. Strictly speaking, we should expect DL_{O_2} estimated by the morphometric model to be equal to DL_{O_2} estimated physiologically. Let us see how the two estimates compare if we study the human lung.

Table 12.2 lists first the basic morphometric data required to calculate DL_{O_2}. We find that, for an average young adult, the alveolar surface area is about 140 m². I should make a few parenthetical remarks about this estimate because it is higher than the figure of 70–100 m² still quoted in most textbooks and taken from my original estimates in 1963. The reason for this difference lies in the methods used and in the significance of the estimate: in 1963 I used low-power light microscopy to estimate a "smooth" alveolar surface, whereas the more recent estimates listed in Table 12.2 are obtained by refined methods on electron micrographs. It is the latest estimates that are relevant for our present purpose because they reflect the actual surface of the air–blood barrier. Just as a winding road is longer than a straight one, a surface estimate that accounts for all wrinkles of the barrier must be larger than one which considers alveoli to be smooth

TABLE 12.2.   ESTIMATE OF DL_{O_2} FOR YOUNG HEALTHY ADULT OF 70 KG BODY WEIGHT, MEASURING 175 CM IN HEIGHT.

Variable	Data
Morphometric	
Total lung volume (60% TLC)	4,340 ml
Alveolar surface area	143 m²
Capillary surface area	126 m²
Capillary volume	213 ml
Air–blood barrier thickness	
Arithmetic mean	2.22 μm
Harmonic mean	0.62 μm
Plasma barrier thickness	
Harmonic mean	0.15 μm
Membrane diffusing capacity DM_{O_2}	567 ml $O_2 \cdot min^{-1} \cdot mm\ Hg^{-1}$
Pulmonary diffusing capacity DL_{O_2}	
$\theta_{O_2} = 1.5$ (desaturated blood)	205 ml $O_2 \cdot min^{-1} \cdot mm\ Hg^{-1}$
$\theta_{O_2} = 0.85$ (effective mean)	137 ml $O_2 \cdot min^{-1} \cdot mm\ Hg^{-1}$
Physiological	
Total lung capacity	7,200 ml
Pulmonary diffusing capacity DL_{O_2}	
At rest	30 ml $O_2 \cdot min^{-1} \cdot mm\ Hg^{-1}$
Heavy exercise	100 ml $O_2 \cdot min^{-1} \cdot mm\ Hg^{-1}$

chambers. By these newer methods we find the capillary surface to be about 10% smaller than the alveolar surface, and the capillary blood volume comes out at about 200 ml. Finally, the effective barrier thicknesses come out at 0.62 μm and 0.15 μm for tissue and plasma, respectively; note that the arithmetic mean thickness of the tissue barrier, the measure of tissue mass, is more than three times larger than the harmonic mean, as commented above.

Using the equations set up in the last section and the physical coefficients listed in Table 12.1 we can now calculate DM_{O_2} and DL_{O_2}. Depending on whether we use a value of θ_{O_2} for desaturated blood or an "effective" mean capillary θ_{O_2} (Fig. 12.10), the estimate for DL_{O_2} comes out at 200 or 137 ml $O_2 \cdot min^{-1} \cdot mm\ Hg^{-1}$.

How does this compare to physiological estimates of $D_{L_{O_2}}$? The standard value for $D_{L_{O_2}}$ of a healthy adult at rest is about 30 ml $O_2 \cdot min^{-1} \cdot mm\ Hg^{-1}$, thus considerably less than what we find by morphometry. Let us briefly have a look at what this means. In Table 10.2 I have listed some functional data from which we see that a resting adult consumes about 270 ml $O_2 \cdot min^{-1}$. With $D_{L_{O_2}} \sim 30$ ml $O_2 \cdot min^{-1} \cdot mm\ Hg^{-1}$ we conclude that the P_{O_2} gradient from alveolar air to the blood must average some 9 mm Hg, a value close to what one has estimated. But if $\dot{V}_{O_2}$ increases to 2420 ml $O_2 \cdot min^{-1}$ in heavy exercise, this means that a P_{O_2} gradient of at least 80 mm Hg would be required to drive O_2 from alveolar air into blood at an adequate rate. This appears clearly impossible for it would require alveolar P_{O_2} to be nearly as high as inspired P_{O_2}; this cannot be because, even in exercise, we inspire fresh air into a substantial cushion of residual air of low P_{O_2}.

This analysis indicates that we have based this comparison on noncomparable data sets. Indeed, we should not even expect the pulmonary diffusing *capacity* to be measurable at rest because, clearly, the lung is capable of increasing O_2 uptake about nine fold upon exercise. In relation to Figure 12.4 we have noted that only a small fraction of the capillary path length is required to saturate blood at rest, whereas we may be needing the entire path length to load O_2 onto blood in exercise; this is because blood flow is higher, leading to shorter transit times, and mixed venous P_{O_2} is lower. There have been a number of estimates of $D_{L_{O_2}}$ in exercising human subjects and they have yielded values of the order of 100 ml $O_2 \cdot min^{-1} \cdot mm\ Hg^{-1}$ (Table 12.2). A $\dot{V}_{O_2}$ of 2400 ml $\cdot min^{-1}$ could now be accommodated with an alveolar–capillary gradient of 24 mm Hg. Such a gradient could well result from increased alveolar ventilation (Table 10.2) combined with a lower mean capillary P_{O_2} (Fig. 12.4).

If we now compare the morphometric with the physiologic estimate of $D_{L_{O_2}}$ obtained on exercise, it is evident that the two numbers are fairly close to each other but the morphometric value is still higher by some 40 to 100%, depending on the value of θ_{O_2} chosen. Why is this? One point is that the gas exchanger may have a built-in safety factor which would ensure efficient gas exchange even if some boundary conditions are not optimal. For example, perfusion of the capillaries may be partly intermittent or even incomplete, perhaps because some capillaries may not be totally expanded, due to the effect of uneven mechanical forces (Fig. 11.19). Furthermore, the alveolar surface may be reduced in air-filled lungs because the barrier is partly folded up beneath the lining layer (Figs. 11.16 and 11.18). In appropriate experiments one finds that this may indeed be the case if the lung is perfused under zone 2 conditions (Fig. 10.17). But at the high flows sustained in exercise, it is likely that all capillaries are well perfused under zone 3 conditions so that the morphometric diffusing capacity should be nearly completely available for gas exchange.

It thus appears, for the time being, that morphometric estimates of human DL_{O_2} are somewhat larger than the physiologic estimates. However, considering the many uncertainties and assumptions that went into either estimate, this difference is actually not very large. The difference also seems to be consistent. We have recently measured DL_{CO} for canids physiologically by a single breath method and have then also estimated it from the morphometric data obtained on the lungs of the same animals; the morphometric estimate was always higher by a factor of 2 (Fig. 12.11a). The reason for this remains obscure; it may be real or due to inadequate assumptions here or there, but the best guess at present is that the design of the

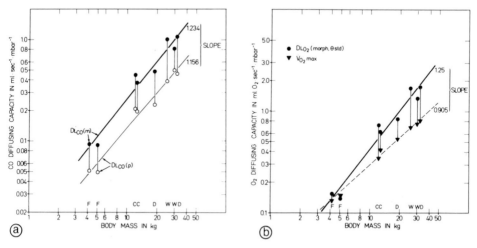

Fig. 12.11 (a) Comparison of morphometric and physiologic CO diffusing capacity of the lung in four species of canids: foxes (F), coyotes (C), dogs (D), and wolves (W). (b) Comparison of morphometric O_2 diffusing capacity with maximal O_2 consumption in the same species. (From Weibel, et al., 1983.)

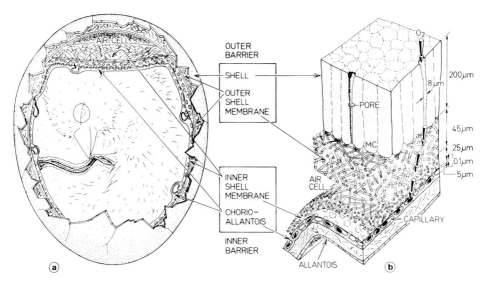

Fig. 12.12 The chicken embryo breathes by means of its chorioallantois which spreads beneath the shell membrane whose air spaces are ventilated through pores in the shell. (From Wangensteen and Weibel, 1982.)

pulmonary gas exchanger respects a certain safety factor and this incorporates a calculated amount of inherent redundancy, a principle observed in many organ systems.

At this point I would like to report a most intriguing recent observation when we studied the chicken egg. The chicken embryo develops a gas exchanger beneath the shell membrane which eventually covers the entire surface of the egg (Fig. 12.12). The gas exchanger consists of a dense capillary network, rather similar to that found in the lung (Fig. 12.13); it takes up O_2 from the air between the fibers of the inner shell membrane which, in turn, is "ventilated" through the pores in the shell. When we estimated, by means of a slight modification of our morphometric model, the diffusing capacity of the chorioallantois of a 16-day egg we came up with a value of 6.8 μl $O_2 \cdot \text{min}^{-1} \cdot \text{mm Hg}^{-1}$, which is almost exactly the value found by physiological measurement. Could this mean that the chicken egg does not need to allow for a safety factor because this gas exchanger will soon be disposed of anyway?

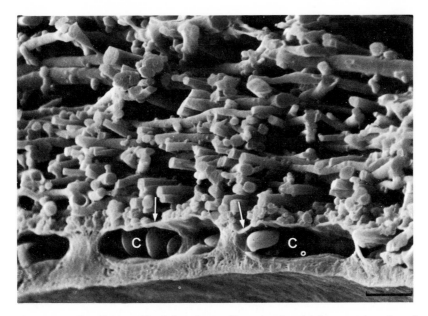

Fig. 12.13 Capillaries (C) of the chorioallantois of a chicken egg incubated for 16 days are shown here in a scanning electron micrograph, together with the inner shell membrane. Note the thin barrier (arrows) which separates the capillary blood from the air between the fibers of the shell membrane. Scale marker: 5 μm.

Matching the Conductance to O_2 Needs: The Emergence of a Paradox

The fundamental question pursued throughout this book is whether the elements of the respiratory system are quantitatively matched to the flow of O_2 they need to support. We should now address this question with respect to the lung's O_2 conductance. In chapter 3 I have introduced the double strategy that we can use to shed some light on this problem, that is, to compare animals of different levels of O_2 needs because of different levels of activity and because of different body size. We shall see that the result of this strategy will be ambiguous, leading in fact to an apparent paradox.

The first approach is to select pairs of species of similar body size but different O_2 needs (see Table 2.1). An obvious pair of this kind is man and his dog; I need not explain that the dog's energetic needs by far exceed those of his master. Another pair is the horse and the cow, which differ by more than a factor of 2 in terms of their O_2 needs per kg body mass. In Figure 12.14 we see that this difference in O_2 consumption is indeed paralleled by a similar difference in DL_{O_2} estimated by morphometry. The same holds if we compare lazy laboratory mice with the Japanese waltzing mouse, which keeps itself continuously in motion because of a hereditary defect in the vestibular apparatus. These findings suggest that DL_{O_2} is proportional to $\dot{V}_{O_2}$. What they do not tell us is whether this proportionality is purely coincidental, simply due to hereditary traits, or whether it

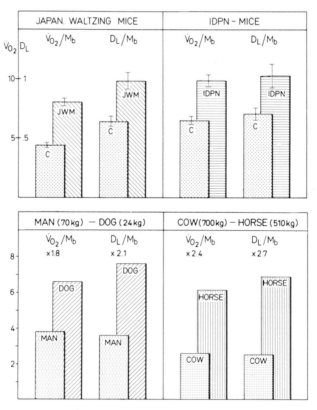

Fig. 12.14 Mass-specific pulmonary diffusing capacity (D_L/M_b) is proportional to mass specific O_2 consumption ($\dot{V}_{O_2}/M_b$) in four pairs of mammals of similar body size: Japanese waltzing mice and drug (IDPN)-induced waltzing mice compared to normal laboratory mice (C), and the pairs man–dog and cow–horse. (From Burri and Weibel, 1977; Weibel, 1979.)

reflects an adaptation of the lung to different O_2 needs of the body. In that respect it is therefore interesting to note that one can induce normal white mice to become waltzers by giving them a drug (IDPN) during the first weeks after birth. One then observes that, as their $\dot{V}_{O_2}$ increases, they enlarge their alveolar surface and by that their DL_{O_2} in proportion to the O_2 needs (Fig. 12.14). This is now rather strong evidence that the lung's diffusing capacity is adapted to the O_2 needs of the body. There is also mounting evidence that this adaptation occurs during growth of the organ and is the result of regulated morphogenesis. How this is achieved and what factors control the process are still unknown.

The second approach is to compare the effects of body size on O_2 consumption and DL_{O_2}. As we have seen in chapter 2, the body-mass-specific metabolic rate falls with increasing body size such that we find $\dot{V}_{O_2}$ proportional to $M_b^{0.75}$. These are large differences: metabolic rate per gram body mass is about ten times greater in the mouse than in the cow.

The question now is whether DL_{O_2} is also relatively larger in small animals. The analytical approach is that of allometry, as explained in chapter 3, where one compares primarily the scaling factor or exponent b in the general allometric relation

$$Y = a \cdot M_b{}^b. \tag{12.14}$$

Remember that on a double-logarithmic plot b is the slope of a linear regression whereas a is the intercept at $\log M_b = 0$ or $M_b = 1$.

In many textbooks one finds the statement that the alveolar surface area, the main determinant of D_L, is proportional to $\dot{V}_{O_2}$, a seemingly happy result which, however, turns out to be incorrect. Figure 12.15 shows that for 36 species of mammals, ranging from cow and horse down to the smallest mammal, a shrew, S_A increases nearly linearly with body mass, more precisely with a scaling factor of 0.95. This graph also shows that the harmonic mean barrier thickness increases with body mass, though only very slightly. When we calculate diffusing capacity from the morphometric data of those species, we find that DL_{O_2} increases with a scaling factor of 0.99, which is clearly and significantly larger than that found for $\dot{V}_{O_2}$ on a similar population of animals (Fig. 12.16). This finding is very troublesome because it suggests that $\dot{V}_{O_2}$ and DL_{O_2} are not proportional to each other when we compare species of different body size. Indeed,

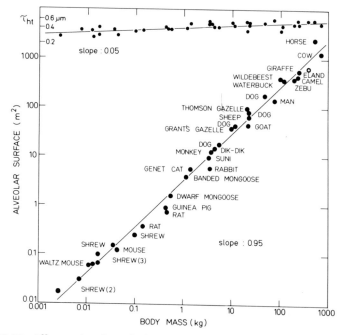

Fig. 12.15 Allometric plot of alveolar surface area and harmonic mean thickness of tissue barrier for 36 mammalian species ranging in body mass from the Etruscan shrew (2 g) to the cow (700 kg). (From Gehr et al., 1981.)

the discrepancy is large: the lung's conductance for O_2 diffusion is ten times greater in the cow than in the mouse when compared to the O_2 flow rates that must be maintained. The first reaction to such a finding is one of skepticism: are the data really correct?

A first reason for doubt is whether the $\dot{V}_{O_2}$ data are correct since most available estimates are obtained on resting animals. However, when we estimated, in a range of animals, maximal $\dot{V}_{O_2}$ by letting them run on a treadmill (see chapter 2) and then obtained morphometric data on the same animals, we confirmed the discordant scaling of $\dot{V}_{O_2}$max and D_{LO_2}.

A second critique could be directed to the model for calculating D_{LO_2} from morphometric data, particularly to the assumption that the physical coefficients are the same for all mammals. This assumption is certainly questionable with respect to θ_{O_2}, but it turns out that possible or even probable differences in θ_{O_2} cannot account for the large difference in the scaling factors for $\dot{V}_{O_2}$ and D_{LO_2}. In that respect

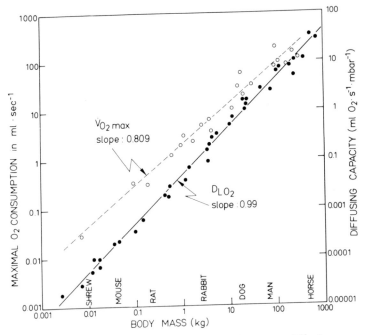

Fig. 12.16 Allometric plot of morphometric pulmonary diffusing capacity for the same species as in Figure 12.15 (full dots), compared with maximal O_2 consumption for a similar set of species. (Data from Taylor et al., 1981; Gehr et al., 1981.)

it is noteworthy that independent studies had shown physiological estimates of DL_{O_2} to scale nearly in proportion to body mass rather than to $\dot{V}_{O_2}$. And when we studied canids (Fig. 12.11), obtaining estimates of physiological and morphometric DL_{CO} as well as of $\dot{V}_{O_2}$max on all animals, we found that the two DL_{CO} estimates were proportional to each other but scaled differently to body mass than $\dot{V}_{O_2}$max. This indicates that the morphometric D_L estimates are valid for that purpose; and thus we conclude that DL_{O_2} is indeed not proportional to $\dot{V}_{O_2}$ when animals are compared across the mammalian size range.

Out of these studies emerges an apparent paradox: why should, on the one hand, the lung adapt its diffusing capacity to the needs for O_2 transfer from air to blood in response to relatively small changes in O_2 demand, when, on the other hand, large variations in O_2 needs, as they occur across the size range of mammals, have no effect on the magnitude of the lung's gas exchange conductance? Does this finding mean that the design of the lung's diffusing capacity is wasteful, that the lung is, after all, not built reasonably? Not necessarily.

Resolving the Paradox: Models and Nature

Let us ask why we actually expect DL_{O_2} to be proportional to $\dot{V}_{O_2}$. One reason is clearly intuitive: we would like to see the conductance adapted to the required flow rate because then the driving force could be kept minimal. But keeping the driving force minimal does not necessarily mean that it should be the same for all animals. Indeed, the paradox could be resolved if the driving force, in our case the P_{O_2} gradient from alveolar air to capillary blood, were body-size dependent. Without making any assumptions, let us see by how much ΔP_{O_2} should vary across the size range in order to account for the paradox. We accept, of course, the basic relation of Bohr by which we had actually *defined* the pulmonary diffusing capacity:

$$\dot{V}_{O_2} = DL_{O_2} \cdot \Delta P_{O_2} \tag{12.15}$$

where

$$\Delta P_{O_2} = (P_{A_{O_2}} - \bar{P}_{C_{O_2}}). \tag{12.16}$$

When we measured $\dot{V}_{O_2}\text{max}$ and DL_{O_2} on a group of mammals ranging from 500 g to 250 kg, we found the following dependencies on body mass:

$$\dot{V}_{O_2}\text{max} = 1.84 \cdot M_b^{0.77}$$
$$DL_{O_2} = 0.055 \cdot M_b^{0.95}. \tag{12.17}$$

By dividing $\dot{V}_{O_2}$ by DL_{O_2} we derive the allometric relation for ΔP_{O_2} as

$$\Delta P_{O_2} = \frac{\dot{V}_{O_2}\text{max}}{DL_{O_2}} = \frac{1.84 \cdot M_b^{0.77}}{0.055 \cdot M_b^{0.95}} = 33.5 \cdot M_b^{-0.18}. \tag{12.18}$$

As shown in Figure 12.17, the results of this analysis look quite reasonable: for an animal the size of adult man, ΔP_{O_2} comes out at

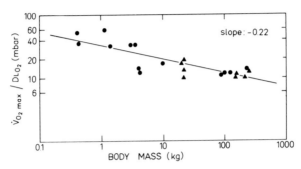

Fig. 12.17 Ratio of $\dot{V}_{O_2}$max/$D_{L_{O_2}}$, estimated on the same animals, falls with increasing body mass. (From Weibel et al., 1981.)

about 7 mm Hg, a value very close to that estimated in man for the P_{O_2} gradient from alveoli to capillaries; for an animal of 500 g the gradient would be about 30 mm Hg.

Is it possible that small animals have a larger P_{O_2} gradient? And if so, how could it come about? Here we have very little hard evidence to go on, but still enough to venture some speculation. A larger ΔP_{O_2} can result from either lowering mean capillary P_{O_2} or from elevating $P_{A_{O_2}}$, or from both occurring simultaneously.

It is well possible that mean capillary P_{O_2} is lower in small species because their cardiac output is relatively larger; it is also proportional to $M_b^{0.75}$. This should cause the transit time for blood in alveolar capillaries to be shorter, particularly since it appears that the capillary path length is shorter in small lungs. These two effects could cut off some of the flat tail of the P_{O_2} toward the end of the capillary path (Fig. 12.4), thus causing *mean* capillary P_{O_2} to be lower.

There are several reasons why $P_{A_{O_2}}$ could be higher in small species. First we should remember that $P_{A_{O_2}}$ is the P_{O_2} in the layer of air immediately adjacent to the air–blood barrier. It depends on alveolar ventilation which brings fresh air into the center of the acinus, but also on diffusion of O_2 through the cushion of residual air. One cause for a higher $P_{A_{O_2}}$ is that alveolar ventilation may be better in small species because they breathe at a higher rate, in fact up to 300 breaths per minute in the smallest mammals as compared to 15 per minute in man. A second reason could be that the distance for O_2 diffusion through air is shorter in small lungs because their acini are considerably smaller (Fig. 12.18). This may not appear to be of great importance because we had seen in chapter 10 that O_2 molecules advance by diffusion at a speed of about 5 cm·sec^{-1}, which means that the few millimeters distance within the acinus are covered almost instantaneously.

But the problem may not be one of diffusion alone. In relation to Figure 10.18 I have mentioned that the perfusion units are much smaller than the ventilation units. All microvascular units are perfused in parallel, each receiving blood of equal P_{O_2}; but they are arranged in series along the alveolar duct pathway through which O_2 moves mostly by diffusion. On the basis of such a model, described as "series ventilation and parallel perfusion" model, one can predict that P_{O_2} should fall along the acinar pathway, not so much because of

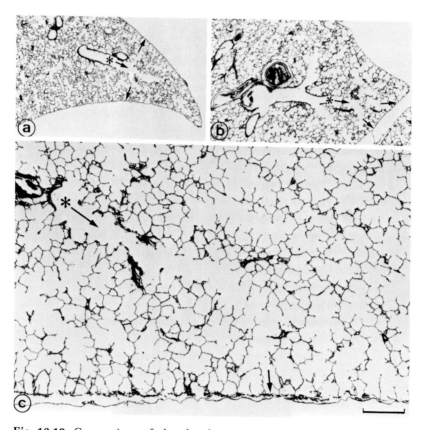

Fig. 12.18 Comparison of alveolar ducts in mouse (a), rat (b), and human lung (c). The length of the acinar pathway from the respiratory bronchiole (*) to the terminal alveolus (arrow) increases with body mass. Scale marker: 500 μm.

diffusion limitation but because O_2 is being extracted from the air all along the pathway. The predicted pattern of P_{O_2} fall is shown in Figure 12.19 for two acini of different length. Without discussing this model in any detail, we note that the total length of the pathway may have a significant effect on the P_{O_2} profile and that consequently the mean $P_{A_{O_2}}$ may be considerably lower in large than in small lungs. Unfortunately, we yet lack the experimental evidence to estimate the magnitude of this effect, except to say that recent measurements in different species reveal that acinar path length increases with about the 0.2 power of body mass, the right order of magnitude.

In conclusion, we note that the paradox in the relation between $D_{L_{O_2}}$ and $\dot{V}_{O_2}$ is probably only apparent, and may be resolved if we can account for a size dependence of the gradient between alveolar air and capillary blood. That alveolar P_{O_2} may be an important determinant of $D_{L_{O_2}}$ is, in fact, demonstrated by the studies in which rats were raised at high altitude. During their growth period they breathed air at an ambient P_{O_2} of 100 mm Hg so that their alveolar P_{O_2}

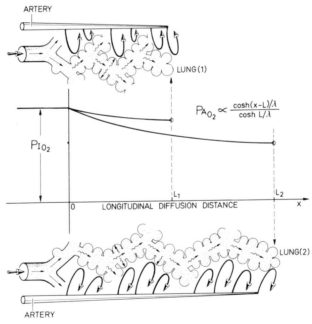

Fig. 12.19 Model to show how the different acinar pathway length could— hypothetically—cause size-dependent differences in mean alveolar P_{O_2}. (After Weibel et al., 1981.)

must have been about 60–70 mm Hg, that is, considerably below normal values. In these animals the driving force for O_2 diffusion into the blood must have been reduced; they responded by increasing their DL_{O_2}, mostly by enlarging the gas exchange surfaces and the capillary volume.

The lesson we have learned is that we must at all times remain critical of our model assumptions from which we derive predictions or expectations on how nature should be made. Any such expectation must be tested by at least two sufficiently different approaches, lest any inconsistencies remain undiscovered and we are left in the happy state of delusion or wishful thinking where our thoughts are free to go astray. There is no scientific progress without often bold hypotheses based on model assumptions, usually grossly simplified. But nature is too complex to be satisfactorily described by any one of our models, however sophisticated they may be. At some time in the critical analysis they will be found to be inadequate and need to be revised. Models are not nature, only our limited view of it. This we must accept, keeping our mind open and skeptical at all times. The very useful model of pulmonary diffusing capacity is no different. We may well have to develop a new model to account for the variable boundary conditions, in particular the effects of a varying driving force, considering not only gas exchange but ventilation and perfusion as well.

Summary

The gas exchange units of the lung are found in the alveoli whose walls are densely populated with blood capillaries. In the human lung some 300 million alveoli establish a surface of about 140 m², nearly the size of a tennis court; their capillaries contain about 200 ml of blood. In terms of ventilation the gas exchange units are grouped into acini, the parenchymal unit that is attached to a first-order respiratory bronchiole and contains some 2,000 alveoli. The microvascular units are much smaller. The barrier separating air and blood is extremely thin, reduced to 0.2 μm over large parts of the capillaries.

Gas exchange between air and blood occurs by diffusion across the air–blood barrier, driven by the P_{O_2} difference between alveolar air and capillary blood. Alveolar P_{O_2} is kept high by alveolar ventilation but never reaches the P_{O_2} in inspired ambient air because of the residual air which remains in alveoli at expiration. Alveolar P_{O_2} is around 100 mm Hg in the human lung. The capillary P_{O_2} varies along the capillary path from venous P_{O_2} (about 40 mm Hg at rest) to arterial P_{O_2} which is equal to alveolar P_{O_2} (100 mm Hg) if the blood equilibrates completely with alveolar air on passage. This depends on the transit time of erythrocytes which is of the order of one second, but may be shorter at the high blood flow rates that occur in heavy exercise. The profile of P_{O_2} increase along the capillary path is nonlinear owing to the shape of the O_2Hb equilibrium curve.

The potential for gas exchange in the lung is estimated by the pulmonary diffusing capacity for O_2. It is a measure of the O_2 flow rate that arises from a P_{O_2} gradient of 1 torr and hence estimates the global conductance of the lung for O_2 transfer to the blood by diffusion. Physiological methods to estimate the diffusing capacity depend on the measurement of gas uptake rate and the partial pressure gradient. This is difficult to perform with O_2 but it can be done with carbon monoxide as a tracer gas which also binds to hemoglobin. The diffusing capacity depends on the permeability of the barrier (often called the membrane) and on the capillary blood available for binding O_2; the latter component is greatly affected by the rate of O_2 binding by the blood.

The pulmonary diffusing capacity can also be calculated from morphometric data since it depends on the gas exchange surfaces, on the blood volume, and on the barrier thickness, parameters that can be estimated by means of stereological methods. This offers the possibility of quantitative structure–function correlation of pulmonary gas exchange. In the human lung the gas exchange surfaces measure 120–140 m², the blood volume is 200 ml, and the effective mean barrier thickness is 0.6 μm. From this the diffusing capacity is estimated at 140–200 ml $O_2 \cdot min^{-1} \cdot mm\ Hg^{-1}$. Physiological estimates range from 30 at rest to 100 ml $O_2 \cdot min^{-1} \cdot mm\ Hg^{-1}$ in heavy exercise, whereby the exercise value must be considered for comparison with the morphometric data. The latter are consistently found to be larger than the physiological estimates by a factor of up to two. This may be explained as an inherent redundancy in the design of the gas exchanger.

The important question is whether the pulmonary diffusing capacity is matched to the O_2 flow rates imposed by the body, particularly under conditions of maximal O_2 consumption. When pairs of animals *of similar size but different O_2 needs are compared (for example, horse to cow, dog to man, or waltzing mouse to normal mouse), the diffusing capacity is found to be proportional to O_2 consumption. The diffusing capacity is also found to be adaptable to match higher O_2 needs imposed experimentally on the animals. The result is different when comparing animals of greatly different body mass using the allometric approach. Whereas O_2 consumption increases with $M_b^{0.8}$, diffusing capacity increases linearly with body mass. The difference is large: per unit body mass, the mouse takes up ten times more O_2 per minute and unit diffusing capacity than the cow. This appears to be a paradox: why should the diffusing capacity adapt to small changes in O_2 needs, when large variations in O_2 demand, as they occur across the size range of mammals, have no effect on the magnitude of the lung's gas exchange conductance? The answer is that the diffusing capacity is not the only factor determining O_2 flow from air to blood in the lung. There are reasons to suspect that the P_{O_2} gradient from alveolar air to capillary blood may not be constant but may be greater in small than in large animals. This may be due to shorter transit times in small animals (which would lower mean capillary P_{O_2}), or to effects of the size of the acinus which is considerably smaller in small animals and could result in higher alveolar P_{O_2}. Gas exchange must be considered in the context of ventilation and perfusion of the gas exchange units.*

Further Reading

Forster, R. E., and E. D. Crandall. 1976. Pulmonary gas exchange. *Annual Review of Physiology* 38:69–93.

Piiper, J., and P. Scheid. 1971. Respiration: alveolar gas exchange. *Annual Review of Physiology* 33:131–154.

Wagner, P. D. 1977. Diffusion and chemical reaction in pulmonary gas exchange. *Physiological Reviews* 57:257–312.

Weibel, E. R. 1973. Morphological basis of alveolar-capillary gas exchange. *Physiological Reviews* 53:419–495.

——— 1979. O_2 demand and the size of respiratory structures. In *Evolution of Respiratory Processes*, ed. S. C. Wood and C. Lenfant. New York: Dekker, pp. 289–346.

West, J. B., and P. D. Wagner. 1977. Pulmonary gas exchange. In *Bioengineering Aspects of the Lung*, ed. J. B. West. New York: Dekker, pp. 361–457.

References

Adaro, F., and J. Piiper. 1976. Limiting role of stratification in alveolar exchange of oxygen. *Respiration Physiology* 26:195–206.

Blomqvist, G., R. L. Johnson, Jr., and B. Saltin. 1969. Pulmonary diffusing capacity limiting human performance at altitude. *Acta Physiologica Scandinavia* 76:284–287.

* Bohr, C. 1909. Ueber die spezifische Tätigkeit der Lungen bei der respiratorischen Gasaufnahme. *Scandinavian Archives of Physiology* 22:221–280.

Burri, P. H., and E. R. Weibel. 1971. Morphometric estimation of pulmonary diffusion capacity. II. Effect of PO_2 on the growing lung: adaptation of the growing rat lung to hypoxia and hyperoxia. *Respiration Physiology* 11:247–264.

―――― 1977. Ultrastructure and morphometry of the developing lung. In *Development of the Lung*, ed. W. A. Hodson. New York: Dekker, pp. 215–268.

Dejours, P. 1981. *Principles of Comparative Respiratory Physiology*. 2nd ed. Amsterdam: Elsevier North-Holland.

Geelhaar, A., and E. R. Weibel. 1971. Morphometric estimation of pulmonary diffusion capacity. III. The effect of increased oxygen consumption in Japanese waltzing mice. *Respiration Physiology* 11:354–366.

Gehr, P., M. Bachofen, and E. R. Weibel. 1978. The normal human lung: ultrastructure and morphometric estimation of diffusion capacity. *Respiration Physiology* 32:121–140.

Gehr, P., C. Hugonnaud, P. Burri, H. Bachofen, and E. R. Weibel. 1978. Adaptation of the growing lung to increased $\dot{V}_{O_2}$. III. The effect of exposure to cold environment in rats. *Respiration Physiology* 32:345–353.

Gehr, P., D. K. Mwangi, A. Ammann, G. M. O. Maloiy, C. R. Taylor, and E. R. Weibel. 1981. Design of the mammalian respiratory system. V. Scaling morphometric pulmonary diffusing capacity to body mass: wild and domestic mammals. *Respiration Physiology* 44:61–86.

Gehr, P., S. Sehovic, P. H. Burri, H. Claassen, and E. R. Weibel. 1980. The lung of shrews: morphometric estimation of diffusion capacity. *Respiration Physiology* 40:33–47.

Holland, R. A. B., W. Van Hezewijk, and J. Zubazanda. 1977. Velocity of oxygen uptake by partly saturated adult and fetal human red cells. *Respiration Physiology* 29:303–314.

Hugonnaud, C., P. Gehr, E. R. Weibel, and P. H. Burri. 1977. Adaptation of the growing lung to increased oxygen consumption. II. Morphometric analysis. *Respiration Physiology* 29:1–10.

Murray, J. F. 1976. *The Normal Lung*. Philadelphia: Saunders.

Piiper, J., A. Huch, D. Kötter, and R. Herbst. 1969. Pulmonary diffusing capacity at basal and increased O_2 uptake levels in anaesthetized dogs. *Respiration Physiology* 6:219–232.

* Roughton, F. J. W., and R. E. Forster. 1957. Relative importance of diffusion and chemical reaction rates in determining rate of exchange of gases in the human lung, with special reference to true diffusing capacity of pulmonary membrane and volume of blood in the lung capillaries. *Journal of Applied Physiology* 11:290–302.

Taylor, C. R., G. M. O. Maloiy, E. R. Weibel, V. A. Langman, J. M. Z. Kamau, H. J. Seeherman, and N. C. Heglund. 1981. Design of the mammalian respiratory system. III. Scaling maximum aerobic capacity to body mass: wild and domestic mammals. *Respiration Physiology* 44:25–37.

Wangensteen, D., and E. R. Weibel. 1982. Morphometric evaluation of chorioallantoic oxygen transport in the chick embryo. *Respiration Physiology* 47:1–20.

Weibel, E. R. 1970/71. Morphometric estimation of pulmonary diffusion capacity. I. Model and method. *Respiration Physiology* 11:54–75.

—— 1972. Morphometric estimation of pulmonary diffusion capacity. V. Comparative morphometry of alveolar lungs. *Respiration Physiology* 14:26–43.

—— 1973. Morphological basis of alveolar-capillary gas exchange. *Physiological Review* 53:419–495.

—— 1979. O_2 demand and the size of respiratory structures. In *Evolution of Respiratory Processes*, ed. S. C. Wood and C. Lenfant. New York: Dekker, pp. 289–346.

—— 1980. Design and structure of the human lung. In *Pulmonary Diseases and Disorders*, ed. A. P. Fishman. New York: McGraw-Hill, pp. 224–271.

Weibel, E. R., and B. W. Knight. 1964. A morphometric study on the thickness of the pulmonary air–blood barrier. *Journal of Cell Biology* 21:367–384.

Weibel, E. R., C. R. Taylor, P. Gehr, H. Hoppeler, O. Mathieu, and G. M. O. Maloiy. 1981. Design of the mammalian respiratory system. IX. Functional and structural limits for oxygen flow. *Respiration Physiology* 44:151–164.

Weibel, E. R., C. R. Taylor, J. J. O'Neil, D. E. Leith, P. Gehr, H. Hoppeler, V. Langman, and R. V. Baudinette. 1983. Maximal oxygen consumption and pulmonary diffusing capacity: a direct comparison of physiologic and morphometric measurements in canids. *Respiration Physiology* 54 (in press).

West, J. B., ed. 1980. *Pulmonary Gas Exchange*, vols. 1 and 2. New York: Academic.

13

THE RESPIRATORY SYSTEM
IN OVERVIEW

WE HAVE NOW LOOKED at the various parts of the mammalian respiratory system, working our way up from the mitochondria, through the circulation of blood, to the lung. We have considered the structural design of each part and its functional performance. What we now need to do is consider these elements as parts of an integral functional system.

We started out with the hypothesis that all parts of the respiratory system are adjusted to needs, dictated by the energy consumer in the cells. Although the immediate energy required to do biological work is drawn from high-energy organic phosphates, oxidative phosphorylation is the ultimate pathway for efficiently making these phosphates. Therefore, oxygen availability to the cells must be the key limiting factor for long-term biological work.

Oxygen availability to the cells depends, however, on a whole sequence of critical events (Fig. 13.1): the lung must be ventilated with air; O_2 must be transferred to the blood; blood must circulate through the lung and through the tissues; O_2 must be discharged into the tissues; and, finally, the cells must be equipped to transfer energy from oxidation to high-energy phosphates. For each of these events we have found a series of determinant factors, some functional and some structural. The question now is whether all these parts in a sequence are adjusted to each other in view of their serving the same ultimate purpose: making energy available for biological work. Indeed, they should be, because a chain is as strong as its weakest link. In a steady state it is necessary that all parts act in concert, well

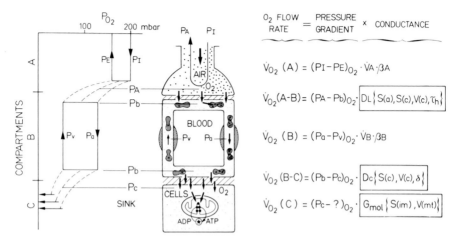

Fig. 13.1 Model of the entire respiratory system where the driving force for O_2 is shown as a P_{O_2} cascade. In a steady state the flow rates through all steps must be equal. (Modified after Taylor and Weibel, 1981.)

balanced to each other; if this were not so there would be no steady state.

In determining whether a system is well balanced as a whole we must ask if it has overcome two problems. The first is the problem of adjusting the performance of the system and its parts to the needs imposed by those parts of the body that are asked to do work. This is a physiological problem, that of regulation of functions to achieve balance or *homeostasis*. This adjustment can occur within the potential of the system, so it will be limited to some maximal value. For example, in all animals, O_2 consumption cannot reach beyond a well-determined value, $\dot{V}_{O_2}$max, although this is reached at levels of biological work that are not the limit of work capacity.

The second problem is adjusting the potential of the system to allow it to reach beyond its limits, that is, to move these limits out. This is not a matter of short-term regulation but one of increasing the scope of the system on a long-term basis, adjusting it to chronically increased needs. It will involve adjustments in the design properties of the system, and is hence largely a morphological problem. The key mechanism will be regulation of morphogenesis, so that the key issue will be whether the principle of *symmorphosis* is operative or not.

Adjusting Performance to Needs

In trying to consider the functional regulation of the processes that transport O_2 from outside air to the mitochondria, we must look at a slightly modified scheme for the respiratory system (Fig. 13.2). From it we see that the various processes which are amenable to physiological control or regulation are intercalated between stores that can serve as buffers of these processes. This construction principle is widely used in organisms: the secretory product of gland cells, for example, is stored in a suitable compartment until it is needed at its site of action. With respect to the respiratory system we have seen three stores of importance located within the cell (compare Fig. 2.2): a high-energy phosphate store from which the cell can draw ATP for immediate use, a small O_2 store from which the mitochondria draw O_2 when they engage in oxidative phosphorylation, and a store for substrates for metabolic processes. Furthermore the blood contains a store for O_2—the hemoglobin within the red cells—and finally our ambient air constitutes a large O_2 store from which we draw O_2 by respiration.

Each of these stores contains a powerful buffer system. In the high-energy phosphate store, ATP is buffered by creatine phosphate;

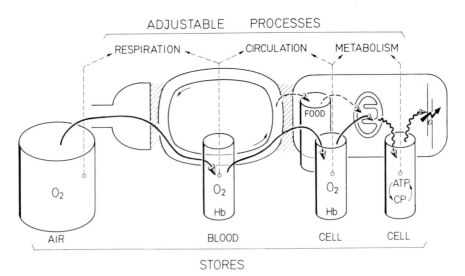

Fig. 13.2 The respiratory system connects a series of stores for O_2 (and substrates) or for high-energy phosphates by means of adjustable processes.

in the blood and in the cell O_2 is buffered by hemoglobin. This is important because the driving forces for O_2 transport, as well as for ATP transfer, are partial pressure differences, and partial pressures are determined only by dissolved O_2 or ATP. Although large quantities of O_2 are exchanged in the lung and in the tissues, the pressure gradient is changed only slowly due to the nonlinear binding properties of hemoglobin (see Figs. 6.7, 7.17, and 12.4), thus allowing the P_{O_2} difference to remain fairly large.

The adjustable processes that determine the transport of O_2 (or of energy), and that are intercalated between the stores, are: *cell metabolism*, which determines the amount of O_2 consumed; *circulation*, which determines the amount of O_2 delivered to the cells; and *respiration*, which determines the amount of O_2 transferred from air to blood. To understand the regulation of any of these processes one has to *look forward and backward*, that is, the conditions in the stores to either side must be considered as boundary conditions for the process. We shall now look at the means for adjusting each of these processes to needs, and then see how the system can be balanced as a whole.

REGULATION OF CELL METABOLISM

Let me limit this discussion to the regulation of oxidative phosphorylation because it is, after all, only this process which determines the O_2 needs. I therefore assume, for the time being, that the substrate stores within the cells, or their supply through the blood, are not limiting factors. I shall also disregard for the moment anaerobic ATP production through glycolysis.

The most widely held view on regulation of oxidative phosphorylation is that it uses the concentration of ADP as a gauge: as ATP is utilized the level of ADP rises and this triggers oxidative phosphorylation. The role of the creatine phosphate pool or shuttle would be to transfer this signal more rapidly to the mitochondrion.

This concept has been derived essentially from experiments with isolated mitochondria, which indeed respond to an addition of ADP by oxidative phosphorylation. It is attractive because the feed-back loop is extremely simple: the need for more phosphate bond energy is signaled by the end product of ATP utilization, so that this would appear to be the most direct way of keeping the pool of immediate energy in the form of phosphate bonds high.

This mechanism is under challenge, however, and there is a fair amount of uncertainty and disagreement among investigators on some points. We therefore need to have a closer look at the relations between the high-energy phosphate store and oxidative phosphoryl-ation. The diagram in Figure 13.3 appears to be the currently most appropriate representation of the situation. The decisive point is that the shift of high-energy phosphate groups between ATP and creatine (C) or between creatine phosphate (CP) and ADP is catalyzed by an enzyme creatine phosphokinase (CPK) which occurs both in the cytoplasm and in the mitochondria, specifically in the intermem-brane space. Some therefore believe that the ATP formed in oxida-tive phosphorylation never leaves the mitochondrion but transfers its phosphate group to creatine in the intermembrane space. By this mechanism the mitochondria would directly feed CP into the phos-phate pool; as ATP is used at a cytoplasmic ATPase to do biological work, the resultant ADP is immediately recharged by transfer of a phosphate group from CP, catalyzed by cytoplasmic CPK, and cre-atine would then go back to the mitochondrion to be stocked up to CP, and so on.

The question now is: who carries the signal that triggers oxidative phosphorylation when the cell needs more ATP? The challengers of

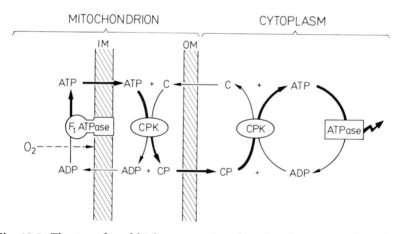

Fig. 13.3 The transfer of high-energy phosphate bonds, generated in the mitochondrion, to the sites where biological work needs to be done involves creatine phosphate (CP) as an intermediate carrier; the reaction is catalyzed by creatine-phosphokinase (CPK). The heavy arrows indicate the flow of energy through the system.

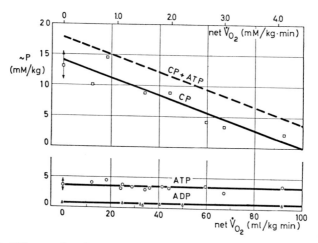

Fig. 13.4 When isolated muscles are made to work at different intensities, ATP and ADP concentrations remain constant whereas creatine phosphate (CP) falls as $\dot{V}_{O_2}$ increases. (From Di Prampero and Margaria, 1968.)

the ADP concept argue that it cannot be ADP because it is immediately converted to ATP in the cytoplasm as well as in the mitochondrion. They postulate instead that creatine must bring the signal to the mitochondrion. Strong arguments in favor of this view derive from experiments with isolated muscles made to contract by increasing electrical stimulation: Figure 13.4 shows that as $\dot{V}_{O_2}$ increases, the content in ATP and ADP remain constant whereas the creatine phosphate pool decreases linearly. From such data it is derived that the change in O_2 consumption, $\Delta\dot{V}_{O_2}$, is inversely proportional to the change in creatine phosphate concentration, $\Delta[CP]$ according to

$$\Delta\dot{V}_{O_2} = -3 \cdot \Delta[CP].$$

The signal therefore appears carried by creatine.

Whatever the final conclusion on that controversy will be, one point is uncontested: oxidative phosphorylation is directly regulated as a function of the need for phosphate-bond energy, be this ATP or CP. In other words, *oxidative metabolism, and by that the O_2 needs of the cells, is regulated to energy demand.*

The question is whether O_2 supply also affects the level of oxidative phosphorylation. There is no strong evidence pointing to this, except when O_2 is in short supply. Under these circumstances not all the NADH produced in glycolysis or in the Krebs cycle can be oxidized to NAD^+ in the respiratory chain; the Krebs cycle is slowed down and lactate is formed from pyruvate. Oxidative phosphorylation then becomes limited due to O_2 shortage although the energy demand of the cell may be higher. It may well be that this happens beyond $\dot{V}_{O_2}$max where we have seen that the cell obtains an increasing part of its ATP anaerobically from glycolysis (Fig. 2.8).

REGULATION OF CIRCULATION

The regulation of O_2 transport by the blood is a complex affair; it involves an adjustment of total systemic blood flow, of the distribution of blood flow to the organs of need, and of the O_2 transport capacity of the blood. Let us look at these factors separately.

Total systemic blood flow is estimated by cardiac output. In Table 10.2 we saw that an increase in O_2 consumption by a factor of 8.6 was accompanied by an increase in cardiac output by a factor of 2.5. Figure 13.5 shows that cardiac output and O_2 consumption increase

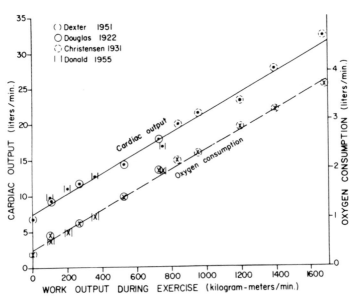

Fig. 13.5 Increase of cardiac output and O_2 consumption with increasing work output in man. (From Guyton et al., 1973.)

in parallel—but not in proportion—when the work output increases during exercise; the parallelism between these two curves is the result of the choice of the two ordinates. What this graph is to show is merely that both $\dot{V}_{O_2}$ and $\dot{Q}_B$ increase linearly as the work load increases.

Cardiac output can be increased by increasing the heart rate, the stroke volume, or, evidently, both in combination. Table 10.2 revealed that an increase in heart rate was by far the dominant factor whereas stroke volume increased relatively little. The intriguing point is clearly that cardiac output increases considerably less than $\dot{V}_{O_2}$, for which we can consider two reasons.

The first reason relates to the distribution of blood flow which is modified in exercise, as shown in Table 13.1. When total blood flow increased from about 6 L·min⁻¹ at rest to 25 L·min⁻¹ in maximal exercise, the major part of exercise blood flow went to skeletal muscle, evidently the organ system in need. The brain retained its absolute blood flow of 750 ml·min⁻¹, while the heart's absolute blood flow increased, though its share, 4%, was the same at rest and in exercise. Both make sense, since the brain does not change its activity in exercise, whereas the heart has to do work in proportion to total blood flow. The other parts of systemic circulation reduced not

TABLE 13.1. ESTIMATED DISTRIBUTION OF CARDIAC OUTPUT IN A NORMAL HUMAN SUBJECT[a] AT REST AND DURING MAXIMAL EXERCISE.[b]

Region	Blood flow at rest		Blood flow in maximal exercise	
	ml/min	% total	ml/min	% total
Splanchnic	1,400	24.1	300	1.1
Renal	1,100	19.0	250	1.0
Cerebral	750	12.9	750	3.0
Coronary	250	4.3	1,000	4.0
Skeletal muscle	1,200	20.7	22,000	88.0
Skin	500	8.6	600	2.4
Other organs	600	10.3	100	0.4
Total	5,800		25,000	

a. Weight = 70 kg.
b. From Wade and Bishop (1962).

only their share, but even the absolute blood flow into the systems, with the exception of the skin whose perfusion is slightly increased in the interest of thermoregulation.

To understand how this redistribution of blood flow and the increased cardiac output come about, let us first look at the mechanisms controlling local perfusion of organs, particularly of skeletal muscle. Regional distribution of blood flow depends essentially on the distribution of vascular resistances since the driving force, the heart beat, is the same for all parts of systemic circulation. Vascular resistance is determined by the tone in the smooth muscle sleeve of arteries, predominantly of the small arteries and arterioles; note that a minute change in diameter causes a large change in resistance because of Poiseuille's law (equation 7.1). Two mechanisms are at hand to regulate vascular resistance—one neural and one local. Peripheral blood vessels are richly supplied with nerve fibers from the sympathetic nervous system, whereby some have vasoconstrictor, others vasodilator activity, depending on whether they discharge adrenaline or acetylcholine, respectively. The increased perfusion of skeletal muscles is apparently due to increased sympathetic vasodilator activity. This neural effect can actually precede muscle work, in anticipation of increased demands. Once the muscles have begun to work, neural control becomes of secondary importance because now local regulatory factors dominate: a decrease in P_{O_2}, an increase in P_{CO_2}, and the accumulation of some metabolites all enhance local blood flow by reducing vascular resistance. In the resting muscle many capillaries are unperfused; with vasodilation these are seen to open up gradually, so that eventually the entire capillary network is perfused. It has been estimated that the number of perfused capillaries can be increased by 10–100 fold in exercise. This evidently has an important regulatory effect on O_2 delivery to the muscle cells since the radius of the Krogh cylinder (or cone) is determined by the distance between perfused capillaries (chapter 7).

The enhancement of muscle blood flow in exercise, initiated by the sympathetic nerves, is accompanied by a number of other changes in the systemic vasculature. Adrenergic nerves cause a constriction of the veins and a reduction of blood flow to the splanchnic circulation (the gastrointestinal organs). This reduces the volume of blood stored in the veins and in the splanchnic vessels and hence increases the volume of circulating blood by over 30%.

As shown in Table 10.2, the increase in cardiac output is due essentially to increased heart rate whereas stroke volume changes little. Stroke volume appears to be determined by the capacity of the ventricles; when the heart becomes enlarged as a result of training, stroke volume will be enlarged both in rest and in exercise. Just as we had observed the blood vessels to the muscles to dilate in anticipation of work, we also find heart rate to increase before work actually begins; this is probably due to impulses from the brain cortex that take their effect through hypothalamic centers and the vasomotor centers in the brain stem, a reaction related to the "fight-or-flight" condition induced by the sympathetic nervous system. It is also noteworthy that adrenergic stimulation which causes vasoconstriction in the peripheral circulation leads to vasodilation in the coronary arteries of heart muscle; this is rather sensible since it prepares the heart for increased work. A second factor important for increasing cardiac output upon exercise is increased venous return of blood which allows the ventricles to be filled more rapidly. This is achieved by the venoconstriction mentioned above, as well as by the restriction of the splanchnic vessels.

We have noted that the increase in blood flow in exercise is considerably less than that of O_2 consumption. Part of the reason is certainly that the blood becomes redistributed to the organs of greater need (Table 13.1), but this does not yet answer the question why total blood flow is not adapted to total O_2 consumption. The reason is that the transport of O_2 through the circulation of blood depends on more than just blood flow. The delivery of O_2 to the tissues by blood flow is given by the Fick equation as

$$\dot{V}_{O_2} = \dot{Q}_B \cdot [Ca_{O_2} - Cv_{O_2}].$$

So, in principle, if $\dot{V}_{O_2}$ increases 8.6 times and $\dot{Q}_B$ 2.5 times, then we must expect the difference in O_2 content between arterial and venous blood to increase by a factor of 3.4. This was, indeed, found: O_2 content of arterial blood increased slightly from 8.63 at rest to 9.08 mmol·L^{-1} in exercise, whereas venous O_2 content fell from 6.65 to 2.24 mmol·L^{-1}. This means that, in exercise, the tissues extracted more than 3 times as much O_2 from the unit volume of blood. This has come about because of a number of adjustments in the blood. First there was a slight increase in hemoglobin content of the blood, as evidenced by higher arterial O_2 content although arterial P_{O_2} did not change. Second, the greater amount of CO_2 produced by the cells in exercise caused a large Bohr shift of the O_2-Hb equilibrium curve (Fig. 6.7); the venous point thus comes to lie on the steepest part of the curve, with the result that moving the point further down releases a lot of O_2 without changing P_{O_2} considerably (Fig. 6.7). As a third factor, the increase in temperature in the working muscle further decreased blood O_2 affinity (Fig. 6.6) and thus assisted the augmented discharge of O_2 into the tissues.

The adjustment of the O_2 transport capacity of blood as a function of demand has thus two roots: (1) the major part is due to greater O_2 extraction in the tissue, aided by the properties of the O_2-Hb equilibrium curve and is thus self-adjusting; (2) in addition, the O_2 binding capacity is increased to some extent by increasing hemoglobin content or rather the hematocrit.

That these adjustments of circulation are a general phenomenon in principle, but that they can be modified in degree, was recently obtained in some experiments of C. R. Taylor on dogs, probably the best "aerobic performers" that can easily outrun their prey. In this group of animals O_2 consumption increased 13-fold between rest and running on a treadmill at $\dot{V}_{O_2}$max (Fig. 2.8). This was accompanied by a 6-fold increase in cardiac output, partly due, in this instance, to increased stroke volume. Hemoglobin content was augmented by over 20% which is possible because the dog maintains concentrated red cell stores in the spleen which he can discharge on demand; as a consequence O_2 content of arterial blood was increased by 20%. Together with the effects of the Bohr shift the amount of O_2 discharged to the tissues could thus be increased by a factor of 2.5, although the arteriovenous P_{O_2} difference changed only from 49 to 62 torr, and although the arterial P_{O_2} actually fell by 5% on running at $\dot{V}_{O_2}$max.

In conclusion, we find that circulation can respond to greater O_2 demands through various mechanisms: by increasing cardiac output and the quantity of circulating blood; by augmenting the O_2 binding capacity of the blood; by redistributing blood flow to regions of need, both through nervous control and in response to local factors. In addition, the O_2 binding properties of blood, the nonlinear O_2-Hb equilibrium curve, and the Bohr and temperature shifts constitute a system of self-adjustment for increased O_2 discharge as a function of local O_2 needs.

Finally, a few words only about "backward regulation," that is, adjustments of circulation and blood to reduced availability of O_2, as it occurs naturally at high altitude. We have already said that O_2 consumption is depressed if O_2 availability is limited, that is, our work capacity becomes limited. If we climb to high altitude, we need a greater cardiac output than at sea level to do the same amount of work; heart rate is increased. After some time—a few days of residence at high altitude may suffice—cardiac output per unit work goes down again, because the blood will have increased its hemoglobin concentration by increasing the number of erythrocytes in the unit blood volume; the blood gets "thicker." In high altitude natives one finds a remarkable adaptation of the O_2 binding properties of the blood (Fig. 13.6): not only is their total O_2 binding capacity increased by 30% due to increased hemoglobin content, but their O_2-Hb equilibrium curve is shifted to the left; in spite of the different P_{O_2} in ambient air, this shift allows them to maintain the same arterial and venous O_2 content as sea-level natives. But this is actually no longer a question of adjusting performance to needs; it is more one of adapting the potential, as discussed below.

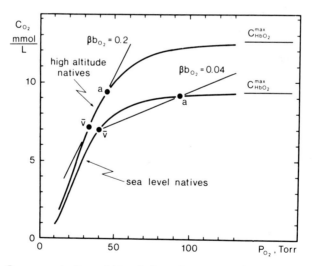

Fig. 13.6 O_2 concentration of blood plotted against ambient P_{O_2} in sea-level and high-altitude residents. High-altitude residents have a higher maximal O_2-hemoglobin concentration ($C_{HbO_2}^{max}$) and their equilibrium curves are shifted to the left. As a result their arterial (a) and mixed venous ($\bar{v}$) O_2 concentrations are the same as in sea-level residents. (From Dejours, 1981.)

REGULATION OF RESPIRATION

Referring back, once more, to Table 10.2, we note that a ninefold increase in O_2 consumption causes total ventilation to be increased tenfold; this is achieved by enlarging tidal volume fivefold and doubling respiration rate. Thus, convective transport of O_2 by ventilation is adjusted about proportionately to O_2 needs. But augmented O_2 consumption also causes CO_2 production to increase proportionately. We have learned how important CO_2 exchange is for the regulation of acid–base balance, so that the question comes up whether respiration responds to O_2 needs or to the (closely related) necessity of discharging CO_2 in order to regulate the milieu intérieur. Our bias would make us assume that respiration responds to O_2 needs, but is this really what happens?

Figure 13.7 shows three graphs in which the effects of P_{O_2} and P_{CO_2} on total ventilation is examined individually and in combination. We see first that the P_{O_2} in inspired air must be dropped to 60 torr or less before ventilation is increased (a); if, however, $P_{A_{CO_2}}$ rises, ventilation goes up about proportionately (b). In the last graph (c) we

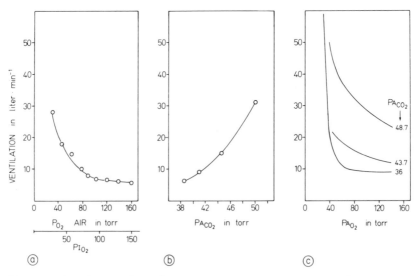

Fig. 13.7   Regulation of ventilation in response to varying P_{O_2} and P_{CO_2} in air. A fall of inspired P_{O_2} below 60 torr causes ventilation to increase (a), as does a rise in alveolar P_{CO_2} (b). At alveolar P_{CO_2} above normal any reduction in alveolar P_{O_2} causes ventilation to increase (c). (Modified after Loeschcke and Gertz, 1958; Lambertsen, 1960.)

observe that a reduction of alveolar P_{O_2} causes ventilation to increase continuously if PA_{CO_2} is above normal. From this type of information we can conclude that respiration is adjusted primarily to keep alveolar P_{CO_2} constant and thus to regulate acid–base balance. This is also shown by a simple experiment: if one takes a deep sigh one washes out a good part of the CO_2 that is retained in the alveoli with the result that the subsequent breaths show a considerable reduction in tidal volume until PA_{CO_2} returns to normal level; conversely if one takes one breath of air enriched with 7% CO_2 the next breaths have increased tidal volume. It is thus evident that alveolar, and by that arterial P_{CO_2}, is the main driving force for short-term adjustment of ventilation.

We may now wonder why P_{O_2} shows such a weak effect on ventilation, why it must be dropped to 60 torr or less before it causes ventilation to increase. This has to do with the O_2 binding properties of blood. Referring back to Figure 6.7 we note that arterial blood will drop its O_2 content to only about 90% if P_{O_2} falls to 60 torr; thus in the upper P_{O_2} range blood has a wide safety margin. Below 60 torr the O_2-Hb equilibrium curve falls rapidly, dangerously reducing O_2 transport capacity. The increased sensitivity to PA_{O_2} when PA_{CO_2} is above normal (Fig. 13.7c) may have to do with the Bohr effect which depresses O_2 binding.

The control of respiration involves groups of neurons located in the pons and the medulla of the brain stem, called the respiratory centers. In the medulla some cells are associated with inspiration, others with expiration; via the spinal cord motoneurons they control the inspiratory and expiratory muscles of the chest, respectively (see chapter 11). Through interactions within the medulla these cells are responsible for a certain spontaneous rhythmicity of respiratory movements which is, however, quite irregular without controlling afferent stimuli. These come either from the pons, from the hypothalamus, or from peripheral receptors via the glossopharyngeal and vagus nerves.

This system responds to changes in arterial P_{CO_2} (or pH) and P_{O_2} through a number of chemoreceptors. One group of chemosensitive cells is located directly in the medulla, close to its respiratory center; they respond to CO_2 and pH changes by increasing ventilation, and may regulate the H^+ concentration in brain fluids. Peripheral chemoreceptors are found associated with the great arteries: near each of the bifurcations of the common carotid one finds a small carotid body, very richly supplied with blood vessels and innervated by a special branch of the glossopharyngeal nerve; two similar aortic bodies, innervated by the vagus nerve, are found at the aortic arch. These peripheral chemoreceptors respond to elevated P_{CO_2} and, to a lesser degree, to reduced P_{O_2} in the arterial blood. A small effect on ventilation is also exerted by afferences from the baroreceptors in the carotid sinus and in the aorta which respond to alterations in arterial blood pressure.

Ventilation is also controlled, to some extent, by peripheral mechanoreceptors. Some stretch receptors are located in the lung; on inflation they send an inhibitory message to the medulla via the vagus nerve, an effect called the Hering-Breuer reflex. The lung may also have receptors that cause an increase of the inspiratory effort when the lung is deflated. And, furthermore, like all skeletal muscles, the ventilatory muscles of the chest and diaphragm contain muscle spindles that control their contraction through reflexes.

How, then, is respiration adjusted to the increased demand for O_2 supply and CO_2 discharge during exercise? Let us first remember that O_2 consumption increases with a certain delay, since the body first operates under O_2 deficit (Fig. 2.3). Nevertheless, the lungs begin to step up their ventilation at the onset of exercise. This seems to be due to reflex stimulation of ventilation originating in the muscles that begin to work. Later on, as CO_2 becomes loaded into the blood and O_2 is being consumed at an increased rate, ventilation will become adjusted to needs, controlled by the basic mechanism of regulating CO_2 and H^+ concentration in the blood, and to a lesser degree by P_{O_2}. That the system responds less to P_{O_2} than to CO_2 is of no consequence, because in exercise CO_2 production is proportional to O_2 utilization, at least if there is no major shift in the substrates burned.

We must further note that the transfer of O_2 from alveolar air to capillary blood also, and importantly, depends on blood flow through the lung. Under steady-state conditions blood flow through the lung is equal to that through the entire systemic circulation; the response of pulmonary blood flow to exercise is therefore the same as that of systemic circulation discussed above.

ADJUSTING THE CASCADE: ACHIEVING HOMEOSTASIS AT DIFFERENT LEVELS OF NEED

It is not sufficient to have each of the parts of the respiratory system adjust its performance to changes in the controlling parameters; they must all do so in concert, gauged eventually to one and the same yardstick, in principle the need for O_2 flow from air to mitochondria. This is the essential postulate of steady-state conditions or homeostasis in the body: if one of the steps in the respiratory system were to transport less O_2 than the others require, the O_2 store following that step would soon be depleted and O_2 flow from there on would have to stop or be reduced; the system could not continue to function. Walter Cannon, for 36 years Professor of Physiology at Harvard Medical School (1906–1942), who coined the term *homeostasis* (Greek for the state of staying similar), remarked, for example: "If a state remains steady, it does so because any tendency toward change is automatically met by increased effectiveness of the factor or factors which resist the change." Let us see how this principle of self-regulation works in our system (Fig. 13.2). Shortly after the onset of muscle work, oxidative phosphorylation begins to draw O_2 from the cellular O_2 store. This will cause the cellular P_{O_2} to fall. As a consequence the P_{O_2} gradient between capillary blood and the cells increases, and this will drive more O_2 from the blood into the cell by diffusion; diffusive O_2 flow, $\dot{V}_{O_2}(B\text{-}C)$ in Figure 13.1, is adjusted to needs. Increased O_2 extraction from blood decreases P_{O_2} in the tissue, and this will cause capillaries to open up, local blood flow and eventually total cardiac output to increase; convective O_2 flow by blood, $\dot{V}_{O_2}(B)$, is adjusted to needs. Increased O_2 extraction from the blood, augmented cardiac output, and greater CO_2 output increase O_2 uptake in the lung by diffusion and also lead to accrued ventilation of the lung; diffusive and convective O_2 transport in the lung, $\dot{V}_{O_2}(A\text{-}B)$ and $\dot{V}_{O_2}(A)$ respectively, are also adjusted to needs.

On the whole, the respiratory system has become adjusted to a steady state at a new level of O_2 flow, matched to the new flow into the O_2 sink determined by the energy needs of the cell. As shown in Figure 13.8 the cascade of driving forces from environmental air to the mitochondria has become steeper, allowing a greater overall O_2 flow rate, both by convective transport and by diffusion. There are two important points to this: (1) the physiological regulation of the adjustable processes discussed above (Fig. 13.2) automatically causes the links between them, the diffusive steps, to be adjusted as well; (2) the signals for the regulation of these processes derive from the changes induced in the forward step, so that the energetic needs of the cells dictate the adjustments of the system as a whole. When the cells' energetic needs regress again, the whole process is reversed: the cascade becomes again more shallow. This is homeostasis at work.

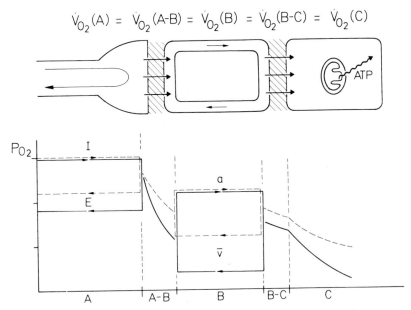

$$\dot{V}_{O_2}(A) = \dot{V}_{O_2}(A\text{-}B) = \dot{V}_{O_2}(B) = \dot{V}_{O_2}(B\text{-}C) = \dot{V}_{O_2}(C)$$

Fig. 13.8 Adjusting the P_{O_2} cascade across the respiratory system from rest (broken line) to work (solid line) causes the overall P_{O_2} gradient from air to the sink to become steeper.

Adjusting Potential to Needs

The respiratory system operates, as we have seen over and over again, within certain limits. Its total performance has a rather well defined upper limit or potential estimated by $\dot{V}_{O_2}$max. One of the central issues of this treatise was that this potential should be intimately linked to the design properties of the system: at each level the design properties which affect the conductance (Fig. 13.1) should be matched to functional needs, that is, to O_2 flow, as a result of regulated morphogenesis; this was the way we have described the principle of symmorphosis.

In order to test the validity of this principle I have formulated, in chapter 3, three hypotheses which we should now examine in overview:

(1) the structural design is a rate-limiting factor for O_2 flow at each level of the respiratory system;

(2) the structural design is adaptable, at least within certain limits;

(3) the structural design is optimized.

The last one of these hypotheses was clearly the most ambitious. It depends essentially on a quantitative assessment of the cost–benefit ratio; but to give a clear answer we lack too much information on what the cost of maintaining a structural system really is. We can therefore answer it only in the most indirect way, by taking recourse, in fact, to the analysis of the two other hypotheses. If we find that the mitochondria of muscle cells set the limit for oxidative metabolism; if we also find that muscle cells augment or reduce their mitochondrial content when energetic needs are increased or decreased, respectively; then we have reasons to believe that the cell considers the cost–benefit ratio in maintaining a mitochondrial population of a given magnitude, in other words, that the system is optimized at that level. We can argue in much the same way with respect to the lung, only there the cost factor is rather complex involving all metabolic functions of the various lung cells, from fibroblasts maintaining the fiber skeleton to the type II epithelial cells synthesizing surfactant. Therefore I shall not try to give a clear-cut answer to this hypothesis; but it remains in the back of our mind as the ultimate measure of "good" or "reasonable" design of the respiratory system.

I will, however, attempt to address the two other hypotheses in overview, starting with the question of adaptability in order to end with that of limitation.

ADAPTATION AND MORPHOGENETIC POTENTIAL

If the functional potential of the respiratory system is quantitatively determined by some design properties, then any adaptation of the functional potential, as it occurs for example in endurance training, must be the result of structural adaptation, at least in part.

The mechanism for achieving this is regulation of morphogenesis to different levels. It is thus evident that adjustment of the potential will be a long-term affair, requiring a minimum of days to weeks for an effect to take place. The capacity to adjust the potential will also depend on the general level of morphogenetic activity of the body: it will clearly be higher during the period of active growth than in the adult where a certain "morphogenetic steady state" has been achieved.

In the adult, adjustment of the potential is relatively easy where the turnover of cells and constituents is high. Thus we have seen in chapter 5 that the mitochondria of muscle cells can be increased in amount if the body requires a higher rate of energy production, as is the case in endurance exercise training. As a consequence maximal O_2 consumption can increase in proportion. We have also seen that the O_2 transport capacity of the blood and circulation can augment in response to accrued needs. Thus at high altitude the hematocrit goes up by adding more erythrocytes from the bone marrow. Strenuous endurance exercise training results in a structural adaptation of the heart's transport capacity in that the ventricles enlarge and their myocardium hypertrophies to allow an increased stroke volume. It also leads to the formation of more capillaries in the muscle, thus reducing the diameter of the functional Krogh cylinder for tissue oxygenation. On the other hand, there is, so far, no positive evidence that suggests an adjustment of the lung's O_2 transport potential through structural modifications in the adult. But maybe longer stimuli would be required to modify this complex and yet delicate structure.

There is a lot of evidence demonstrating the adjustability of the potential of the respiratory system during the growth period. It responds to increased energetic needs by adjusting the morphometric properties of the system at all levels, from the mitochondria to the lung. The lung also responds during growth to altered O_2 availability in ambient air: animals raised at high altitude develop a larger pulmonary diffusing capacity thus compensating for the reduced driving force for O_2 uptake. Furthermore, a loss of lung tissue during the growth period is compensated by augmenting the growth rate of the remaining tissue until the lost gas exchange units are replaced, which demonstrates the adaptability of the lung very clearly.

The adjustability of the potential of the respiratory system is very prominent when one compares different mammalian species which differ in terms of their energetic needs for behavioral reasons or because of size; this adaptation also occurs during growth of the organism, but it is, to a large extent, determined by genetic traits rather than by secondary effects directly imposed by energetic needs. The question clearly is why the dog is such a good endurance runner: is it because "something" tells him to run harder causing more mitochondria to be formed, or does his genetic make-up cause more mitochondria to be built into his muscles, allowing him to perform aerobically at a higher level than other animals of similar size? We don't know yet, but it should be possible to design experiments to answer this question.

In summary, the evidence accumulated so far indicates that the respiratory system is, indeed, adaptable to functional needs at all levels, but that this is limited by the morphogenetic potential of the structures involved, a feature which is different in adulthood than during the growth period.

ARE THE STRUCTURES OF THE RESPIRATORY PATHWAY RATE-LIMITING FACTORS FOR O_2 FLOW?

How far is the first hypothesis validated by the findings reported in the previous chapters? All evidence shows that the O_2 flow rate through the system is dictated by the "consumer," by the O_2 sink in the mitochondria. The study of animals running on a treadmill has shown that $\dot{V}_{O_2}$ increases linearly with running speed up to a certain level, called $\dot{V}_{O_2}max$. At higher speeds this level of $\dot{V}_{O_2}$ is maintained, but the additional ATP required is now generated anaerobically by glycolysis. Oxidative phosphorylation in the mitochondria must therefore have an upper functional limit, probably set by the maximal rate at which the respiratory chain units, or some other elements of mitochondria, can operate. All evidence accumulated indicates that the amount of mitochondria in the working muscle sets the limit for $\dot{V}_{O_2}$: as well within size classes as across the mammalian size range we have found the mitochondrial volume to be proportional to $\dot{V}_{O_2}max$. This is because oxidative phosphorylation in mitochondria is the only, the unavoidable pathway for ATP production by oxidative metabolism, and the number of units that perform this function is limited by the size of the compartment in which they are housed. In addition, the potential for homeostatic adaptation of mitochondrial function is limited, particularly by the stoichiometry of the process which determines that 6 mol ATP are formed for every mol O_2 consumed. The structural design of the mitochondrial compartment is thus clearly a limiting factor for O_2 consumption.

Things are not quite as simple at the other levels of the respiratory system. In principle, the structural design affects only, or mostly, the conductance (Fig. 13.1) whereas the driving forces for O_2 flow are importantly affected by homeostatic regulations, as discussed in the previous section (Fig. 13.8). But now, if the partial pressure difference across a diffusion conductor is doubled, O_2 flow is doubled without changing the conductance. This must have an effect on the relation between the O_2 flow rate and the diffusion conductance in the lung and in the microvascular units. We must therefore give the potential for homeostatic regulation of the driving forces due consideration along with the potential set up by structural design.

Looking first at the microvascular unit of muscles we note that the driving force for O_2 delivery into the cells is essentially determined by the capillary P_{O_2}; since its value is somewhere between arterial and venous P_{O_2} the potential for its homeostatic adaptation is limited, because arterial P_{O_2} is limited by O_2 uptake in the lung. Our findings on the design of the microvasculature suggest that the conductance for O_2 delivery into the cells is closely adapted to the size of the O_2 sink: we have found consistently that there is about 1 μm^3 of blood for every 3 μm^3 of mitochondria in muscle cells. It is therefore well possible that the design of the microvascular unit is a limiting factor for O_2 flow into the cells. This statement must, however, be regarded with caution. We have noted that capillary density in muscle shows a large variation which is only in part due to variations in mitochondrial density. We have interpreted this in terms of the multiple functions that capillaries must serve: the delivery of substrates and the removal of wastes and heat, to mention only a few.

If we finally consider the lung as a gas exchanger, we note that the potential for homeostatic regulation of the driving force for O_2 flow is greater (Fig. 13.8): the P_{O_2} gradient from alveolar air to capillary blood depends importantly on ventilation and perfusion. Increased ventilation can elevate the alveolar P_{O_2}, whereas the mean capillary P_{O_2} will fall if the perfusion rate is increased with the result that the P_{O_2} gradient across the air–blood barrier becomes larger. These effects will occur as a consequence of homeostatic regulation of the performance of the respiratory system to higher levels of O_2 needs, as seen in the preceding section. But it appears that this occurs to quite a variable degree in different species; thus the dog seems to have an unusually high potential of homeostatic regulation of this system, since he can augment his cardiac output by nearly sixfold from rest to maximal exercise, or twice as much as most other mammals including man. Unfortunately, we still know very little about the potential for homeostatic regulation as a limiting factor for pulmonary gas exchange. In consequence, we cannot come up with a definitive answer whether the design of the lung's gas exchanger is a limiting factor for gas exchange.

Two pieces of very recent evidence suggest that this may yet turn out to be the case. The first one relates again to the peculiarities of the dog with his unusually high capacity for aerobic metabolism. In a recent study of the physiology of the dog running on a treadmill C. R. Taylor has found that the P_{O_2} of arterial blood falls as $\dot{V}_{O_2}$max is approached. The analysis of these data suggests that the extraordinary augmentation of the dog's cardiac output causes the blood to traverse the lung at such a velocity that its P_{O_2} cannot become equilibrated with that in the alveoli; there remains a difference between alveolar and arterial P_{O_2}. Clearly, gas exchange in the lung is limited by diffusion in this case, and the design properties of the gas exchanger are limiting factors for O_2 flow.

A similar result has recently been obtained by J. B. West and his colleagues during the 1981 American Scientific Mt. Everest Expedition. Two scientist-climbers reached the top of Mt. Everest without supplemental O_2. There they recorded barometric pressure and took a sample of alveolar gas. The analysis of the data revealed that Pa_{O_2} was 35 and Pa_{O_2} 28 mm Hg. Hence there was a marked alveolo-arterial P_{O_2} difference which could only be explained by diffusion limitation of O_2 uptake: the head pressure for driving O_2 across the air−blood barrier was too small, and the design of the pulmonary diffusion conductance became a limiting factor.

In summary, all this evidence taken together suggests strongly that design properties of the respiratory system are potential limiting factors for O_2 flow at all levels of the O_2 pathway. The evidence is strong and unambiguous for the limiting role of mitochondria in the last step which leads into the O_2 sink. It is less tight at the other levels because the limiting effect of design features can often be overcome by appropriate homeostatic adjustment of the boundary conditions which determine the driving forces. The limitation of the process by structural design features then becomes apparent only under extreme conditions.

The Limits to Potential: The Smallest Mammal

Let me now address a final question: whether there is an absolute limit for the potential of the mammalian respiratory system. If the potential of the respiratory system is adjusted to functional needs, then it should be largest in the smallest mammal in existence, the Etruscan shrew (Suncus etruscus), weighing about 2 g (Fig. 13.9), for it

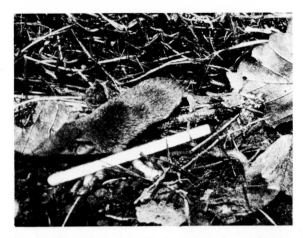

Fig. 13.9 The smallest mammal, the Etruscan shrew (*Suncus etruscus*), weighing 2.5 g, is shown beside a match.

is known to have the highest metabolic rate of all mammals (Fig. 2.6) with an *average* $\dot{V}_{O_2}$ of the order of 0.2 to 0.3 ml $O_2 \cdot min^{-1} \cdot g^{-1}$.

Figure 13.10 shows that the Etruscan shrew's heart rate is over 1000 min^{-1} at rest and its respiratory rate over 300 min^{-1}; the heart rate can go up to 1300 min^{-1} during running! The muscles of heart and diaphragm (Fig. 13.11) are particularly rich in mitochondria and

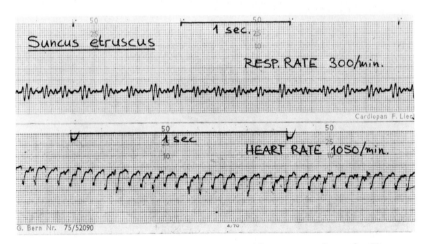

Fig. 13.10 Recordings of the respiratory and heart rates from the Etruscan shrew at rest. (From Weibel, 1979.)

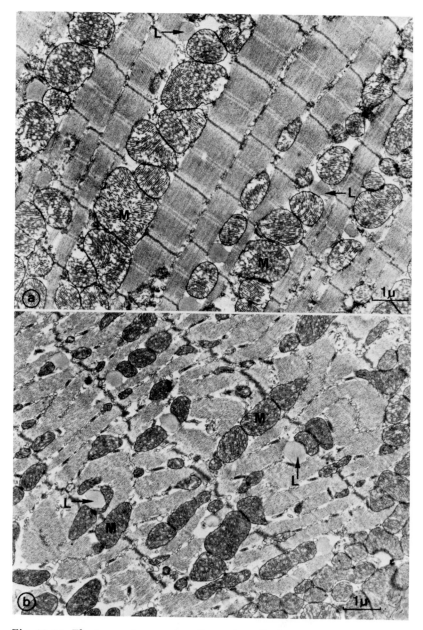

Fig. 13.11 Electron micrographs of muscle cells from (a) myocardium and (b) diaphragm of Etruscan shrew show unusually high densities of mitochondria (M), related to the high work output of these muscles required by the high metabolic activity of the animal. Note the lipid droplets (L). Scale marker: 1 μm.

in capillary supply—indeed the diaphragmatic muscle cells contain 34% mitochondria in volume, the heart muscle cells even as much as 45%. In the diaphragm one finds about 4600 capillaries per mm² of cross-section, in the heart even 6400! These figures are way above all other data recorded for mammals. Nevertheless, the matching between mitochondria and capillaries, as worked out in chapter 7 (compare Figs. 7.9 and 7.10), holds also for these extreme values: there are about 3 μm³ of mitochondria for each μm³ of capillary blood. The shrew's heart is, by the way, a comparatively enormous structure: it fills about half the left chest cavity, leaving little space for the left lung (Fig. 13.12).

Finally, the shrew's lung is an extraordinary structure (Fig. 13.13): its alveoli are very tiny chambers around narrow alveolar ducts. When comparing this figure to the human lung, shown in Figure 12.1 at somewhat lower power, one sees that the density of gas exchange surface in this lung is, with 2800 cm²·cm⁻³, some eight times larger than in the human, four times larger than in the rat, and still three times larger than in the mouse. Indeed, one wonders whether the term "alveolus" is at all an appropriate description, whether the shrew lung would not be better described as an interlaced maze of air

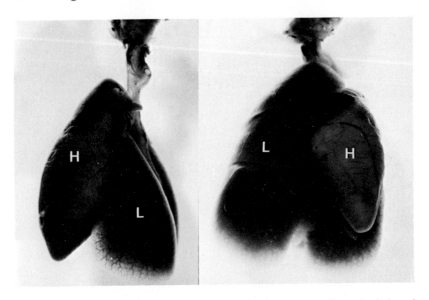

Fig. 13.12 The Etruscan shrew's lung (L) and heart (H) seen from the left and from the front. The unusually large heart occupies the major part of the left chest cavity.

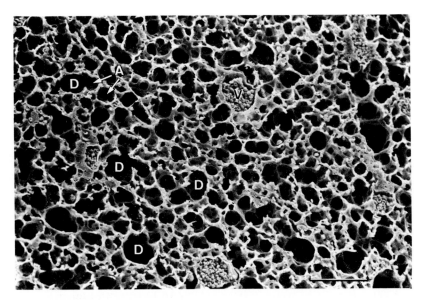

Fig. 13.13 Scanning electron micrograph of Etruscan shrew lung shows tiny alveoli (A) around alveolar ducts (D) together with some larger vessels (V). Note the dense capillary network (arrows). Scale marker: 50 μm. (From Gehr et al., 1980.)

and blood "capillaries," similar, in a way, to what one finds in a bird's lung (compare Fig. 1.14). And, finally, we find the air–blood barrier in the Etruscan shrew lung to be extremely thin (Fig. 13.14), its harmonic mean thickness measuring no more than 0.25 μm, about half that found in the rat. This could be achieved only by reducing all tissue layers to a minimum: over large parts of the barrier, the cell sheets of epithelium and endothelium are each reduced to just a pair of cell membranes, and the type I epithelial cells are much reduced in number, forming excessively complex epithelial sheets with many branches, as discussed in chapter 9 as a means to effectively reduce tissue mass in the gas exchange barrier.

There is no mammal smaller in size than *Suncus etruscus*, none more demanding in terms of energetic needs. Could this be because the potential of the respiratory system has been pushed to extremes at all levels? Indeed, if nearly half the space of heart muscle cells is taken up by the machinery generating the fuel for the heart beat; if the heart occupies a third of the chest cavity; and if the size of the air

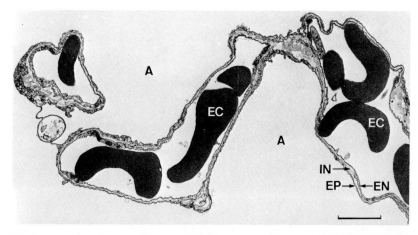

Fig. 13.14 Alveolar capillaries (C) of Etruscan shrew lung are separated from alveolar air (A) by a very thin barrier made of extremely attenuated endothelium (EN), type I epithelium (EP1), and interstitium (IN). Scale marker: 2 μm. (From Weibel, 1979.)

spaces in the pulmonary gas exchanger is so small that enormous potential surface forces due to high surface curvature must be compensated or sustained to maintain a large air–blood contact surface; then it may well be that a limit of bioengineering feasibility has been reached, that the potential of the respiratory system has been adjusted to its limit.

Summary

All parts of the respiratory system (lung, blood, circulation, mitochondria) serve the same ultimate purpose: making energy available for biological work. According to the hypothesis of symmorphosis we postulate that all parts should be adjusted to the needs of maintaining the O_2 flow required for oxidative phosphorylation, and they should all be adjusted to each other. Two problems must be overcome: the system must adjust its performance by regulating functions to homeostasis; the system must adjust its potential to move the limits of performance to higher levels if needed.

The adjustable functional processes of the respiratory system are buffered by operating against a number of stores: a phosphate store in the cells, an O_2 store in the cells and in the blood, and some stores of substrates. The processes are regulated by adjusting their perform-ance to the boundary conditions set by the stores to either side of the process.

In the cells the high-energy phosphate store is buffered by creatine. The enzyme creatine phosphokinase (CPK) catalyzes the transfer of high-energy phosphate groups between ATP and creatine to make creatine phosphate (CP) and between CP and ADP to make ATP. The first process occurs in the mitochondrial intermembrane space; CP diffuses to sites of energy utilization where CPK transfers its phosphate back to ATP. High-energy phosphates are stored in the cell mostly as CP, but a small amount of ATP is stored in the cytoplasm for immedi-ate use. When ATP is utilized the resultant ADP is immediately stocked up to ATP by CPK. The signal for triggering oxidative phos-phorylation and adjusting it to the cell's needs is carried by creatine; the change in O_2 consumption in working muscles is inversely pro-portional to the change in the CP concentration. O_2 supply affects oxidative phosphorylation only when it is in short supply by limiting the amount of NAD^+ available as a cofactor for the Krebs cycle.

The regulation of O_2 transport by the blood involves an adjustment of total systemic blood flow (cardiac output), of the distribution of blood flow to the organs of need, and of the O_2 transport capacity of the blood. During work, cardiac output increases with O_2 consumption, but only by a factor of 2.5 for a ninefold increase in O_2 consumption. This is achieved mostly by increasing heart rate; stroke volume changes less. Cardiac output increases less than O_2 consumption during exercise because blood flow is distributed preferentially to the working muscle groups by regulating the resistance of the arteries through the action of the sympathetic nervous system on arterial smooth muscle: arteries to working muscles are vasodilated, those to other organs (the intestinal tract, for example) are vasoconstricted. These same mechanisms also increase the quantity of circulating blood. The perfusion of muscle capillaries is thus increased consider-ably, improving O_2 discharge to the muscle cells. These changes (increased heart rate, redistribution of blood flow) can occur even before work actually begins, because the sympathetic nerves prepare the body for the "fight-or-flight" condition. The O_2 transport capacity of the blood depends on the O_2 content difference between arterial and venous blood. In exercise this difference becomes considerably in-creased owing to the greater O_2 extraction by the muscle cells. When, at high altitude, O_2 is in short supply, heart rate and cardiac output are higher than at sea level for the same amount of work. Reduced O_2 availability limits work capacity at high altitudes until the O_2 transport capacity of the blood can be increased by augmenting the concentration of red blood cells.

Regulation of O_2 uptake in the lung involves an adaptation of ventilation and perfusion. Ventilation is regulated from the respiratory centers in the medulla of the brain stem which influence the spinal cord motoneurons that drive the inspiratory and expiratory muscles. Ventilation is adjusted to both the needs of O_2 uptake and CO_2 discharge; it is regulated primarily to keep alveolar P_{CO_2} constant and thus to regulate acid–base balance. The P_{O_2} of arterial blood becomes a driving force for ventilatory response when it falls below 60 torr. During work the needs for O_2 uptake and CO_2 discharge are equal. At the onset of work ventilation is stepped up by reflex stimulation, although O_2 uptake increases only with a certain delay (O_2 deficit). Pulmonary blood flow increases with cardiac output. The lower venous O_2 content increases O_2 uptake into the blood. Homeostasis requires that O_2 transport through each step of the respiratory system be adjusted to the needs of the consumer. During work the P_{O_2} cascade from the air to the cells becomes steeper.

Adjusting the potential of the respiratory system to needs requires adaptation of design properties by regulating morphogenesis. This is a long-term affair, requiring days to weeks; it depends on the morphogenetic capacity, which is greater during growth than in the adult and is greater in cells with a high turnover than in whole organs. In endurance training the potential of muscle cells for oxidative phosphorylation is augmented by increasing their mitochondrial content, even in the adult; capillaries can also increase and the heart develops a larger stroke volume by enlarging the ventricles. There is no evidence yet that the lung can adapt its diffusing capacity to higher needs in the adult, but this does occur during the growth period. The evidence accumulated indicates that the respiratory system is adaptable to functional needs at all levels, at least during the growth period. The structures of the respiratory pathway are limiting factors for O_2 flow, but to a different degree depending on the potential for homeostatic regulation. The evidence is strong that mitochondria set the limit for O_2 consumption. At the other levels the results are less conclusive, because the limiting effects of design features can often be overcome by homeostatic adjustments. Gas exchange in the lung is *normally determined mostly by perfusion, but under extreme conditions diffusion becomes a limiting factor as well.*

The importance of design features as a limit to functional potential becomes evident when studying the smallest mammal, the Etruscan shrew, which has the highest metabolic rate. The muscles contain the highest amount of mitochondria (nearly 50% in the heart), the heart is very large, and the lung is made of extremely small alveoli. The potential of the respiratory system has been adjusted to its limit.

Further Reading

Dejours, P. 1979. Respiratory controls: oxygenation, CO_2 clearance, or acid–base equilibrium? In *Claude Bernard and the Internal Environment*, ed. E. D. Robin. New York: Dekker, pp. 161–177.

———— 1981. *Principles of Comparative Respiratory Physiology*. 2nd ed. Amsterdam: Elsevier North-Holland.

Dempsey, J. A., and H. V. Forster. 1982. Mediation of ventilatory adaptation. *Physiological Reviews* 62:262–346.

Guyton, A. C., C. E. Jones, and T. G. Coleman. 1973. *Circulatory Physiology*. Vol. 1: *Cardiac Output and Its Regulation*. 2nd ed. Philadelphia: Saunders.

McArdle, W. D., F. I. Katch, and V. L. Katch. 1981. *Exercise Physiology*. Philadelphia: Lea & Febiger.

Rothstein, H. 1982. Regulation of cell cycle by somatomedins. *International Review of Cytology* 78:127–232.

Weibel, E. R. 1979. Oxygen demand and the size of respiratory structures in mammals. In *Evolution of Respiratory Processes*, ed. S. C. Wood and C. Lenfant. New York: Dekker, pp. 289–346.

References

Adams, R. P., L. A. Dieleman, and S. M. Cain. 1982. A critical value for O_2 transport in the rat. *Journal of Applied Physiology* 53:660–664.

Bouverot, P. 1978. Control of breathing in birds compared with mammals. *Physiological Reviews* 58:604–655.

* Cannon, W. B. 1929. Organization for physiological homeostasis. *Physiological Reviews* 9:399–431.

Dejours, P. 1981. *Principles of Comparative Respiratory Physiology*. 2nd ed. Amsterdam: Elsevier North-Holland.

Di Prampero, P. E., and R. Margaria. 1968. Relationship between O_2 consumption, high energy phosphates and the kinetics of the O_2 debt in exercise. *Pflügers Archiv* 304:11–19.

* Farhi, L. E., and H. Rahn. 1955. Gas stores of the body and the unsteady state. *Journal of Applied Physiology* 7:472–484.

Gehr, P., S. Sehovic, P. H. Burri, H. Claassen, and E. R. Weibel. 1980. The lung of shrews: morphometric estimation of diffusion capacity. *Respiration Physiology* 40:33–47.

Guyton, A. C., C. E. Jones, and T. G. Coleman. 1973. *Circulatory Physiology.* Vol. 1: *Cardiac Output and Its Regulation.* 2nd ed. Philadelphia: Saunders.

Lambertsen, C. J. 1960. Carbon dioxide and respiration in acid–base homeostasis. *Anesthesiology* 21:642–651.

* Loeschcke, H. H., and K. H. Gertz. 1958. Einfluss des O_2-Druckes in der Einatmungsluft auf die Atemtätigkeit des Menschen, geprüft unter Konstanthaltung des alveolaren CO_2-Druckes. *Pflügers Archiv* 267:460–477.

Schmidt-Nielsen, K. 1979. *Animal Physiology: Adaptation and Environment.* 2nd ed. Cambridge: Cambridge University Press.

Taylor, C. R., and E. R. Weibel. 1981. Design of the mammalian respiratory system. I. Problem and strategy. *Respiration Physiology* 44:1–10.

Wade, O. L., and J. M. Bishop. 1962. *Cardiac Output and Regional Blood Flow.* Oxford: Blackwell Scientific.

Weibel, E. R. 1979. Oxygen demand and the size of respiratory structures in mammals. In *Evolution of Respiratory Processes,* ed. S. C. Wood and C. Lenfant. New York: Dekker, pp. 289–346.

Weibel, E. R., and C. R. Taylor, eds. 1981. Design of the mammalian respiratory system. *Respiration Physiology* 44:1–164.

Weibel, E. R., C. R. Taylor, P. Gehr, H. Hoppeler, O. Mathieu, and G. M. O. Maloiy. 1981. Design of the mammalian respiratory system. IX. Functional and structural limits for oxygen flow. *Respiration Physiology* 44:151–164.

Wood, S. C., and C. Lenfant, eds. 1979. *Evolution of Respiratory Processes: A Comparative Approach.* New York: Dekker.

UNITS OF MEASUREMENT
GENERAL REFERENCES
INDEX

UNITS OF MEASUREMENT

THE UNITS by which measurements are expressed and the symbols used to express them must be standardized. By tradition different types of units have evolved: in the United States distances are still measured in miles or inches, whereas the rest of the world uses the meter as a basic unit, to mention only one example. In science the metric system has been adopted because of its consistency and ease of calculation. The General Conference on Weights and Measures has developed a coherent International System of Units, commonly known as the SI System (for "Système International" because the "Conférence" is located in Paris), which has been internationally adopted.

The SI System uses seven *base units* for the seven dimensionally independent quantities and several *derived units*, which are given special symbols for reasons of simplicity, although they can be fully expressed in terms of the base units (Table A.1). Unduly large or small numbers are avoided by using prefixes to write units enlarged or reduced by decimal multiples. Centimeter ($cm = 10^{-1}$ m) and micrometer ($\mu m = 10^{-6}$ m) are familiar units, for example; similarly $kPa = 10^3$ Pa.

The SI System is very convenient for purposes of calculation because all units have a common base. Eventually all other units should be abandoned. At present, however, it appears impractical and didactically difficult to express all physiological quantities in SI units only. One reason is that a widely known body of existing information is in daily use, particularly in clinical medicine. Thus the normal systolic blood pressure in man is known to be 120 mm Hg = 120 torr, whereas the corresponding value in SI units, namely 16,000 Pa = 16 kPa, is very unfamiliar. I have therefore retained some such traditional units in this text. Table A.2 presents some of the formulas needed to convert one unit into the other.

TABLE A.1   SI SYSTEM OF UNITS.

Physical quantity	SI unit	Symbol	Definition in terms of base units
Base units			
length	meter	m	
mass	kilogram	kg	
time	second	s	
thermodynamic temperature	kelvin	K	
amount of substance	mole	mol	
electric current	ampere	A	
luminous intensity	candela	cd	
Derived units (selection)			
force	newton	N	$m\ kg\ s^{-2}$
energy	joule	J	$m^2\ kg\ s^{-2}$
power	watt	W	$m^2\ kg\ s^{-3}$
pressure	pascal	Pa	$m^{-1}\ kg\ s^{-2}$
viscosity	poise	P	$m^{-1}\ kg\ s^{-1} \times 10^{-1}$
frequency	hertz	Hz	s^{-1}

TABLE A.2 CONVERSION OF SOME TRADITIONAL UNITS INTO SI UNITS.

Volume

1 liter = 1 dm^3 = 10^{-3} m^3

1 ml = 1 cm^3 = 10^{-6} m^3

Temperature

The unit 1° C (degree Celsius, sometimes called "centigrade") equals the unit of 1 K.

The temperature in ° C is the thermodynamic temperature in K minus 273.15 K.

The melting point of ice at 1 atm is 0° C = 273.15 K; the boiling point of water at 1 atm is 100° C = 373.15 K.

Amount of substance

1 mol O_2 = 22.39ℓO_2 STPD

at temperature 0° C and 1 atm (see p. 54)

Force

1 dyn = 1 cm g s^{-2} = 10^{-5} N

Energy

1 kcal = 4.184 J

Pressure

1 atm = 1.013 · 10^5 Nm^{-2} = 101.3 kPa

1 mm Hg (at 0° C) = 1 torr = 1.333 · 10^2 Nm^{-2} = 133.3 Pa

1 cm H_2O = 1 mbar = 10^2 Pa

GENERAL REFERENCES

Altman, P. L., and D. S. Dittmer. 1971. *Biological Handbooks: Respiration and Circulation*. Bethesda: Federation of American Societies for Experimental Biology.

Åstrand, P. O., and K. Rodahl. 1977. *Textbook of Work Physiology*. 2nd ed. New York: McGraw-Hill.

Dejours, P. 1981. *Principles of Comparative Respiratory Physiology*. 2nd ed. Amsterdam: Elsevier North-Holland.

Kleiber, M. 1961. *The Fire of Life: An Introduction to Animal Energetics*. New York: Wiley.

Lenfant, C., ed. 1976–83. *Lung Biology in Health and Disease*. New York: Dekker. (20 volumes on biochemistry, morphology, development, physiology, pharmacology, immunology, and pathology of the lung.)

Loeppky, J. A., and M. L. Riedesel. 1982. *Oxygen Transport to Human Tissues*. New York: Elsevier North-Holland.

McArdle, W. D., F. I. Katch, and V. L. Katch. 1981. *Exercise Physiology*. Philadelphia: Lea & Febiger.

Murray, J. F. 1976. *The Normal Lung*. Philadelphia: Saunders.

Prosser, C. L. 1973. *Comparative Animal Physiology*. 3rd ed. Philadelphia: Saunders.

Schmidt-Nielsen, K. 1964. *Desert Animals: Physiological Problems of Heat and Water*. New York: Oxford University Press.

—— 1979. *Animal Physiology*. 2nd ed. Cambridge: Cambridge University Press.

Taylor, C. R., K. Johansen, and L. Bolis, eds. 1982. *A Companion to Animal Physiology*. Cambridge: Cambridge University Press.

Weibel, E. R., and C. R. Taylor, eds. 1981. Design of the mammalian respiratory system. *Respiration Physiology* 44:1–164.

Wood, S. C., and C. Lenfant, eds. 1979. *Evolution of Respiratory Processes: A Comparative Approach*. New York: Dekker.

INDEX

Acetyl CoA, 92, 93–94

Acid-base balance, 153–156, 390–391

Acidosis, 154

Acinar pathway, 280, 370–372, *371*, *372*

Acinus(i), 273, 310; number of, 280; size of, 280, 310; ventilation of, 283, 284, 295; capillary sheet, 292; ventilation–perfusion matching in, 298, *298*; construction of, 310–311, *312*; fiber system of, *324*

Actin, 118–120

Activity levels, 61–62

Adaptation: to oxygen needs, 60–61, 366; experimental, 65; of muscles, 126–131; and morphogenetic potential, 395–397

Adenosine diphosphate, *see* ADP

Adenosine triphosphatase, *see* ATPase

Adenosine triphosphate, *see* ATP

Adjustability: of processes, *380*, 381; of potential, 396

ADP: in energy transfer, 30, *31*, 98, 98–99; chemical structure of, *85*; in energy storage, 85–86; in metabolic regulation, 381–383

Aerobic capacity, *see* $\dot{V}_{O_2}$ max

Air-blood barrier, *see* Tissue barrier

Air breathing, 19–23

Air flow: with minimal energy loss, 277; velocity of, 284–285; resistance to, 285–287

Air sacs, 21–22, *22*

Air space stability, 318

Air volume, *see* Lung volume

Airways: origin of, 213; development of, 217; conducting, 221, 273; epithelium of, 233–237, *236*; branching of, 273–280, *274*, *275*; irregular dichotomy of, 274, *275*, 279–280; generations of, 275–276, 277; diameter of, 277–278, *278*, 286; ventilating unit of, 280; physiology of, 282–287; oxygen transport in, 285; resistance of, *286*, 287

Alkalosis, 154

Allometry, 62–64; for oxygen consumption rates, *40*; for maximal oxygen consumption, *45*; for diffusing capacity, 366

Alpha-stat regulation, 156

Altitude, *see* High altitude

Altmann, Richard, 106

Alveolar air, 346

Alveolar capillary network, *290*, 290–292, 340–341, *341*, *342*

Alveolar cells, *see* Type I cells; Type II cells

Alveolar corners, 328–330, *329*, *330*

Alveolar ducts, 339–341, *340*, *371*; pathway, 298, 371

Alveolar epithelium, *see* Alveolar lining layer

Alveolar gas volume, 281–282

Alveolar lining layer: cells of, 237, 253, *254*; surfactant on, 325, *326*; in gas exchange, 342

Alveolar septum: interlobular, 311; fiber system of, 311, 313–315, *314, 315*; surface tension on, 318–320, *319*; mechanics of, 325–331, *327*; stable configuration of, 331; hydrostatic pressure gradients in, 332–333; interstitial spaces of, 333–334

Alveolar surface area: estimates of, 340, 359; and tissue barrier thickness, 352, 354; allometric plot of, 366, *367*

Alveolar ventilation, 283; with exercise, 284; distribution of, 295

Alveolar wall, *see* Alveolar septum

Alveolus(i), 20–21, *20, 21*; formation of, 226, *226*; growth of, *227*; number of, *227*, 228; macrophages in, *243*, 243–245, *245*; open vs. collapsed, *323*; in gas exchange, 339–343, *340, 341*

Amino acids, in Krebs cycle, 94–95

Amniocentesis, 223–224, 265

Amniotic fluid, 223, 265

Amphibia: gills in, 15–16, *16*; lungs in, 19–21, *20, 21*

Anatomic dead space, 281; ventilation of, 283, 284

Anemia, 144

Angiotensin, 238

Animals: in oxygen cycle, 3; cold-blooded vs. warm-blooded, 36–37

Anoxic region, 197–198, 199

Aorta, 176

Aortic bodies, 392

Apoprotein, 260, 262

ARDS, 265–266

Arteries: branchial, 17, 215; design of, 157–158, 176–178; bronchial, 218; pulmonary, 287–290, *288, 289*, 313; caliber of, 292–295

Arterioles, 158; pressure in, *177*, 179; pulmonary, 289

Asbestosis, 244

Asthma, 286

ATP: energy storage in, 30–32, 85–86, 98–99; chemical structure of, *85*; buffering of, 380

ATPase: F_1–, 112, 114; myosin, 122, *195*; myofibrillar, 123; cytoplasmic, 382

Atrioventricular node, 165

Axial fiber system, 307–308, *308*

Bacteria, oxidation by, 4

Barrier, *see* Tissue barrier

Basal lamina, 233

Basement membrane, 182

Benda, Carl, 106

Bernard, Claude, 14

Bertalanffy, L. von, 63

Bicarbonate buffer system, 153

Bicarbonate ion, 151, 152

Biological time, 40

Biological work, 30, 35–36

Bird lung, 21–22, *22, 23*

Blood: oxygen capacity of, 12–13, 56, 143–146; structure of, 140–144; characteristics of, 143–144, *145*; oxygen content of, 144–148, *146*; as oxygen carrier, 144–151; oxygen binding properties of, 147–151, 391; carbon dioxide transport by, 151–153, *152*; mixed venous, 167–168; oxygen transport by, 170–171, 388; end-capillary, 348

Blood flow: through muscles, 70–71, *71*, 386–387; resistance to, 176, *177*, 292–294, 386; sheet-flow concept of, 291; pulmonary, 292–294, 345; in exercise, 294. *See also* Cardiac output; Circulation

Blood flow distribution: with exercise, 161, 169, 385–388; vascular resistance in, 176–178, *177*, 293; regional, 178, 386; uneven, *296*, 296–297; neural control of, 386

Blood plasma: lactate concentration in, *43*, 43–44; conductance of, 355

Blood pressure, 176

Blood vessels, *see* Arteries; Capillary(ies); Veins

Blood volume, in capillaries, 349–350, 356, 360

Body building, 126

Body size: effect on metabolic rate, 38–40, 44–45, 63–64, 366; and maximal oxygen consumption, 44–45, *45*; and P_{O_2} gradient, 369–372

Bohr, Christian, 148, 346

Bohr effect, 149; fixed acid, 149; oxygen delivery in tissue and, 150–151, 199–200, *200*; and gas exchange, 346

Bohr integration, 346

Bohr shift, 388

Branching ratio, 276

Bronchial buds, 217
Bronchial pathway length, 280, *280*
Bronchial tree, *273*
Bronchioles: branching of, *274*, *312*;
    terminal, 277; first order respiratory,
    310
Bronchoarterial units, 287
Bronchopulmonary segments, *309*, 310
Brush cells, 235
BTPS conditions, 67
Buffer system, 153, 380–381
Bulk flow, 55–57

Canalicular stage, 221
Cannon, Walter, 393
Capacitance coefficient, 56
Capacity: oxygen, 12–13, 56, 143–146;
    total lung, 282; vital, 282; functional
    residual, 282–283
Capillary(ies), 179–180; lung, 159; wall
    structure of, 180–182, *181*; muscle,
    181; distances between, 184; model of,
    186; number of, 186; surface area of,
    187, 354, 360; preferred orientation of,
    189, 189–190; to glycolytic fibers,
    194–195; oxygen flow from, 195–206,
    197, *198*; endothelial cells of, 249;
    pressure drop in, 293, 297; permeable
    epithelium of, 332; blood volume in,
    349–350, 356, 360; perfusion of, 386
Capillary density, 184–187; descriptors
    of, 187–191; variability of, 191–193;
    and oxygen needs, 193–195, *194*, 202
Capillary distending pressure, 326–328,
    327, *328*, *329*
Capillary length density, 188
Capillary network: architecture of,
    182–184; geometry of, 183; alveolar,
    290, 290–292, 340–341, *341*, *342*;
    support by fibers, 313–315, *314*; pits
    in, 325, 332–333
Capillary path, *344*, 345–347, 357, 370
Capillary transit time, 345, 370
Capillary volume density, 187, 189
Carbon dioxide: production of, 91;
    transport by blood, 151–153, *152*;
    discharge in lung, 346–347
Carbon dioxide equilibrium curve, 153
Carbon dust, 244
Carbon monoxide, to measure diffusing
    capacity, 348–349
Carbonic anhydrase, 151, 152

Cardiac catheterization, 168
Cardiac muscle, *see* Heart muscle
Cardiac output, 164, 165–169, *170*; and
    oxygen consumption, *384*, 384–385;
    distribution of, 385–386; and heart
    rate, 385, 387; and stroke volume, 385,
    387; in exercise, 386–387; at high
    altitude, 389
Carotid body, 391
Cascade model, *9*, 9–10, 51–52, *379*,
    392–394
Catabolism, oxidative, 91, 100, 101
Catheterization, cardiac, 168
Cell(s): evolution of, 4; metabolic
    pathways of, *31*, 87–88, *88*; metabo-
    lism of, *81*, 111; energetic balance
    sheet of, 99–102; mitochondrial
    content of, 117; diffusion into,
    197–198; oxygen availability to, 378
Cell junctions, 233–235, *234*
Chemiosmotic theory, 112, *113*
Chemoreceptors, 391–392
Chest wall, 303, *304*
Chicken embryo, 363, *363*, *364*
Chorioallantois, 363, *363*, *364*
Ciliated cells, 236, *237*
Circulation: basic design of, 156–161,
    157; in fish, *157*, 158–159; in frogs,
    157, 159; in birds and mammals, *157*,
    159–161, *160*; systemic, 159; pulmo-
    nary, 159, 213, 216, 292–294; heart as
    pump in, 161–165, 176; changes with
    exercise in, 284; pressure drop in,
    293; regulation of, 384–389
Citric acid cycle, *see* Krebs cycle
Clara cell, 237
Clements, John, 320
Closed chamber method, 68–69
Coenzyme A (CoA), *86*, 86–87; acetyl,
    92, 93–94
Coenzyme Q, 97
Cold-blooded animals, 36–37
Cold exposure, 42
Collagen fibers, 239, 316
Colloid osmotic pressure, 331, 332
Combustion, of glucose, 80–82
Conductance, diffusive, 6–7; in oxygen
    flow rate, 50–51, *51*, 398; in oxygen
    exchange, 52–55; for oxygen
    transport by bulk flow, 55–57, *56*; for
    oxygen flow into sink, 57–58, *58*; of
    tissue barrier, 353–355; of blood

Conductance (*Continued*)
plasma, 355; of erythrocytes, 355–358;
total, 358; matched to oxygen needs,
364–369
Conducting airways, 221, 273
Conducting blood vessels, 221
Conducting zone, 212
Connective fiber tracts, 308
Convection, oxygen transport by, 5–6,
7, 7–8
Corticosteroids, 264
Cost-benefit ratio, 395
Costodiaphragmatic recess, 305, *306*
Countercurrent system, 17–19
Coupling: chemical, 112; conformational,
112; chemiosmotic, 112–115, *113*
Coupling factor, 112, 114
Cournand, A., 168
Creatine phosphate (CP), 31–32, 122,
380, 383
Creatine phosphokinase, 382, *382*
Cross-bridge cycling, 120
Cytochrome oxidase, 98
Cytochromes, 97–98
Cytoplasmic plates, nonnuclear,
253–255

Dead-space, 281; ventilation of, 283, 284
Defense: nonimmune, 243–245;
immune, 246
Defense cells, 242–248
Density: volume, 74–76, 115–117, 128,
130–131, 187, 189; surface, 74–76,
116–117, 128, 189; capillary, 184–195,
202; transsection, 189
Desmosomes, *234*, 235
Diaphragm, 191, 303, *304*
Diastole, 164
Dichotomy, 217; irregular vs. regular,
274, *275*, 279–280
Dichotomy model, 276–277
Diffusing capacity, 347; of carbon
monoxide, 348–349; physiological
estimates of, 348–350, 359–363; in
exercise, 349, 350, 361–362; membrane, 349, 359; morphometric model
for, 352–359, 361–363; in canids, *362*,
362–363; of chorioallantois, 363, *363*,
364; and oxygen consumption,
365–369
Diffusion: oxygen transport by, 5, *6*,
6–7; oxygen exchange by, *8*, 8–9,

52–55, *53*; measurement of, 188; into
cells, 197–198; radial, 198; facilitated,
204–206; resistance to, 351–352
Diffusion barrier, *see* Tissue barrier
Diffusion coefficient, 53–54, 55, 197
Dipalmitoyl lecithin, *see* Dipalmitoyl-
phosphatidylcholine (DPPC)
Dipalmitoylphosphatidylcholine
(DPPC), 257–262, *258*, 321
2,3 Diphosphoglycerate, 149, 150
Dissociation curves, physiological vs.
physicochemical, *150*, 151
Distending pressure, in capillaries,
326–328, *327, 328, 329*
DL_{CO}, 348–349
DL_{O_2}, *see* Diffusing capacity
Dog, energetic needs of, 364–365
Double strategy, 65–66
2,3 DPG, 149, 150
DPPC, 257–262, *258*, 321
Ductus arteriosus Botalli, 217

Economical construction, principle of,
59–60
Edema: alveolar, 265–266; interstitial,
334; pulmonary, 334
Efficiency: energy transduction to ATP,
99–102
Elastic fibers, 239, 316
Electron acceptors, 82; terminal, 84
Electron carriers, *83*, 83–84, 96–98
Electron transfer, 82, *84*, *98*, 98–99
Electron transport, 95
Electron-transport chain, 112, 114
Emphysema, 312
End-capillary blood, 348
Endosymbiosis, 4–5
Endothelial cells: capillary, 180–182,
249; of lung, 238
Endurance training, 128–129, 396; and
enlarged heart, 169
Energetic cost, of biological work, 36
Energetic demands, of exercise, *33*,
33–36, 42–44
Energetic equivalent, of oxygen, 101
Energetic needs, 33–36, 42–44, 364–365
Energy: solar, 3; transfer of, 30, *31, 84,
98*, 98–102; storage of, 31, 85–86, 95,
380; by combustion, 80–87; drop in,
98; standard free, 100
Energy balance sheet, 99–102
Energy metabolism, 102

Environmental condition, 14
Enzymes: in Krebs cycle, 109–110; in mitochondria, 110–111; marker, in cell metabolism, 111
Epithelium, of airways, 233–237, *236*
Erythrocytes: hemoglobin in, 140; formation of, 140–141; immature, 141; mature, 141; structure of, *141*; mammalian, *141*, 141–144, 145; size of, 141, 144; shape of, 141–143; of camel, *142*, 143; number of, 143–144; conductance of, 355–358
Erythropoiesis, 140–141
Esophagotracheal fistulae, 215
Etruscan shrew, 399–404
Eukaryotes, oxidation in, 4
Exercise: energetic demands of, *33*, 33–36, 42–44; blood flow distribution in, 161, 169, 385–388; ventilation changes with, 284; blood flow in, 294; P_{O_2} in, 345; diffusing capacity in, 349, 350, 361–362; cardiac output in, 386–387; oxygen extraction in, 387–388; Bohr shift in, 388
Expiratory muscles, 303

FAD, 90, 93, 97
F_1-ATPase, 112, 114
Fatty acids: entrance into Krebs cycle, 94; β-oxidation of, 94, 110; energy balance sheet for, 100–102
Fermentation, 84–85
Fetus: lung morphogenesis in, *214*, 214–220; lung histogenesis in, 220–224; lung secretions of, 223
Fiber continuum, 307–313; development of, 218; surface tension on, 293–294, 322; axial, 307–308, *308*; peripheral, *308*, 308–309; support of blood vessels by, 313–315, *314*; mechanical properties of, 316
Fiber rings, 310, *313*
Fibers: muscle, 122–129; glycolytic, 194–195; collagen and elastic, 239, 316
Fibroblasts, 239, *239*
Fibrosis, of lung, 313
Fick, A., 70
Fick principle, 70–71, 167
Fight-or-flight condition, 168, 387
Filtration coefficient, 331
Fish: gills in, 16–19, *17*, *18*; circulation in, *157*, 158–159

Fistulae, esophagotracheal, 215
Flavine adenine dinucleotide, 90, 93, 97
Flight muscle, *11*
Foramen ovale, 217
Force training, 126
Forssmann, W., 168
Forster, R. E., 350
Fractal trees, 218–220, *220*
FRC, 282–283
Functional needs, 59–60; adaptation of muscles to, 126–131; adjusting performance to, 380–393; adjusting potential to, 394–399
Functional residual capacity, 282–283
Functional system, integral, 378

Gap junction, 234–235
Gas exchange: two-compartment model of, *332*; physiological basis for, 343–347; limiting factor for, 398
Gas exchange barrier, *see* Tissue barrier
Gas exchange units, 339
Gas exchanger(s): evolution of, 13–23; differentiation of, 221; design of, 339–343
Gills: tadpole, 15–16, *16*; fish, 16–19, *17*, *18*
Glucose: combustion of, 80–82; energy liberated from, 81; glycolytic breakdown of, 88–91, *89*; catabolism of, 100; energy balance sheet for, 101
Glycogen, 88
Glycolysis, 32, 87, 88–91, *88*, *89*; efficiency of, 102; reversion to, 102
Glycolytic fibers, 194–195
Goblet cells, 235, *237*
Growth period, 396

Haldane effect, *152*, 152–153
Harmonic mean barrier thickness, 354, 366, *367*
Hasselbalch, K. A., 148–149
Head pressure, 196
Heart: design of, 157–158, *158*; in fish, 158–159; in frog, 159; in mammals and birds, 159–161; as pump, 161–165, 176; size of, 164; Starling law of, 168, 331; enlarged, 169
Heart failure, 334
Heart muscle, 162–164, *162*, *163*; mitochondria of, 117; cells of, 162, *162*; fibers of, 163

Heart rate, 164, 294, 385, 387

Hematocrit, 143–144, 145, 357–358

Heme, 97, *97*, *139*, 139–140

Hemocyanin, 12, 139

Hemoglobin: and oxygen capacity, 12–13, 140; structure of, 139, *139*; concentration of, 146; oxygen saturation of, *146*, 146–147, 148, 151–152; binding capacity of, 149–150; deoxygenated, 152; as buffer, 381

Henderson-Hasselbalch equation, 154

Hepatocytes, mitochondria of, 117

Hering-Breuer reflex, 392

Hibernation, 37, 156

High altitude: hypoxic vasoconstriction from, 297–298; and pulmonary hypertension, 298; and diffusing capacity, 345, 372–373; and circulatory regulation, 389, *389*; and respiratory system potential, 396; at Mt. Everest, 399

High-energy intermediate state, 112

High-energy phosphate bonds, 30–32, *31*, 85

Hill, A. V., 34, 35

Histogenesis, of lungs, 220–224

Homeostasis, 379, 392–393, 398

Homeotherms, 36–37

Howald, H., 129

Huxley, J. S., 63

Hyaline membranes, 264

Hydrogen ion acceptor, terminal, 84

Hypertension, pulmonary, 298

Hypophase, 325

Hypoxic vasoconstriction, 297

Insects, respiratory system of, *10*, 10–12

Inspiratory muscles, 303

Integral functional system, 378

Integument, 14–15

Intercapillary pits, 325, 332–333

Intercostal muscles, 303, *304*

Interdependence, mechanical, 318, 322–323

Interlobular septa, 311

Intermembrane space, 106–108, *108*

Interstitial cells, 238–242

Interstitial fluid drainage, 333

Intrapleural pressure, 307

Johnson, W. A., 93

Kennedy pathway, 258–260, *259*

Kernlose Platten, 253

Kinocilia, 233, 235–236, *237*

Kleiber, Max, 1, 62, 63

Kölliker, Albert, 253

Krebs, Hans, 93

Krebs cycle, 87, *88*, 91–93, *92*; entrance into, 93–95; enzymes in, 109–110; mitochondrial matrix in, 110

Krogh, August, 149, 184

Krogh cylinder, 186; radius of, 188–189; mitochondrial content of, 191–193, *193*; P_{O_2} profiles in, *199*, *200*, 200–201; oxygen delivery into, 199–206

Krogh cone, 201–202, *202*

Krogh's permeability constant, 53–54

Lactate: concentration in blood plasma, 32, *43*, 43–44, 90–91; formation of, *89*

Lactic acid, 35

Lamellar bodies, 257, 259–260, *260*

Length density, of capillaries, 188

Limiting factor, *see* Rate-limiting factor

Lining layer, alveolar, *see* Alveolar lining layer

Liquid exchange, three-compartment model of, *332*

Liver, mitochondria from, *107*

Lobes, *309*, 310

Lobule, 310, *311*

Locomotion, *see* Running

Long-distance runners, 127

Low, Frank, 248

Lung(s): primitive, 19; in amphibia and reptiles, 19–21, *20*, *21*; alveolar, 20–21, *20*, *21*, 225–228, *340*; bird, 21–22, *22*, *23*; design of, 211–212; basic structure of, 212; respiratory zone of, 212, 273; functional zones of, 212, 272–273, *275*; development of, 213–224; morphogenesis of, *214*, 214–220; fetal, 214–224, *219*; anlage for, 215; vasculature of, 217–218; mesenchyme of, 218; histogenesis of, 220–224; differentiation for gas exchange in, 221; at birth, 224; postnatal maturation of, 224–228, *225*, *226*, *227*; nonrespiratory functions of, 232; lymphatics of, 246–248, *247*; in shock, 265; capacity of, 282; regional perfusion of, 295–296; perfusion zones of, 296–297, 328, *329*; recoil

Lung(s) (*Continued*)
  force of, 306, 318; fiber continuum of,
  307–313; units of, *309*, 310; morphometric data on, 360
Lung buds, *214*, 215
Lung cells: functions of, 231–232;
  epithelial, 233–237; endothelial, 238;
  interstitial, 238–242; defense,
  242–248; volume of, 249; at gas
  exchange barrier, 249–255; characteristics of, 250; alveolar secretory,
  255–265; vulnerability of, 265–266
Lung segments, *309*, 310
Lung volume: distribution of, 280–282;
  measurement of, 282–283
Lungfish, 19
Lymph nodes, *247*, 247–248
Lymphatics, 221, 246–248, *247*, 333
Lymphocytes, 246
Lysosomes, 243–244

Macrophages, *243*, 243–245, *245*
Macula adhaerens, *234*, 235
Mandelbrot, Benoit, 218
Marathon runner, 127
Mead, Jere, 317
Mean capillary P_{O_2}, 345
Mean corpuscular volume, 144, 145
Mean curvature, 318
Mediastinum, 214, 305
Membrane diffusing capacity, 349, 359
Metabolic debt, *33*, 33–35
Metabolic pathways, *31*, 87–88, *88*
Metabolic rate: total, 30; temperature
  effect on, 36–38, *38*, 42; specific, 38,
  40; allometric plots of, 38–39, *41*;
  body size effect on, 38–40, 44–45,
  63–64, 366; and biological time,
  40–41; standard resting, 40–41. *See
  also* Oxygen consumption
Metabolism: of cell, *81*, 111; anaerobic,
  84–85, 88–91; aerobic, 84–85, 91–92;
  oxidative, *88*; regulation of, 381–384
Microscopic observation, 72
Microvascular unit, 178–180, *180*,
  182–183; parallel perfusion of, 371; as
  limiting factor for oxygen flow, 398.
  See also Capillary(ies)
Milieu intérieur, 14
Minimal tissue barrier, *252*, 315, *315*, 354
Minute volume, 283
Mitchell, Peter, 112

Mitochondrial mass, and oxygen
  consumption, 118
Mitochondrial matrix, 108, *108*, 110
Mitochondrial membranes, 106–108,
  108; as hydrogen ion barrier, 112;
  elementary particles of, 114; surface
  area of, 115; surface density of,
  116–117, 128
Mitochondrial number, 117
Mitochondrial volume, total, 130–131,
  131
Mitochondrial volume density:
  descriptor of, 115–117; and $\dot{V}_{O_2}$ max,
  128, *129*, 130–131, *130*, *131*; and
  capillary density, 191–193, *193*, 194
Mitochondrion(dria), 4–5; as oxygen
  sinks, 5–10; structure of, 106–108,
  107, *108*; protein synthesis by,
  108–109; enzymes in, 110–111; and
  aerobic capacity, 115–118; distribution
  of, 120–122, *121*; interfibrillar (core),
  121; sarcolemmal, 122, 124; and limits
  of oxygen consumption, 132; in
  myocardial cells, 165; inhomogeneity
  of, 202–203, *203*, *205*, 206
Morphogenesis: of lungs, *214*, 214–220;
  regulation of, 379, 394, 395–397
Morphologist, 24–26
Morphology, quantitative, *see* Morphometry
Morphometry, 26, 72; in estimating
  diffusing capacity, 352–359, 361–363
Mt. Everest, 399
Multivesicular bodies, 257, 259, *260*
Muscle(s): oxygen consumption in, 70;
  blood flow through, 70–71, *71*,
  386–387; adaptation to functional
  needs, 126–131; needle biopsy of, 127,
  128; red vs. white, *192*; capillary
  perfusion in, 386
Muscle cells: structure of, 118–120, *119*;
  cardiac, 162, *162*; smooth, 239–242,
  240
Muscle contraction, 120, 240
Muscle fiber types, 122–126; histochemistry of, *124*, 124–125; differentiation of, 125–126; in weightlifters
  vs. marathon runners, 126–127; in
  marathon runners vs. sedentary
  people, 127–129
Muscle work, 33–36
Myelin, tubular, 260, 262, *262*, 325

Myocardial cells, 162, *162*, 165, *166*

Myofibrils, 118–120

Myofibroblasts, *241*, 242, 334

Myoglobin, 122, 124–125; in oxygen delivery, 203–204

Myosin, 118–120

Myosin-actin bridges, *120*

Myosin ATPase, 122, *195*

NAD, 82–84, *83*

NADH: in oxidation-reduction reaction, 83–84; in Krebs cycle, 94; free energy stored in, 95; in respiratory chain, 95, 96, 98

Neuroendocrine cells, 235

Nexus, 234–235

Nicotinamide adenine dinucleotide, 82–84, *83*

Occupational diseases, 244

Oncotic pressure, 332

Open circuit method, 68

Optimization, of design, 60

Orientation parameter, 190

Osmiophilic granules, 257

Oxidation, 3, 4; of substrate, 82, *83*, 83–84; β–, 94, 110

Oxidation-phosphorylation coupling, 111–115

Oxidation-reduction reactions, 82–85, *83*, 95–99

Oxidative catabolism, 91, 100, 101

Oxidative phosphorylation, 4, 30–32, *31*; in respiratory chain, 95, 99–100; efficiency of, 100; location of, 110; chemiosmotic coupling, 114; regulation of, 381–384; upper functional limit of, 397

Oxidoreductases, 112

Oxygen: energetic equivalent of, 101; solubility of, 138–139, 144–146; bound to hemoglobin, 146; availability of, 378

Oxygen binding: properties of blood for, 147–151, 391; rate of, 349–350, 356–358, *357*

Oxygen capacity, 12–13, 56; and number of erythrocytes, 143–144, 145; and hemoglobin concentration, 146

Oxygen carrier(s), 12–13, 139–140; bulk flow of, 55–57, *56*; blood as, 144–151

Oxygen concentration, 67; fractional, 68

Oxygen consumption: and energetic needs, 33–36, *33*, *35*, 42–44, *43*; allometric plots of, 38–39, *41*; limits of, 41–45, 132; summit, 42; measurement of, 66–71, *69*, *71*; in muscles, 70; mitochondrial mass and, 118; inhomogeneity of, 202–203, *203*, *205*, 206; diffusion capacity and, 365–369; cardiac output and, *384*, 384–385. *See also* Metabolic rate; $\dot{V}_{O_2}$ max

Oxygen cycle, *2*, 2–3

Oxygen debt, *33*, 33–35

Oxygen deficit, *33*, 33–36, *35*

Oxygen dissociation curve, 147–151, *148*, *149*, *150*

Oxygen equilibrium curve, 147–151, *148*, *149*, *150*

Oxygen exchange, diffusive, *8*, 8–9; conductance for, 52–55

Oxygen extraction, in exercise, 387–388

Oxygen flow: rate of, 49–52, 398; driving force for, 51; by diffusion, 52–55, *53*; structural parameters of, 52–58; into sink, 57–58, *58*; rate-limiting factors for, 60, 397–399; from capillary blood, 195–206, *197*, *198*; model of, 197–198, *197*, *198*

Oxygen needs, 1–2; adaptation to, 60–61; modifying, 64–65; capillary density and, 193–195, *194*, 202; conductance matched to, 364–369

Oxygen sinks, 5–10; mitochondrial, 57–58, *58*

Oxygen stores, 204, 380, *380*

Oxygen toxicity, 265

Oxygen transport: by diffusion, 5, *6*, 6–7; by convection, 5–6, *7*, 7–8; basic pathway for, 9–10; by bulk flow of a carrier, 55–57; by blood, 170–171, 388; in airways, 285; regulation of, 384–389; capacity for, 388

Oxyhemoglobin dissociation curve, 147–151, *148*, *149*, *150*

Oxyhemoglobin equilibrium curve, 147–151, *148*, *149*, *150*

Palade, G. E., 106

$P_{A_{O_2}}$, 343–344, *344*, 370–372

Pa_{O_2}, 344

Parabronchi, 21, *23*

Parenchyma, of lung, 340, *340*

Parenchymal cells: volume of, 249; characteristics of, 250

Parietal pleura, 305
Partial pressure, see P_{O_2}, P_{CO_2}
Pattle, R. E., 319
P_{CO_2}, 345–347
Performance, and functional needs, 380–393
Perfusion: of lungs, 295–296; parallel, 371; of muscles, 386
Perfusion fixation of tissue, 72
Perfusion unit, 298, 371
Perfusion zones of lung, 296–297, 328, 329
Pericardium, 214
Pericytes, 182
Peripheral fiber system, 308, 308–309
Permeability, of alveolar tissue, 331–332
Permeability coefficients, 52–55, 331
Permeability constant, 53–54
pH, 154–155, 155
pH gradient, 113, 114
pH stat regulation, 155–156
Phagocytosis, 243, 243–244
Phosphate bonds, high-energy, 30–32, 31, 85
Phosphate stores, 31, 85–86, 95, 380
Phospholipase A_2, 258, 263
Phosphorylation, see Oxidative phosphorylation
Photosynthesis, 3
Phrenic nerve, 304
Physical exercise, see Exercise
Physiological methods, 66–71; for estimating oxygen consumption, 66–71; for estimating diffusing capacity, 348–350, 359–363
Physiologist, 24–26
Plants, in oxygen cycle, 3
Plasma, see Blood plasma
Plasma cells, 246
Pleural adhesions, 306
Pleural cavities, 305–307, 306
Pleural mesothelium, 213
Pleural recesses, 305
Pleural space, 305–307, 306
Pneumothorax, 307
P:O ratio, 102
P_{O_2}: mixed venous, 161; alveolar, 343–344, 344, 370–372; arterial, 344; capillary, 344, 345–347, 356; in exercise, 345; in high altitude, 345, 372–373
P_{O_2} cascade, 9, 9–10, 51–52, 379, 392–394

P_{O_2} gradient, 6–7, 51–52; alveolar-capillary, 344–346, 398; estimating, 347–348; and body size, 369–372
Poikilotherms, 36–37
Point-counting methods, 75–76
Poiseuille's law, 176, 286, 292
Pores of Kohn, 254
Potential: standard reduction, 96; and functional needs, 394–399; limits to, 399–404
Power function, 63
Precapillaries, 179; pulmonary, 289
Premature infants, surfactant production in, 264
Pressure: blood, 176; transmural, 293; intrapleural, 307; capillary distending, 326–328, 327, 328, 329; colloid osmotic, 331, 332; oncotic, 332. See also P_{O_2}
Pressure-volume curves, 317, 322
Professionalism, in science, 24
Proton acceptors, 82
Proton gradient, 112
Proton-motive force, 114
Protozoa, mitochondria in, 5
Pseudoglandular stage, 220
Pulmonary diffusing capacity, see Diffusing capacity
Pulmonary fiber system, see Fiber continuum
Pyruvate, 89, 90, 93–94
Pyruvate dehydrogenase, 110

Q_{10}, 37
Quantitative morphology, see Morphometry

Rate-limiting factor: structural design as, 60, 397–399; mitochondria as, 132; absolute, 399–404
Reaction rate, for oxygen binding, 349–350, 356–358, 357
Recoil force, 306, 318
Red blood cells, see Erythrocytes
Redox couple: NAD-NADH, 96–97; FAD-FADH$_2$, 97
Redox reactions, 82–85, 83, 95–99
Reducing equivalents, 83
Reduction potential, standard, 96
Reflection coefficient, 331
Regulation: of acid-base balance, 153–156, 390–391; pH stat, 155–156; alpha-stat, 156; of regional blood flow,

Regulation (*Continued*)
178; of surfactant, 264; of airway
caliber, 286; of functions, 379,
380–381; homeostatic, 379, 392–393,
398; of morphogenesis, 379, 394,
395–397; of cell metabolism,
381–384; of oxidative phosphorylation, 381–384; of circulation,
384–389; of oxygen transport,
384–389; backward, 389; of ventilation, *390*, 390–392; of respiration,
390–392; of pulmonary blood flow,
392; signals for, 393
Reptile lungs, 19–21, *20, 21*
Residual volume, 282
Resistance: vascular, 176–178, 292–294,
386; to diffusion, 351–352
Respiration: in water, 15–19; in air,
19–23; and energy metabolism, 102;
regulation of, 390–392; control of,
391–392
Respiratory centers, 391
Respiratory chain, 87, *88*, 95–99, *98*;
oxidoreductases of, 112
Respiratory distress syndrome: of
newborn, 264, 324–325, 334; of adult,
265–266
Respiratory failure, 265
Respiratory quotient, 69–70
Respiratory system, mammalian, 23–26;
structure-function correlation of,
24–26; cascade model of, 49, *50*,
51–52, *379*; potential of, 394–404
Respiratory zone, 212, 273
Reticulocytes, 141
Rib cage, 302–303, *304*
Richards, D. W., 168
Root effect, 149
Roughton, F. J. W., 350
Running: treadmill, 42–43, 127;
long-distance, 127

Saccular stage, 221–223, *223, 224*
Sarcomeres, 118–120
Scaling, 63; of volume density, 130–131,
130, 131
Scaling factor, 63
Scholander, P., 204
SDH stain, 124
Secondary lobule, 310, *311*
Sectioning, 73
Self-regulation, *see* Homeostasis

Semitendinosus muscle, 191
Septum, *see* Alveolar septum
Series ventilation and parallel perfusion
model, 371
Serotonin, 293
Sheet-flow concept, 291
Shock lung, 265
Shrew, Etruscan, 399–404
Silicosis, 244
Sinus node, 165
Sjöstrand, F., 106
Skeletal muscle: mitochondria in, *107,
121*; structure of, *118–119*; muscle
fiber types in, 122–126; microvascula-
ture of, *179*
Smooth muscle cells, 239–242, *240*
Solar energy, 3
Solubility coefficient, 54, 55
Spiracles, *10*, 10–12
Splanchnopleura, 215
Squamous lining cells, 249–253
Stability, of air spaces, 318
Standard free energy, 100
Standard reduction potential, 96
Starling, E., 168
Starling law, 168, 331
Steady-state conditions, 393
Stereology, *73–77, 74*
STPD conditions, 67
Strahler method, 276
Stress, adaptation to, 129
Stretch receptors, 392
Stroke volume, 164, 294, 385, 387
Structure-function correlation, 24–26;
models of, 25; testing of, *62, 64*; in
diffusing capacity, 364–369
Substrate, oxidation of, 82, *83*, 83–84
Succinyl dehydrogenase, 93, 110, 123
Suncus etruscus, 399–404
Surface area: of tissue barrier, 53, 354;
measurement of, 73–76; of mitochon-
drial membranes, 115; of capillaries,
187, 354, 360; alveolar, 340, 352, 354,
359, 366, *367*
Surface balance, 320, *321*
Surface density, 74–76; of inner
mitochondrial membrane, 116–117,
128; of capillaries, 189
Surface law, 39
Surface tension, 317–325, *319, 321*
Surfactant, 257; synthesis of, 257–260,
263, 264; in fetal lung, 259, 264;

Surfactant (*Continued*)
   secretion of, 260, *261*, *263*; turnover
   of, 262–263; removal of, *263*;
   regulation of, 264; in surface tension,
   319–322; inadequate, 323–325; in
   alveolar surface lining, 325
Surfactant apoprotein, 260
Surfactant phospholipid, 257–258
Symmorphosis, 59–60, 379, 394
Systole, 164

θ_{O_2}, 349–350, 356–358, *357*
Tadpole gills, 15–16, *16*
Taylor, C. R., 388, 399
Temperature effects: on metabolic rate,
   36–38, *38*, 42; central body, 37;
   critical, 37, *38*; ambient, 37–38; on
   oxygen binding, 148, 151; and
   physiological pH, *155*
Terminal bar, 182, 233–234, *234*
Thermoneutral zone, 38, *38*
Thorax, 302–305
Tidal volume, 282
Tight junction, 182, 233–234, *234*
Tissue barrier: surface area of, 53, 354;
   cells of, 249–255; minimal, *252*, 315,
   315, 354; thick, *315*; gas exchange
   across, 342, *342*; thickness of, 352, 353,
   354, 360; conductance of, 353–355
Tissue fixation, 72–73
TLC, 282
Tonus, 241
Total lung capacity, 282
Total ventilation, 283, 284
Trachea(e): of insect, *10*, 10–12; anlage
   for, 215; mammalian, 272
Training effect, 65, 126–129
Transit time, through capillaries, 345,
   370
Transmural pressure, 293
Transsection density, 189
Treadmill running, 42–43, 127
Tricarboxylic acid cycle, *see* Krebs cycle
Tubular myelin, 260, 262, *262*, 325
Type I cells: differentiation of, 221, *222*;
   design of, 249–252, *251*, 253–255,
   254; complex shape of, 255
Type II cells: differentiation of, 221, *222*;
   structure of, 255–257, *256*; synthesis
   of surfactant by, 257–265; cytoplasmic
   organelles of, *260*

Ubiquinone, 97

Vascular perfusion, *see* Perfusion
Vascular resistance, 176–178, 292–294,
   386
Vasculature, *see* Arteries; Capillary(ies);
   Veins
Vasoconstriction, hypoxic, 297
Veins, 157; pulmonary, 287, *288*, 313
Venous return, 387
Ventilation, 283; dead-space, 283; total,
   283; alveolar, 283, 284, 295; changes
   with exercise, 284; series, 371;
   regulation of, *390*, 390–392
Ventilation rates, 67, 283
Ventilation-perfusion matching,
   294–298
Ventilation-perfusion ratio, 297
Ventilatory unit, 280
Visceral pleura, 305; rupture of, 307
Vital capacity, 282
Volume: measurement of, 73–76; total
   mitochondrial, 130–131, *131*; mean
   corpuscular, 144, 145; stroke, 164,
   294, 385, 387; lung cell, 249; lung,
   280–283; alveolar gas, 281–282;
   residual, 282; tidal, 282; minute, 283
Volume density, 74–76; of mitochondria,
   115–117, 128, *129*; scaling of,
   130–131, *130*, *131*; of capillaries, 187,
   189
V_{O_2} max: and body mass, 39; calculation
   of, 43–45; allometry of, *45*; morphometric parameters of, 115–118;
   mitochondrial volume density and,
   128, *129*, 130–131, *130*, *131*; capillary
   density and, 193–195, *194*; as
   estimate of respiratory potential, 394;
   limit for, 397
von Neergaard, K., 317

Waltzing mice, *365*, 365–366
Warm-blooded animals, 36–37
Water breathing, 15–19
Weightlifter, 126
West, J. B., 399
Wilhelmy balance, *321*

Zonula occludens, 182, 233–234, *234*